||| **PERSPECTIVES**
||| ON CRIME AND JUSTICE

Joseph A. Schafer,
Series Editor

Crime, Corrections,
and the COVID-19 Pandemic

Crime, Corrections, and the COVID-19 Pandemic

Responses and Adaptations in the U.S. Criminal Justice System

Edited by Breanne Pleggenkuhle
and Joseph A. Schafer

Southern Illinois University Press
Carbondale

Southern Illinois University Press
siupress.com

First printed July 2025.

Publication of this book has been underwritten by the Elmer H. Johnson
and Carol Holmes Johnson criminology fund.

Jacket/Cover illustration: Human Rights Law in the Time of the
Coronavirus, iStock image 1251456134 by 101cats (cropped).

ISBN 978-0-8093-3970-9 (cloth)
ISBN 978-0-8093-3969-3 (paperback)
ISBN 978-0-8093-3971-6 (ebook)

Printed on recycled paper ♻

SĬU
Southern Illinois University System

Contents

Illustrations

Crime, Corrections,
and the COVID-19 Pandemic

Introduction: COVID-19, Crime, and Criminal Justice

Breanne Pleggenkuhle and Joseph A. Schafer

In late fall of 2019, news broke of a spreading virus that originated in Wuhan, China. The highly infectious SARS-CoV-2, the virus that causes COVID-19, quickly spread through the winter months and, by spring 2020, had global impacts. Governments around the world issued "stay at home" orders and restricted domestic and international travel. Educational institutions and workplaces faced shutdown. Throughout 2020, 2021, and into 2022, nations sought to identify and enact public health policies to mitigate the spread of the virus and to reduce the consequences of infection, including masking policies, vaccination requirements, and various degrees of quarantine. These responses varied enormously across place and time. By mid-2022 international and domestic travel restrictions began to relax, as vaccination access and usage increased. Many nations began lifting masking requirements in 2022, and by 2023 many nations were concluding their public health declarations connected with COVID-19. Despite the ongoing presence of the virus and continued infection and death, the pandemic phase of life with COVID-19, from the viewpoint of politics and policy, was winding down globally by 2023. Collectively, the events of the pandemic had a tremendous social, economic, and behavioral impact.

Crime and criminal justice were part of the swift societal changes. Within months of the emergence of COVID-19, researchers and policymakers alike realized there would be shifts in human behavior related to criminal victimization and perpetration; subsequently, shifts were needed in the operations of the criminal justice system. Early research indicated changes in the frequency and type of calls for service to law enforcement and other social service agencies (Bradbury-Jones & Isham, 2020; Koziarski, 2021), pointed out challenges for first responders and institutions in managing the pandemic (Martin et al., 2022), and observed the potential for drastic shifts in crime trends (Jackson et al., 2021). For instance, stay-at-home orders might decrease certain forms of crime, such as residential burglary, as individuals remaining close to their homes and property were better able to serve as capable guardians. Conversely, intimate partner violence, alcohol consumption, and the use of illicit substances might be expected to increase as individuals found themselves in prolonged contact with others while under continual stress. The criminal justice system had to consider what aspects of its operations to maintain (e.g., police responding to calls for service), to modify (e.g., parole and probation officials conducting community supervision appointments via videoconference), or to halt (e.g., courts suspending activities such as jury trials).

The COVID-19 response coincided with another massive social movement spurred by the death of George Floyd in May 2020. In the midst of a pandemic, continued calls for social justice echoed prior incidents of the past decade that questioned the police's use of force, disparities in the criminal justice system, and overall responses to crime in society. Amid pandemic policies and efforts of social distancing, protests erupted that further strained embattled public agencies yet necessitated their immediate response. The protests of the summer of 2020 complicate the ability of researchers to ascertain how COVID-19 influenced rates of crime and how it shifted some operations of the criminal justice system and the efficacy of those shifts.

Throughout 2020 and beyond, the spread of COVID-19 generated substantial social and legal policy change. This occurred in tandem with other reform efforts and demands that cast light on crime, criminal justice practices, and justice-related policies and legislation. This edited volume broadly considers both crime and criminal justice effects of, and responses to, the COVID-19 pandemic. Its contributors evaluate how policies meant to protect public health may have impacted crime, how a global pandemic changed sentencing and community supervision strategies, and how many of those within the criminal justice system—responders and supervised alike—faced change, strain, and possibilities for reform.

Crime Considerations

The policy and public health responses to COVID-19 reached into virtually all aspects of society. These responses changed where and how people lived, worked, and learned. They influenced how people interacted with family and loved ones, coworkers, and government service providers. Stay-at-home orders radically changed the ways in which citizens did (or did not) move through their geographic and social world. Some workers found their employment suddenly change to a work-from-home arrangement, while others found themselves forced to continue going in to work, often having to worry about exposing themselves and their family to COVID-19. Still others found themselves furloughed or unemployed as a result of the shuttering of businesses. The multitude of events and policies prompting changes to behavioral patterns, household dynamics, and interpersonal relationships, in the midst of economic failures and heightened mental health strains, raised many issued for criminologists.

Early speculations considered how COVID-19 could impact criminal activity, with an expectation that shifts in guardianship, targets, strains, and lifestyles would influence crime patterns. Many scholars, drawing from neoclassical schools of thought, predicted that widespread stay-at-home orders were likely to increase residential guardianship and limit outside activities, thereby decreasing property crimes and opportunities for violence (Hawdon et al., 2020). This circumstance could either increase (Kim & Phillips, 2021) or decrease (Kaukinen, 2020) various types of crime. More time spent at home would increase opportunities for intimate part-ner violence (Machlin et al., 2022) or cybercrime (Hawdon et al., 2020), whereas street crimes, such as burglary or robbery, were likely to decrease with less population mobility through public spaces (Felson et al., 2020; Lopez & Rosenfeld, 2021).

In addition to shifting patterns of vulnerability and guardianship, mobility restrictions designed to limit the spread of COVID-19 changed interpersonal dynamics, introducing negative stimuli or weakening social bonds through isolation, quarantine, and fear of contagion. Income and employment disruptions, health impacts, abrupt changes to daily life, and the uncertainty that came with the pandemic produced negative strain for many (Kim & Phillips, 2021; Murray & Davies, 2022). As Bradbury-Jones and Isham (2020) noted, the United Kingdom refrain of "Stay Home; Protect the National Health Service (NHS); Save Lives" would ring false if lockdown measures increasing contact between family members and romantic partners led to more intimate partner violence, child abuse, or elder abuse. Even more concerning, instances of such violence might not generate the same scrutiny or consequence. When victims do not leave home for school, work, or other obligations, then a friend, teacher, or coworker has less chance of observing injuries and choosing to intervene.

Stay-at-home orders also limited potentially negative influence from peers. For example, youth who were no longer attending school in person and having unsupervised interactions with peers outside school might have less exposure to negative peer influence, which in turn might lead to a reduction in delinquent behavior. However, as Buchanan and colleagues (2020) noted, despite efforts to divert individuals from confinement, opportunities for peer interaction may ultimately have led to rises in delinquency.

Scholars immediately recognized the opportunity to study crime in the natural experiment created by the COVID-19 pandemic (Miller & Blumstein, 2020; Stickle & Felson, 2020). While much speculation occurred over how pandemic responses might alter crime patterns and opportunities, the empirical evidence on outcomes varied widely, with findings and conclusions being heavily dependent on timing, place, measurement, and operationalization. Part of the challenge in studying the pandemic's effects on crime stems from the fact that mitigation strategies, such as stay-at-home orders or school closures, were not enacted equally in all places or enforced for equal durations of time. In addition, not all criminal conduct has the same correlates and drivers, so the effects of public health policies would be expected to vary by offense type. Piquero and colleagues (2021) demonstrated this by comparing trends prior to and after the implementation of stay-at-home orders and documented the variable nature of calls for service and reporting to police. Mohler and colleagues (2020) compared cities and types of crimes and found that crime trends were difficult to untangle and had varied effects. Despite this variability, some general patterns did emerge from this research literature.

Decreases in Crime

Some early studies of the pandemic's effects on crime found that some types of crimes decreased in the spring of 2020, with early evidence of widespread drops in drug crimes, larceny, residential burglaries, and many violent crimes: sexual assault, simple assault, and homicide (Abrams, 2021; Payne et al., 2020; Piquero, 2021). Lopez and Rosenfeld (2021) extended this examination and substantiated a decline in property crimes, drug crimes, robbery, and homicide throughout 2020 and into 2021, though these patterns varied as the pandemic persisted and stay-at-home orders fluctuated. While their findings modestly suggest that increased time spent at home (by large segments of the population) was tied to some reductions in violent crime, this finding did not tend to uphold over time (particularly as researchers looked into crime in 2021 and beyond) and varied by geography. Researchers have struggled to disentangle geographic variation to determine whether the inconsistency in observed crime declines was a function of public health policies (which placed diverse restrictions on population mobility) or was otherwise influenced by latent social, economic, cultural, or geographic drivers.

Increases in Crime

Another line of research demonstrated the theoretical expectation that COVID-19 policies and social changes would result in crime remaining stable or increasing in some cases. Despite social distancing and stay-at-home orders, Jeffrey Brantingham and colleagues (2021) suggested that gang-related crimes neither increased nor decreased but rather persisted through time. Others saw an evolution in the commission of crimes, such as the emergence of new fraud-related crimes both broadly and specific to the pandemic (Kennedy et al., 2021) or the commission of crimes geographically closer to home (Lentz et al., 2022). As another example: although residential burglaries tended to decrease, Felson and colleagues (2020) suggested that burglary shifted to commercial targets, a finding substantiated by others.

Risks of emergent types of crime and coping rose with the spread of COVID-19. Kennedy and colleagues (2021) found close to half of their sample respondents felt themselves at risk or targeted for fraud related to COVID-19 health and safety products, such as cures, vaccines, or financial aid, and nearly a quarter purchased products related to the pandemic, such as purported COVID-19 cures (oils, minerals) or financial offers for small business loans. Many noted the possibility for a rise in online crimes. Halford (2022) highlighted survey results of policing that illustrated greater reporting of online criminality demands on the profession. In contrast, Hawdon and colleagues (2020) indicated no difference in self-reported cybervictimization, including identity theft, online fraud, or harassment in personal communications. Substance use may have evolved during the pandemic, as deliveries of alcohol and cannabis increased, and changes in access occurred in tandem with lockdown orders. This has the potential to affect longer-term patterns of behavior and addiction (Matthay & Schmidt, 2021). Usage of other drugs also shifted in step with stay-at-home orders, with some noting an uptick in opioid overdosing (King et al., 2021). Other research found a rise in calls for mental health needs (Koziarski, 2021) and other calls for service that may have long-term behavioral and responsive effects.

Of concern also were threats of violence in a situation of stay-at-home orders, increased strain, and changed opportunities. As Boman and Gallupe (2020) pointed out, although minor and property-related offenses may have declined overall in the early months of the pandemic, more serious and violent crimes (such as homicide and intimate partner violence) either remained stable or in some cases increased. Kim and Phillips (2021) found some evidence of a short-term increase in lethal gun violence that extended to greater nonfatal gun violence (with and without injury) as well as gang-related firearm violence. The mix of health, social, and economic factors was thought to have contributed to an early-pandemic spike in homicides (Murray & Davies, 2022).

Crime Patterns: A Focus on Intimate Partner Violence

Most research found general increases in incidents of intimate partner violence or calls for service (Machlin et al., 2022; Nix & Richards, 2021; Piquero et al., 2021; Richards et al., 2021), although some noted exceptions to this (see A. R. Miller et al., 2022). In a systematic review, Bhuptani and colleagues (2022) determined that the majority of empirical evidence showed at least a short-term increase in calls for service related to intimate partner violence (see also Hsu & Henke, 2021; Piquero et al., 2021; Sorenson et al., 2021). Increases in instances of intimate partner violence appeared to be stronger in places of greater economic disparity, and these incidents occurring during a pandemic seemed to have substantial mental health impacts on victims (Bhuptani et al., 2022). Families already at high risk for, or with prior incidence of, violence saw sustained and increased violence (Machlin et al., 2022). Other forms of domestic or intimate partner crimes were also observed to increase in the early months of the pandemic, including stalking behaviors (Short et al., 2022). In contrast, Sorenson and colleagues (2021) found that help-seeking calls for rape and other forms of assault initially fell in the early months of the pandemic. However, as Nix and Richards (2021) noted, these patterns varied by locality and tended to decrease as stay-at-home policies receded and then to increase with new lockdown orders as infection rates resurged (Machlin et al., 2022; Piquero et al., 2021).

Criminal Justice Measures: Evidence of Change

COVID-19 provided challenges and opportunities in responses to crime. From street-level bureaucrats to service provision, the pandemic drastically disrupted the ability to respond in traditional ways. As Jennings and Perez (2020) noted, there was "no existing 'play book' for law enforcement" (p. 699), which also extended to other service and justice-related agencies that were wholly unprepared for the disruption and duration of the pandemic. Great variation emerged in terms of protocols and requirements regarding COVID-19 and also in changes in how to execute duties within the system (Piquero, 2021). In some cases, this prevented adequate service provision. In others, this altered and expanded the ways in which criminal justice workers were able to communicate and carry out the routine aspects of their occupations. As Altheimer and colleagues (2020) pointed out, COVID-19 prevented access to victims or incidents of violence and led organizers to develop distancing strategies to facilitate responsiveness and communication between victims and responders.

Resource distribution and responses dramatically shifted. Some noted the potential for broad structural change, with releases from prison of individuals incarcerated for substance-related crimes having the potential to become more permanent in nature (Del Pozo & Beletsky, 2020). Specifically, opportunities for a "lighter touch" by the justice system emerged across agencies through shifts in strategies and presence (Jackson et al., 2021). The pandemic motivated new conversations about health and safety protocols among criminal justice actors (Jennings & Perez, 2020) and a reconsideration of resource allocation, training protocols, and the demand for interaction with the public previously taken for granted. The lack of planned and executed policies across crime and justice systems was well documented (Piquero, 2021), with innovative responses leaving open an opportunity for reform.

Policing and Law Enforcement

Policing strategies often demand face-to-face contact with communities, victims, and those accused of crimes (Lum et al., 2023). As a result, law enforcement officers had a high rate of exposure and infection through the early months of the pandemic (Halford, 2022). This not only increased the stress of performing law enforcement duties but also limited the available workforce in times of uncertainty (Halford, 2022). The demands placed on law enforcement agencies changed with evolving COVID-19 restrictions in terms of enforcement of policies, consideration of public health strategies, and the general approach to policing (Lum et al., 2023; Maskály et al., 2021; Nix et al., 2021; White & Fradella, 2020). Many noted policy adaptations that decreased community-based and preventive efforts (Lum et al., 2023). The need to shift working practices led many agencies to explore ways to minimize public interaction, at times by implementing the remote handling of less serious and nonemergency calls (Jennings & Perez, 2020). Demir and Cassino (2024) observed modest decreases in traffic stops and arrests during the pandemic, while Lum and colleagues (2023) found an overall decrease in calls for service to the police.

Additionally, policing strategies and interactions with the public shifted, and this had the potential of increasing the strain on police-community relations. Many studies documented increased anxiety experienced by law enforcement personnel, with officers reporting stress from both the threat of infection and the organizational changes they were experiencing (Brown & Fleming, 2022; De Camargo, 2022; Martin et al., 2023; Stogner et al., 2020). Browning and Fleming (2022) reported about half of their sample of frontline officers perceived an increase in work difficulties and cited changing workloads, increased out-of-office responsibilities, and a sense of isolation due to distancing protocol. Others noted that communication and policy changes decreased their feelings of value and indicated perceptions of failed leadership or diminished organizational legitimacy (Martin et al., 2023). Law enforcement officers provided rich narratives that illustrated considerations of the risk of contracting COVID-19 and the increased stress associated with managing health, uncertainty, and putting their own loved ones at risk (De Camargo, 2022).

Court Proceedings

While the Bill of Rights guarantees citizens' right to a speedy trial and due process in criminal justice proceedings, the pandemic and associated policies transformed the way in which courts operated. From social distancing and virtual courtroom settings (Baldwin et al., 2020; Thornburg, 2020; Viglione et al., 2023), to clustering and backlogged cases (Buchanan et al., 2020; Viglione et al., 2023), and to changing strategies of release and supervision during pretrial (Thornburg, 2020; Viglione et al., 2023), court procedures faced a number of challenges while at the same time courts found opportunities during the pandemic.

Rossner (2021) highlighted some limitations of virtual court proceedings, including the potential for distraction and technological difficulties. Basics such as identity confirmation and electronic record keeping are not formalized or guided by official protocols, making virtual court proceedings and courtroom security difficult to carry out (Baldwin et al., 2020). Courtroom considerations of space, privacy, and communication can be complicated by the use of virtual settings (Baldwin et al., 2020; Gagnon & Alpern, 2021; Rossner, 2021) in addition to limited accessibility and the instability of technology (Jackson et al., 2021). Essential court functions such as questioning, real-time answers, and jury selection may be complicated or altered in a virtual setting (Baldwin et al., 2020).

Despite its changing how courtrooms operated at a basic level, the pandemic response also offered the opportunity for reform and evolution. COVID-19 presented a setting for increased or changed discretion in the judiciary, while allowing the opportunity to implement creative diversionary tactics in sentencing decisions (Gagnon & Alpern, 2021). Alternatives to in-person court appearances can be extended beyond COVID-19 protocols (Collica-Cox & Molina, 2020; Piquero, 2021; Viglione et al., 2023). Court appearances often place demands on those who are system-involved; thus opportunities for remote engagement with the court may help some people navigate employment or childcare requirements that make it difficult to attend court in person. This has the potential to create greater access to justice and more positive outcomes.

Institutional Corrections

It was expected—and found—that COVID-19 had a tremendous impact on corrections institutions, which tend to have close space by design, limited health care infrastructure, and limited strategic plans in place (Byrne et al., 2020; Marcum, 2020; Puglisi et al., 2023; Wetzel and Davis, 2020). Transmission of the coronavirus inside institutions was exponential, with both staff and incarcerated individuals alike testing positive at high rates (Hummer, 2020; Novisky et al., 2021) and incarcerated persons having increased mortality rates as a result of COVID-19 infections (Puglisi et al., 2023). Despite recommendations from the U.S. Department of Justice and the Federal Bureau of Prisons for institutions to prioritize testing and isolation to mitigate spread, to limit transfers, and to emphasize alternatives to institutional detention, infection rates remained high (Hummer, 2020; Marcum, 2020), though efforts to decarcerate made mitigation strategies easier to implement (Puglisi et al., 2023). Impossible to separate from broader health challenges in carceral institutions, the pandemic has highlighted the need for health protocols that extend beyond the COVID-19 crisis (Byrne et al., 2020; Collica-Cox & Molina, 2020; Piquero, 2021; Puglisi et al., 2023).

In some cases, the primary measure remained diversion or release from incarceration, with more emphasis on community corrections (Buchanan et al., 2020; Marcum, 2020; Nowonty & Piquero, 2020; Puglisi et al., 2023). Federal and state institutions worked to decrease prison populations (Sharma et al., 2020), which increased the responsibilities of community supervision agents and agencies. Others proposed greater release and efforts at sustained decarceration (Abraham et al., 2020), a result spurred by existing overcrowding, cost considerations, and the risk of infection. Considerations of *whom* to release impelled suggestions of more systematic evaluations or tools to guide release decisions, notably considering risk, need, and vulnerability (Vose et al., 2020). Piquero (2021) and others have pointed out that the pandemic might have had the short-term effect of restricting the use of incarceration to those deemed a true threat to public safety, as opposed to incarceration being a solely retributive strategy.

While carceral institutions generally suspended visits and limited any inmate programming, improved accessibility to technology for telecommunications with family or educational training emerged (Collica-Cox & Molina, 2020; Marcum, 2020). In some cases, the cost of phone calls or other communication-related fees were suspended or reduced to support communication and offset potential threats to the mental and emotional health of incarcerated persons (Marcum, 2020; Novisky et al., 2020). However, loved ones outside the institutions were still left with high levels of worry over the health of the incarcerated individuals. They reported increased levels of self-blame for the circumstance and existed in states of denial regarding risky carceral circumstances (Testa & Fahmy, 2021).

Community Supervision

While much is made of reducing prison and jail populations, a lot of criminal justice supervision and enforcement happens within communities. Experimentation and innovation were also evident in community corrections strategies at the height of COVID-19. Community corrections organizations experienced difficulties in sustaining both rehabilitative services and the supervision accountability of clients due to social distancing, closures or program suspensions, and changed work strategies for probation officers (Lockwood et al., 2023; Viglione et al., 2021). Supervision strategies drastically changed during the pandemic, with increased reliance on virtual meetings in place of face-to-face meetings (Schwalbe & Koetzle, 2021; Viglione et al., 2020). This added longer-term benefits with consistent—but less intrusive—contact being made, and it provided an opportunity to integrate more case management within supervision efforts.

These shifts all occurred at a time when challenges increased in frequency and intensity for clients under community correctional supervision who faced job loss, childcare demands, increases in drug and alcohol use and mental health concerns, and food and housing insecurities (Schwalbe & Koetzle, 2021). These challenges to daily demands paralleled the experiences of the non-system-impacted population as well, but they particularly changed the demands and success of supervision for those who were already system-involved.

COVID-19 also changed the nature and response of supervision violations and subsequent court proceedings, though some alternatives and video accessibility were introduced (Lockwood et al., 2023). Many agencies continued face-to-face contact in some capacity, with texting, videoconferencing, and other technological advances allowing community officers to maintain contact through normative activities such as drug testing and community service requirements, and revocations/violations decreased in frequency (Schwalbe & Koetzle, 2021; Viglione et al., 2020). This led some supervising officers to feel as though they were unable to hold persons under supervision accountable and were facing consequences for failures (Viglione et al., 2021). However, high-risk caseloads were given priority, with fewer contacts for moderate and low-risk individuals, following evidence-based practices (Viglione et al., 2021). Agencies reported the benefit of adapting to telecommunications that allowed more flexibility and diminished traditional barriers of contact, and they sought to extend such efforts beyond the nominal end of the COVID-19 pandemic (Viglione et al., 2021).

COVID-19, Crime, and Justice

The purpose of this book is to advance the conversation about how the social, economic, cultural, legislative, and policy responses to COVID-19 affected crime and justice, with a primary focus on the United States. The public health responses to the pandemic created a natural experiment that will allow criminologists to test theories of crime for years to come. What is apparent from the research published soon after the pandemic's peak is that determining the pandemic's effects on crime is complicated and nuanced.

In chapter 1, Ibrahim and Nasirudeen explore aspects of the complex and, at times, contradictory research on whether and how COVID-19 influenced offending and criminal victimization. As is traditionally the case with criminological research, our understanding of crime, its causes, and its correlates varies across space, time, and by offense type. In chapter 2, Stickle and Plank conduct a detailed analysis of how the pandemic influenced aspects of larceny when public health strategies shifted behavioral routines; these shifts either accelerated or inhibited the possibility of property theft at various sites and within different contexts. Criminological research seeks to explain the commission of crime, as well as vulnerability and victimization. In chapter 3, Christensen, Gerry, and Bennett provide an in-depth examination through the lens of intimate partner violence to identify opportunity change, trends, and policy and support in response to COVID-19. In chapter 4, Heil and Nichols report on a pilot study of how pandemic responses created new opportunities for labor trafficking exploitation, while complicating the ability of criminal justice and social service agencies to detect and intervene in this offense and provide services to victims.

Understanding how societies respond to crime is a key aspect of the study of criminal justice. The onset of a global pandemic forced criminal justice organizations and personnel to quickly shift their policies, approaches, and operations, while also creating the impetus for radical experimentation and innovation that might not have occurred under normal circumstances. While court systems were able to modify or reduce operations to keep personnel safe and healthy, frontline employees in policing and institutional corrections had to continue to be physically present to perform their duties. Such a mandate likely created significant stressors for these employees, as they worried about their own safety and well-being, along with the health of their family members. White and Hartung, in chapter 5, explore how the pandemic influenced aspects of police officers' job commitment and satisfaction in the midst of the pandemic. They focus on campus police officers. Because the pandemic occurred at the same time as public protest and calls to defund the police, it is important to explore how these events intersected in the experiences of police personnel. In chapter 6, Gaub and Koen report findings from a series of interviews they conducted with officers during and after these overlapping experiences.

While the slowing of court operations during the pandemic served to protect the health of many court workers (attorneys, judges, bailiffs, clerks, and citizens serving as witnesses or jurors), it had the additional effect of delaying justice for those charged with crimes. One possible outcome of these delays may have been an increased tendency among detained defendants awaiting adjudication to engage in more plea bargaining, including the possibility of making a false guilty plea to secure release from jail. Forston, Yan, Wilford, and DiFava consider this possibility in chapter 7. The pandemic created a substantial public health crisis within institutional corrections facilities. The design and operations of jails and prisons impeded the use of public health strategies that were undertaken in society, such as social distancing, sanitization methods, and quarantining. Vanden Bosch examines these public health challenges in chapter 8. The pandemic led many jurisdictions to try expedited or alternative release practices to reduce jail and prison populations in the hope of creating healthier institutional environments. Murolo considers how parole decision-making was influenced by COVID-19 in chapter 9. Community supervision also faced a great deal of challenges during the pandemic. Alward, Lockwood, Macleod, Ackerman, and Viglione consider this in chapter 10 in their examination of probation officers' stress and burnout during the pandemic. Finally, in chapter 11, Lee, Ayerza, Lee, Jadidi, and Holt offer an analysis of online crime and victimization trends at the height of COVID-19.

Conclusion

Understanding the effects of the COVID-19 pandemic on crime and justice is a complicated process. A century of criminology and criminal justice research has clearly demonstrated that there are myriad types, degrees, and motivations in the commission of crime, the experiences of criminal victimization, and the responses to crime and to those involved. There are challenges to drawing broad conclusions given the variation in crime patterns and responses by geography and over time.

For example, rural policing and correctional response trends during the pandemic showed differences in efficacy and efforts of response (Hansen

& Lory, 2020; Martin et al., 2022), and the policies for early release or targeted enforcement continued to expand or minimize as the pandemic progressed. Even efforts at preventing and responding to crime changed. Segura and colleagues (2023) pointed out that though programs for preventing sexual and dating violence were shifted to online delivery instead of being suspended, this limited the establishment and sustainability of trust between participants and service providers, while uneven access to technology compromised program integrity. At the same time, the shift to online service delivery provided benefits that allowed programs to expand and created flexibility in scheduling.

It remains unclear to what extent pandemic-prompted innovations will be sustained within criminal justice. New programs and adaptations are never completely successful or free of undesirable consequences. Whether criminal justice shifts initiated by COVID-19 produce a better mix of advantages and disadvantages will have to be determined in time. Further complicating matters, even policy shifts that are objectively advantageous must often be weighed against social and cultural beliefs about crime and justice. Though efforts to decarcerate might save money and reduce custodial populations without compromising public safety, these policies may be challenged by social and political calls to remain "tough" on crime and not to be "soft" on those found guilty.

The intention of this volume is not to provide a definitive conclusion on how the pandemic has affected crime and justice but rather to advance evidence-based conversations about how this chapter in American history connected with crime and criminal justice and how innovation born of necessity might offer possibilities for more just and effective policies and practices.

1. Trends: A Consideration of Crime and COVID-19

Rasheed Babatunde Ibrahim and
Ismail Ayatullah Nasirudeen

Introduction

The COVID-19 pandemic, caused by severe acute respiratory syndrome coronavirus 2 (SARS-CoV-2), has left an indelible mark on global health. In response to its threat to health, nations implemented containment measures and public health strategies to curb the virus's spread (Mervosh et al., 2020; Nivette et al., 2021). These measures included stay-at-home (SAH) orders, lockdowns, border controls, travel restrictions, limitations on gatherings, quarantines, social distancing, mandatory mask usage, and closure of schools, services, and businesses (Boman & Gallupe, 2020; Education Week, 2020; Nivette et al., 2021). Of these measures, SAH orders and mass lockdowns significantly curtailed social interactions, mobility, and normal life for millions worldwide (Estévez-Soto, 2021; Lewnard & Lo, 2020). The enforcement of these measures had immediate economic repercussions, altering work routines and leading to unemployment and business closures (Boman & Gallupe, 2020; Piquero et al., 2021). Furthermore, COVID-19 policies influenced nonmarket activities, including criminal behavior (Hoehn-Velasco et al., 2021), human rights, and mental well-being. The pandemic reshaped policing, criminal opportunities, and penalties, with adjustments to other justice system policies and practices, such as releasing inmates from jails and prisons (Abrams, 2021; Surprenant, 2020). Courts deferred cases, potentially resulting in fewer prosecutions (Abrams, 2021; Melamed & Newall, 2020). Job losses due to business closures influenced the probability of crime, surveillance, capture, arrest, prosecution, and punishment (Chetty et al., 2020).

This unprecedented situation prompted inquiries from public safety officials, politicians, criminologists, media, and the public into the influence of COVID-19 and its countermeasures on criminal behavior and crime trends (Boman & Mowen, 2021; Estévez-Soto, 2021). The alterations in social structures, processes, and organizations related to crime led many to question how the pandemic would affect crime patterns and victimization. This chapter explores these dynamics and reviews crime trends during the COVID-19 pandemic.

COVID-19 and Crime

Governments worldwide responded to the COVID-19 crisis by implementing SAH orders to curb the virus's spread. These orders, designed to constrain public movement, were expected to reduce opportunities for offending and victimization and were the subject of early studies in the pandemic that examined their impact on crime rates (Meyer et al., 2022). While numerous studies have documented changes in crime rates in response to COVID-19 movement restrictions (Langton et al., 2021b), the evidence for the impacts of SAH orders and lockdown policies on crime has been mixed.

In the short term, particularly in early- to mid-2020, crime rates showed a substantial decline across many countries (Langton et al., 2021a; Meyer et al., 2022; Nivette et al., 2021; Stickle & Felson, 2020). Notably, a significant global study by Nivette and colleagues (2021) explored the effects of SAH orders on six types of police-recorded crimes in 27 cities across the Americas, Europe, the Middle East, and Asia. Their findings revealed an overall drop of 37% in crime rates worldwide. Other studies too found that the extraordinary circumstances associated with the pandemic led to a significant overall decline in crime rates (Ashby, 2020; Boman & Gallupe, 2020; Fattah, 2020; Stickle & Felson, 2020).

Further investigations by Abrams (2021), Ashby (2020), and Campedelli and colleagues (2021) delved into the impact of the COVID-19 pandemic on crime in major cities in the United States. Abrams (2021) estimated the pandemic onset's impact on crime in major U.S. cities, while Ashby (2020) utilized police-recorded crime data to understand changes in crime frequency in 16 large cities or urban counties. Campedelli and colleagues (2021) investigated the immediate impact of COVID-19 containment policies on crime trends specifically in Los Angeles. Some studies found increases in particular types of crime, such as homicide (Rosenfeld & Lopez, 2020) and domestic violence (Bullinger et al., 2021; Miller et al., 2020; Piquero et al., 2021), with mixed findings on associated predictors (Campedelli et al., 2020; Campedelli et al., 2021). These varied findings underscore the complexity of the relationship among the pandemic, containment measures, and crime dynamics.

COVID-19 and Crime Rate Changes in the United States

The profound impact of COVID-19 on crime rates in the United States reflects the global response to the pandemic, notably through containment measures (Boman & Gallupe, 2020). Anticipation arose concerning potential spikes in various crime categories, including violent crime, organized crime, intimate partner violence, and cybercrime, juxtaposed with expected declines in opportunistic and property crimes (Eisner & Nivette, 2020; Halford et al., 2020; Pfitzner et al., 2020; Van Gelder et al., 2020). With exceptions, the general speculation was that COVID-19, alongside lockdowns and SAH orders, would lead to a decline in crime rates globally, including in the United States (Stickle & Felson, 2020).

City-level time-series analyses, such as those conducted by Campedelli and colleagues (2020), revealed a decrease in various crime rates after implementing COVID-19 containment or lockdown policies. Major urban centers experienced early declines in crime rates, including Los Angeles, New York City, Dallas, Chicago, Detroit, Indianapolis, San Francisco, St. Louis, Miami-Dade, Philadelphia, and Oakland (Brantingham et al., 2021; Bullinger et al., 2021; Campedelli et al., 2021; Felson et al., 2020; Moise & Piquero, 2023; Piquero et al., 2020). Most evidence pointed toward a drop in the general frequency of crimes, with mixed effects observed across different crime types (Stickle & Felson, 2020). Notable patterns emerged through empirical studies, revealing three main effects of COVID-19 lockdowns and SAH orders on crime (Balmori de la Miyar et al., 2021a): a consistent decline in property crimes (theft, robbery, burglary); mixed evidence for assault, battery, drug crimes, and homicides; and a return to normal crime rates after an initial decline caused by COVID-19 lockdowns (Andresen & Hodgkinson, 2020; Borrion et al., 2020).

Ashby (2020) investigated the pandemic's effects on crime in its early months by focusing on 16 cities and six crime types and utilizing police-recorded open crime data. The results demonstrated variations in crime patterns, including significant declines in residential burglaries, inconsistent changes in nonresidential burglary, and divergent patterns in theft from and of motor vehicles. Abrams's (2021) examination of crime data from the

25 largest U.S. cities several months into the pandemic revealed a general immediate decline in crime reports and arrests, particularly for theft, drug crimes, residential burglary, and most violent crimes. The study suggested that changes in crime rates preceded SAH orders, indicating voluntary alterations in behavior. After SAH orders went into effect, significant declines were observed in theft, residential burglaries, and violent crime, with increases in nonresidential burglary and car theft and no decline in homicide and shootings in most cities. Meyer and colleagues (2022) examined crime changes across three periods of the pandemic, revealing mixed but significant changes in crime rates. Homicide rates increased significantly, while larceny and robbery rates declined, indicating complex patterns during the pandemic.

In sum, the impact of COVID-19 on crime rates in the United States was multifaceted, with diverse effects across time periods, crime types, and geographic locations. Studies also utilized different data sources, which could contribute to the complex and sometimes contradictory findings. The trends suggest a nuanced relationship among the pandemic, containment measures, and crime dynamics. There is some evidence that COVID-19 and SAH orders resulted in decreases in crimes of opportunity, while contributing to an increase in some forms of violent crime.

Crime Rates before COVID-19 and after the Pandemic's Onset

Numerous studies have delved into the relationship between crime rates and the onset of the COVID-19 pandemic, often making comparisons with pre-pandemic periods. Boman and Gallupe (2020) noted a substantial nationwide decrease in crime rates during the early months of COVID-19 compared with the pre-pandemic year of 2019. In contrast, Abrams (2021) reported an immediate decline in crime reports and arrests across various cities, highlighting a potential lack of significant correlation between the pandemic's SAH orders and the observed decline. The decline was particularly notable in drug crimes, theft, residential burglary, and most violent crimes. Meyer and colleagues (2022) observed an increase in homicide and auto theft rates, a decline in larceny and robbery rates, and some indications of reduced burglary frequency during the pre-pandemic periods of 2020 across the United States.

Examining pre-pandemic crime patterns, Ashby (2020) found no consistent pattern in the frequency of major crimes when comparing three distinct periods: pre-pandemic, early pandemic, and later pandemic. Boman and

Gallupe (2020) reported that, generally, the most common finding was a lack of change in crime rates before and after the first wave of COVID-19 from March to June 2020. Where changes were identified, they varied and appeared to be influenced by the city or county under study.

Mixed Findings on the Pandemic's Effect on Crime

The collection of studies reviewed presents a complex picture, and several factors may contribute to their varied observations:

1. Measurement of trends (pre/post): Discrepancies in measuring trends before and after the onset of the pandemic might contribute to diverse findings. The reported outcomes could be influenced by different methodologies and time frames for assessing pre-pandemic and pandemic periods.
2. Type of data: Variation in the types of data analyzed across studies may also contribute to divergent results. Reliance on official crime reports, self-report surveys, or other data sources could impact the observed patterns.

It is imperative to acknowledge the limitations and inconsistencies inherent in these studies. Geographic restrictions, conceptual variations, and the temporal dimensions of the examined periods introduce complexities. Andresen and Hodgkinson (2020) and Borrion et al. (2020) underscore the temporal aspect, noting a return to normal crime rates after the initial decline, suggesting the dynamic nature of crime trends over time. In essence, this exploration of crime trends during the COVID-19 pandemic emphasizes the dynamic and multifaceted nature of the relationship, urging a nuanced understanding of evolving patterns across time, place, and crime types.

Crime Types and Patterns of Change

The intricacies of crime dynamics during the COVID-19 pandemic create a complex tapestry, influenced by various factors. Examining crime by types offers a nuanced perspective on the evolving landscape of criminal activities.

Violent Crimes

Regardless of the cities studied or the duration of examination, empirical studies consistently revealed an overall downward trend in the volume of most violent crimes in the United States during the pandemic (Abrams, 2021). This trend encompassed homicide, robbery, and vandalism (Mohler et al., 2020; Malpede & Shayegh, 2022). Notably, Malpede and Shayegh (2022) reported a decline in the frequency of sex crimes during March 2020 in Oakland and San Francisco. However, amid this general decline, Meyer et al. (2022) found a significant spike in homicide rates throughout all three pandemic periods examined, challenging the overall trend. Additionally, Ashby's study (2020) found no significant changes in the rate of serious assaults during the early months of 2020, illustrating the complexity and heterogeneity of violent crime patterns.

Property Crimes

Empirical studies suggested a general decline in the frequency of property crimes across North America, including theft/larceny (Abrams, 2021; Campedelli et al., 2021; Malpede & Shayegh, 2022; Meyer et al., 2022), burglaries (Abrams, 2021; Campedelli et al., 2020), residential burglaries (Abrams, 2021; Ashby, 2020; Felson et al., 2020), shoplifting (Campedelli et al., 2021), and theft from motor vehicles (Ashby, 2020). However, divergent findings complicate the picture. For example, evidence shows that while there was no decline in residential burglary in the cities of Minneapolis, Indianapolis, and San Francisco (Ashby 2020; Mohler et al., 2020), in the city of Los Angeles, the change was not significant (Campedelli et al., 2021). Empirical evidence further shows that while there were no significant changes in nonresidential burglary in most urban counties (see Ashby 2020; Mohler et al., 2020), there were significant increases in other places largely due to SAH orders, which rendered nonresidential buildings unmanned (Abrams, 2021). Similarly, while there was a reported spike in auto theft in major metropolitan cities (Abrams, 2021), specifically between summer and the end of 2020 (McDonald & Balkin, 2020; Meyer et al., 2022), there were no significant changes in places such as Los Angeles or Vancouver, Canada (Campedelli et al., 2021; Hodgkinson & Andresen, 2020). These conflicting trends underscore the complexity of property crime dynamics during the pandemic.

Domestic Violence and Simple Assault

Research on domestic violence during the pandemic yielded mixed findings. There is support for an overall increase in domestic violence in major cities in the United States during the initial weeks of the lockdown (Leslie & Wilson, 2020). Specifically, studies showed a significant increase in calls for police service for domestic violence in Los Angeles and Indianapolis (Mohler et al., 2020), Chicago (Bullinger et al., 2021), and some other major cities (Ashby, 2020; Sanga & McCrary, 2021). However, Bullinger et al. (2021) found that official reports by police officers and arrests for domestic violence in Chicago dropped by 6.8% and 26.4%, respectively, but they contend that around a thousand cases of domestic violence were unreported in Chicago between March and April of 2020. Piquero and colleagues (2020) observed a spike in the rate of domestic violence in Dallas; however, the increase was transient, appearing only in the first two weeks after lockdown, following which there was a drop in the volume of these offenses.

Conversely, studies in Los Angeles, Oakland, and San Francisco suggested a largely unchanged incidence of domestic violence (Campedelli et al., 2021; Malpede & Shayegh, 2022). With respect to assault and battery crimes, studies generally reported either a reduction (such as Campedelli et al., 2020, in Los Angeles; Campedelli et al., 2021, in Chicago; and Halford et al., 2020) or an insignificant change (such as Mohler et al., 2020, for Los Angeles and Indianapolis). The patterns for these crimes, especially in domestic violence, are multifaceted, influenced by factors such as prolonged interpersonal proximity due to lockdowns and variations in reporting behaviors.

Drug, Substance Abuse, and Narcotic-Related Crimes

There was an overall decline in the rate of drug crimes throughout the United States (Abrams, 2021; Campedelli et al., 2020). However, a sharp and unprecedented increase in drug overdoses and overdose mortality rates was reported following the onset of the pandemic in the United States (Currie et al., 2021; Friedman & Akre, 2021; Friedman & Hansen, 2022; Glober et al., 2020). Currie and colleagues (2021) found in Ohio a 70.6% increase from March to the end of May 2020. Friedman and Akre (2021) found the largest increases in drug overdoses in Kentucky, Tennessee, and West Virginia. These findings might suggest changes in police enforcement behaviors, which are important drivers of drug and narcotics crime data in the United States. Because drug and narcotics crime data are largely reflections of police arrest activities, they might not truly reflect the level of substance use or abuse. A global pandemic that shifted police enforcement efforts, coupled with the protest movements that took place in the summer of 2020, may have diverted police personnel and priorities away from drug and narcotics enforcement. The increase in overdoses and overdose mortality might suggest that substance use and abuse was stable or increased during the pandemic period.

Gang-Related Crime, Gun Shootings, and Weapons Possession

Brantingham and colleagues (2021) found no statistically significant change in the overall frequency of gang-related violent crimes, robberies or assaults, or gang-related violent gun crimes in Los Angeles. No significant change was discovered in the rates of shootings in the major U.S. cities examined by Abrams (2021). For the illegal possession of weapons, Malpede and Shayegh (2022) reported a decline during March 2020 in Oakland and San Francisco.

Traffic and Sidewalk Crimes

Malpede and Shayegh (2022) reported a decline in the rate of traffic and sidewalk crimes in March 2020 in Oakland and San Francisco. Bullinger et al. (2021) reported a decline or no significant change in police service calls for traffic crimes in Chicago. Preliminary evidence showed an increase in risky driving behaviors (such as speeding, distracted driving, drinking and driving, and drugged driving) and resultant severe crashes during the pandemic due to a reduction in traffic volumes (Adanu et al., 2021; Vanlaar et al., 2021). However, there was an average decline in non-severe traffic crashes during the pandemic (Hughes et al., 2023; Katrakazas et al., 2020; Saladié et al., 2020; Shilling & Waetjen, 2020). In Louisiana, a decline was reported in the frequency of traffic accidents involving injury, distracted drivers, and ambulances (Barnes et al., 2020, 2022).

Cybercrime

Reports on the frequency of cybercrimes have a general implication for the United States. Although cybervictimization may have remained largely unchanged in the early months of the pandemic (Hawdon et al., 2020), studies have revealed a general increase in the rate of cybercrimes during SAH periods. This includes a likely increase in data theft and attacks from hackers (Kashif et al., 2020). The overall rise has been generally attributed to the increased unemployment generated by lockdown measures or the shutdown of businesses. It is likely that some unemployed individuals resorted to cybercrimes to support themselves (Lallie et al., 2021).

Policing Activities and Crime Trends amid the COVID-19 Pandemic

It is impossible to isolate changes in crime trends from concurrent shifts taking place in police activities and strategies. COVID-19 influenced the behaviors and activities of both crime victims and lawbreakers, but it also altered the behaviors and activities of police organizations and individual officers. The intricate relationship between policing activities and crime rates during the COVID-19 pandemic underscores the need for a comprehensive analysis. Anecdotal evidence supports the claim that some communities experienced decreased police presence and enforcement, possibly influencing criminal activities (Elinson & Chapman, 2020; Melamed & Newall, 2020). Because the police are a major source of crime detection, changes in police behaviors would significantly impact reported crime rates, particularly for traffic offenses, drug-related crimes, and gang-related activities (Abrams, 2021; Brantingham et al., 2021; Mohler et al., 2020).

A decline in policing activities, especially in traffic enforcement and proactive patrols, has multifaceted consequences. It can affect the reported rates of traffic crimes and may have implications for other offenses. Abrams (2021) suggests that the decline in drug and narcotic-related crime rates may be linked to reduced police presence and changes in deployment attitudes toward crime detection. Understanding the dynamics of these shifts in policing activities is crucial for interpreting true crime rates, which may differ significantly from the recorded rates.

Another critical aspect of crime detection lies in reports from the public and victims. Abrams (2021) points out that the curtailing of people's mobility during the pandemic might well have resulted in a drop in public observations and reports of crime. This anticipated decrease is likely to influence the rates of crimes for which the primary detection source is the victim or the public. Bullinger et al. (2021) noted declining traffic crime rates due to reduced traffic volume during lockdown. However, this reduction simultaneously enhances the chance of police detection for specific crime types, emphasizing the interplay between enforcement dynamics and crime trends (Abrams, 2021).

An Integrated Theoretical Perspective on COVID-19 and Crime Rate Changes

Understanding the shifts in crime rates during the COVID-19 pandemic involves a multifaceted exploration, blending empirical insights with theoretical frameworks to offer a comprehensive perspective. The primary reason behind the overall decline in crime rates is attributed to SAH orders and movement restrictions in response to COVID-19. However, a single theory or perspective cannot adequately explain the variations in the timing and magnitude of change across different crime types. Hence, a nuanced examination reveals varied trends across different crime types.

Routine Activities

Empirical insights emphasize that changes to routine activities, marked by shifts in daily life patterns, contribute significantly to alterations in crime rates (Estévez-Soto, 2021; Hodgkinson & Andresen, 2020). Estévez-Soto (2021) suggested that changes in mobility might partially be connected to observed declines in the rate of some crimes and could correlate with crime type. The decline in routine economic and social activities during the pandemic corresponded with a decrease in the opportunity for criminal activities (Balmori de la Miyar et al., 2021a, 2021b; Hoehn-Velasco et al., 2021; Miller & Blumstein, 2020), in line with the routine activity theory.

Routine activity theory posits that crimes occur when motivated offenders encounter suitable targets in the absence of capable guardians (Cohen & Felson, 1979; Felson, 1986). This convergence underscores the relevance of routine activities in shaping crime dynamics during the pandemic (Estévez-Soto, 2021; Felson et al., 2020; Lallie et al., 2021; Mohler et al., 2020). Lockdown measures disrupted regular routines, leading to variations in criminal behavior across different crime types (Campedelli et al., 2021; Cheung & Gunby, 2022; Hodgkinson & Andresen, 2020; Payne & Morgan, 2020).

Opportunities

Both empirical and theoretical perspectives underscore the pivotal role of opportunities in influencing crime rates. The reduction in opportunities due to lockdowns and changes in routine activities was associated with a decline in various crime types (Campedelli et al., 2020; Campedelli et al., 2021; Hodgkinson & Andresen, 2020; Meyer et al., 2022; Nivette et al., 2021). For example, a decline in robbery rates could result from the reduction of people out in public, particularly at night (Meyer et al., 2022). Explanations of opportunities align with theoretical perspectives such as crime pattern theory, which posits that a massive reduction in opportunities contributes to changes in crime rates (Brantingham & Brantingham, 1984).

Opportunity theories, including routine activity theory, have been instrumental in explaining observed shifts in crime rates. These theories highlight the significance of situational factors and the availability of targets, emphasizing how changes in routine activities and lockdown measures directly impact criminal opportunities. The pandemic-induced alterations in mobility and social interactions reshaped the landscape of criminal opportunities, influencing the overall patterns of criminal behavior. In line with the opportunity perspectives, the modern economic theory of crime—much like rational choice theory—argues that crime rate is a function of expected gains and risked penalties from crime (Becker, 1968); it was used to explain changes in property crime during the pandemic (see Abrams, 2021; Cheung & Gunby, 2022).

Social Learning

Empirically, insights from Boman and Gallupe (2020) suggest that peer-group-based crimes, such as domestic violence (which may or may not include homicide), may also be largely responsible for the overall decline in crime rates during the pandemic. The government-issued lockdowns limited associations among deviant peer groups, thus preempting crimes that deviant peers would have ordinarily influenced. Theoretical perspectives, including social learning theories, further contribute to understanding how peer influences shape criminal behavior (Balmori de la Miyar et al., 2021a, 2021b; Hoehn-Velasco et al., 2021). Social learning theories delve into the influence of peers on criminal behavior, positing that individuals learn deviant behavior from their social environment. The disruption of social interactions during the pandemic, including limitations on peer interactions and gatherings, altered the dynamics of social learning. As a result, the decline in peer-based crimes, such as domestic violence, can be linked to changes in social learning patterns influenced by lockdown measures.

Strains

Stickle and Felson (2020) attempted to explain what likely did and did not change during the lockdown periods, suggesting numerous important factors such as poverty, social inequality, stress, anomie and fear, and societal disorganization. Empirically, factors related to strain, including fear of infection, economic impacts, and changes in alcohol consumption, are identified as contributors to shifts in crime rates (Balmori de la Miyar et al., 2021a, 2021b; Boman & Gallupe, 2020; Hoehn-Velasco et al., 2021). Theoretical perspectives, particularly general strain theory, align with these observations by connecting negative emotional states to increased criminal behavior (Campedelli et al., 2020; Campedelli et al., 2021). General strain theory sees crime as a function of negative emotional states that result from individual and structural strains, and crimes tend to increase with higher levels of negative emotions such as anxiety, disappointment, fear, frustration, rage, and anger (Agnew, 1992, 1999, 2006).

Strain-related explanations offer valuable insights into the psychological and economic consequences of the pandemic on criminal behavior. The fear of infection and the economic fallout created heightened emotional states, potentially triggering criminal activities. General strain theory provides a theoretical framework for understanding how individual and structural strains contribute to increased negative emotions, which, in turn, may manifest as criminal behavior.

Social Disorganization

Both empirical and theoretical viewpoints converge in the relevance of social disorganization for explaining changes in crime rates. Disruptions to social order during exceptional events like the pandemic contribute to increased crime rates (Hodgkinson & Andresen, 2020; Stickle & Felson, 2020). Social disorganization theory highlights the role of societal breakdown in fostering criminal activities. Disruptions to social order during the pandemic, including strains on community relationships, economic hardships, and increased fear, collectively contributed to an environment conducive to criminal behavior.

Prosocial Theories

Prosocial theories (also known as social cohesion or altruism) and antisocial theories are twin theories that have been offered as an explanation for general changes in crime rates (whether an increase or decrease in different crime types) (see Balmori de la Miyar et al., 2021a, 2021b; Foran & O'Leary, 2008; Hoehn-Velasco et al., 2021). While prosocial theory predicts a decline in crime rates after a catastrophic event because of the altruistic behaviors of criminals (Fritz, 1996; Zahran et al., 2009), antisocial theory predicts an increase in crime rates after a catastrophic event due to the opportunistic behaviors of criminals or a change in routine activities (Curtis et al., 2000; Davila et al., 2005).

Theoretical Synthesis

An integrated synthesis bridges the empirical and theoretical realms, offering a unified understanding of the complex interplay of factors influencing crime rate changes during the COVID-19 pandemic. By merging the notions of routine activities, opportunities, social learning and peers, and strain-related explanations, this comprehensive perspective lays the foundation for a nuanced analysis that transcends traditional dichotomies and embraces the holistic nature of crime dynamics in unprecedented times.

Methodological Approaches in Examining the Interplay of COVID-19 and Crime

Numerous studies, spanning diverse geographic areas and populations, have primarily relied on official and/or police crime data, reports, records, count data, and statistics specific to the counties, cities, states, or countries under investigation (Abrams, 2021; Balmori de la Miyar et al., 2021a, 2021b; Brantingham et al., 2021; Campedelli et al., 2020; Campedelli et al., 2021; Hoehn-Velasco et al., 2021; Felson et al., 2020; Langton et al., 2021a, 2021b; Moise & Piquero, 2023; Nivette et al., 2021; Syamsuddin et al., 2021). This conventional approach directly examines crime trends through authoritative channels, offering a foundation for robust empirical analysis. However, the implications of relying solely on official crime data warrant consideration, as it may not capture the entirety of criminal activities, especially those underreported or affected by law enforcement biases.

In addition to direct crime data, researchers have applied a spectrum of data methodologies to enrich their analyses. Studies drawing from published literature and public statistical reports from newspapers, government agencies, and criminal justice sources contribute valuable insights to the broader contextual understanding of the pandemic's impact on crime (Boman & Gallupe, 2020; Boman & Mowen, 2021; Zhang,

2022). This approach taps into existing knowledge, providing a historical backdrop and facilitating comparisons over time. However, the reliance on secondary sources introduces potential biases present in the original studies, demanding cautious interpretation.

Cell phone block-level activity and administrative 911 data (calls for police service) offer innovative avenues for comprehending changes in human mobility and law enforcement responsiveness during the pandemic (Bullinger et al., 2021). Such data sources provide real-time, granular insights into behavioral shifts, aiding in the exploration of nuanced patterns that traditional crime data might overlook. Yet challenges related to privacy concerns and potential sampling biases associated with mobile phone data must be acknowledged.

Victimization reports, as utilized by Cheung and Gunby (2022), present a crucial departure from traditional crime data by directly tapping into individuals' experiences. This approach captures incidents regardless of law enforcement involvement, offering a more comprehensive view of criminal victimization. However, victimization reports are susceptible to issues like memory biases and varying perceptions of criminal events.

Justice, security, and mobility datasets, as employed by Estévez-Soto (2021), broaden the scope of analysis by integrating multifaceted dimensions of societal activities. These datasets encompass diverse aspects of the justice system and societal behavior, contributing to a holistic understanding of the pandemic's ripple effects on crime. Nevertheless, challenges associated with data integration, standardization, and potential selection biases need careful consideration.

Internet questionnaires, as exemplified in Kashif et al. (2020), signify an innovative foray into capturing public perceptions and experiences related to crime during the pandemic. This method allows for a direct exploration of community sentiments, providing a qualitative layer to complement quantitative crime data. However, issues like response bias and the inability to generalize findings to broader populations should be acknowledged.

Conclusion

Undoubtedly, the global landscape of crime underwent a seismic shift after the arrival of the COVID-19 pandemic. The profound impact of this unprecedented event was intricately interwoven with the array of governmental responses worldwide, characterized by the implementation of lockdown measures and stay-at-home orders aimed at mitigating the spread of the formidable virus. While the literature examining the effects of these measures on crime rates yielded mixed evidence, a prevailing theme emerges: a pervasive decline in crime rates spanning cities, states, countries, and continents, with the United States standing as no exception.

Though a noteworthy departure from pre-pandemic levels, this overarching reduction in crime rates does not necessarily characterize the impact as uniformly positive. The mitigated crime rates during the pandemic, while providing a temporary respite, are nuanced and transient. As lockdown measures and SAH orders eased, the resurgence of crime rates to prepandemic levels emerged as a disconcerting reality. The multifaceted impact of COVID-19 and its associated containment measures on crime trends becomes evident, revealing divergent trajectories across different crime types.

Empirical investigations aimed at deciphering the intricacies of these variations both within and outside the confines of lockdowns have added depth to our understanding. Criminological theories, particularly routine activity theory, have been pivotal in interpreting the underlying dynamics. However, the complexity of the observed changes demands a more comprehensive approach, acknowledging that no single theory can fully encapsulate the intricacies of global crime trends during the COVID-19 era.

An amalgamation of criminological theories emerges as the key to comprehensively elucidating the global shift in crime patterns. Notably, studies have underscored the necessity of considering a spectrum of theories to account for variations by crime type. For instance, a decline in residential burglary coinciding with a surge in nonresidential burglary underscores the need for a nuanced theoretical framework. Similarly, the static levels of certain violent crimes, a general decline in property offenses, and a concerning rise in domestic violence crimes collectively defy a singular explanatory paradigm.

In conclusion, the impact of COVID-19 on global crime trends is undeniably substantial, with far-reaching consequences. The evolving nature of crime rates, influenced by myriad factors intricately tied to the pandemic, necessitates a holistic understanding. As societies grapple with the aftermath of the pandemic, the insights garnered from empirical studies and criminological theories will be instrumental in crafting thoughtful policies and responses to address the dynamic and multifaceted landscape of post-pandemic crime.

2. Property Crime Considerations: The Impact of COVID-19 on Theft

Ben Stickle and James A. Plank

Introduction

COVID-19 had a profound impact around the world and in all societies. However, its impact was not experienced evenly across all communities in time or scope, thus creating an opportunity to examine criminological theories of crime and prevention methods. With the implementation of lockdowns (e.g., stay-at-home orders) and other government-directed actions intended to control the movement of people and thereby lessen the spread of disease, the daily routine activity of entire populations shifted dramatically. For example, as more individuals stayed home, many stores closed, and retail purchases moved to online sales. As a result, shoplifting increased at gas stations and pharmacies while decreasing at department stores. Furthermore, the theft of delivered packages from stoops and porches increased dramatically as the rate of retail home delivery increased. Similarly, burglary shifted from residential areas to commercial and business districts as people abandoned businesses and stayed home.

Public orders passed during the COVID-19 pandemic significantly impacted crime rates as day-to-day travel dropped off significantly (Stickle & Felson, 2020). Changes in theft rates varied depending on the nature of the theft. For example, retail theft rates dropped as people remained at home after stay-at-home orders went into effect in their locale (Abrams, 2021; Borrion et al., 2020; Ceccato et al., 2022; Cheung & Gunby, 2022; Langton et al., 2021a, 2021b; Meyer et al., 2022; Payne et al., 2021; Schleimer et al., 2021). Conversely, commercial burglaries increased as businesses shuttered and employees stayed home (Abrams, 2021; Felson et al., 2020; Jackman, 2020). These results have allowed criminologists to study crime in society as never before, influencing future strategies for crime reduction (Miller & Blumstein, 2020).

This chapter examines the impact of COVID-19 on various types of theft within a routine activity and situational crime perspective framework, emphasizing the relation of these events to time and space as well as the implementation of policies aimed at restricting movement in public places. The findings indicate that an overall crime drop occurred in most communities during the initial months of COVID-19. However, as the response to the pandemic continued, crime shifted in different ways, rising in some aspects while dropping in others (i.e., place, type, and time). This chapter focuses on COVID-19's impact on theft and discusses the relationship between the COVID-19 pandemic and retail theft, burglary, vehicle theft, storage locker theft, metal theft, and package theft.

COVID-19 and Lockdowns

The COVID-19 pandemic shook the world as it became the most significant public health crisis in over a century (Chattopadhyay et al., 2022). Across the globe, different nations had divergent responses to the virus and its rampant spread. It was quickly learned that the virus spread mainly from person to person, so isolating, social distancing, and quarantining were initially identified as optimal measures to slow its advance (Edwards, 2020).

The first lockdown of an entire population in response to COVID-19 occurred in Wuhan, China, on January 23, 2020. In the United States, the implementation of lockdowns was uneven by state, county, and city. On February 3, 2020, the Trump administration declared a public health emergency due to the growing number of outbreaks, but lockdowns did not begin in the United States until March 19, 2020, when Governor Gavin Newsom enacted a stay-at-home order in California. This order allowed people to leave their homes for necessary trips (Onyeaka et al., 2021). Soon after, aside from Oklahoma and Utah, every other state began implementing its version of lockdown. Oklahoma ordered its older and vulnerable citizens to stay home, but mayors in cities such as Ardmore, Claremore, Edmond, Moore, Oklahoma City, Sallisaw, Stillwater, and Tulsa ordered all their citizens to shelter in place (Mervosh et al., 2020). Utah responded similarly by county, with the counties of Davis, Salt Lake, and Summit issuing stay-at-home orders to all their citizens. Table 2.1 provides a timeline of lockdowns enacted by U.S. states.

Table 2.1 Timeline of Lockdowns by U.S. State

State	Start of lockdown in 2020
California	March 19
Illinois, New Jersey	March 21
New York	March 22
Connecticut, Louisiana, Ohio, Oregon, Washington	March 23
Delaware, Indiana, Massachusetts, Michigan, New Mexico, West Virginia	March 24
Hawaii, Idaho, Vermont, Wisconsin	March 25
Colorado, Kentucky	March 26
Minnesota, New Hampshire	March 27
Alaska, Montana, Rhode Island, Wyoming	March 28
Kansas, Maryland, North Carolina, Virginia	March 30
Arizona, Tennessee	March 31
District of Columbia, Nevada, Pennsylvania	April 1
Maine, Texas	April 2
Florida, Georgia, Mississippi	April 3
Alabama	April 4
Missouri	April 6
South Carolina	April 7

Adapted from Mervosh et al. (2020)

Worldwide, most countries were under lockdown in the initial months of the pandemic, except South Korea and Sweden. Sweden opted against lockdown measures and adopted a voluntary approach that encouraged social distancing and good hygiene as the Swedes sought herd immunity in their population (Reuters, 2022). South Korea focused on contact tracing and artificial intelligence while keeping its economy open (Bhatia et al., 2021). The lockdowns of 2020 altered the lifestyles of entire populations as more people began working remotely and avoided mass gatherings. Criminologists who observed an overall crime drop in most communities during this time saw an opportunity to test criminological theories as never before (Stickle & Felson, 2020).

Crime Opportunity Structure and Routine Activity Theory

Crime opportunity structure explains crime as the result of a rational choice made by an offender who chooses targets based on how valuable the expected reward will be relative to the effort and risk. This criminological perspective was developed by Cloward and Ohlin (1960), who originally sought to understand why young people commit crimes and how beliefs about the opportunities made available to them determine their choices. Similarly, routine activity theory complements this explanation of crime by viewing crime as the "convergence in time and space of three minimal elements: a likely offender, a suitable target, and the absence of a capable guardian against crime" (Cohen & Felson, 1979, p. 588). According to Felson and Clarke (1998), this theory of crime rests on the single principle that "easy or tempting opportunities entice people into criminal activity" (p. 2). This principle is found in both opportunity theories of crime and the routine activity approach, and Felson and Clarke conclude that opportunity is a cause of crime.

COVID-19 created plentiful opportunities for crime to occur that were both "easy" and "tempting." The daily routine activity of entire populations shifted dramatically when their governments implemented lockdowns to stop the spread of disease. Inadvertently, opportunities were increased for motivated offenders seeking to take advantage of the disruption brought on by the pandemic. At the same time, other opportunities were reduced or eliminated. The literature on COVID-19's impact on theft is reviewed in the next section through the lens of crime opportunity structure and routine activity to understand how changed opportunity structures impacted crime during the early stages of the pandemic.

Theft and Burglary during COVID-19

Retail Theft
Retail theft, defined as "the act of removing a product or item from a retail establishment without presenting the proper payment" (Hicks &

Stickle, 2021, p. 1), has been a constant nuisance for retailers, forcing them to shift the costs of lost profits to customers. The documentation and research available on retail theft during the pandemic are abundant, whereas studies of other types of crime during this time frame were more exploratory, especially storage locker theft. Multiple published studies show how lockdowns impacted retail theft in different countries (see Stickle et al., 2023). The COVID-19 pandemic created unique circumstances for retailers as shoplifting patterns changed significantly worldwide. Most notable were decreases in retail theft that coincided with stay-at-home orders and other government-directed initiatives early in the pandemic. These orders and initiatives were aimed at reducing population movement in countries like Australia (Payne et al., 2021; Wang et al., 2021), China (Borrion et al., 2020), England and Wales (Agrawa et al., 2022; Langton et al., 2021a, 2021b), New Zealand (Cheung & Gunby, 2022), and the United States (Abrams, 2021; Ceccato et al., 2022; Meyer et al., 2022; Schleimer et al., 2021). As a result, researchers can compare retail theft with orders restricting movement in light of routine activity theory and a situational crime perspective.

In Queensland, Australia, Payne et al. (2021) examined shoplifting and retail theft rates in April, May, and June 2020, noting that rates were significantly lower than forecasted. These forecasted rates came from quantitative models that employ regression analysis and are used by researchers to predict future crime rates. When mobility restrictions were implemented nationwide in April 2020, shoplifting rates decreased 49% more than expected. Soon after, retail theft rates trended upward in May and June 2020 but were still well below forecast. Wang et al. (2021) used an advanced statistical approach (called ARIMA) to examine data from New South Wales, Australia, from January 2, 2017, to June 28, 2020. Their analysis observed a reduction in retail theft of more than 30% immediately following the April 2020 lockdown restrictions.

In an anonymous city in China, Borrion et al. (2020) found that retail thefts in January 2020 dropped almost to zero when government lockdowns began. Several months later, as the restrictions loosened, the daily number of retail thefts returned to expected rates. In broad terms, Borrion et al. attributed the finding to COVID-19 and the measures taken to reduce infections, but a closer analysis revealed a general trend of decreasing annual crime levels. For example, there was a 20% decrease in crime levels between 2018 and 2019 during this same period (para. 42). They also noted similar patterns in the past, coinciding with the annual spring festival held in the city each January. To remedy this, Borrion et al. generated a realistic counterfactual time series to capture secular trends and seasonal components that accurately estimated the net effect of the pandemic and the measures taken to slow its spread. They concluded that increased security by store managers during the government-imposed restrictions, coupled with increased surveillance by authorities and social distancing measures, had a suppressing effect on levels of theft as thieves had fewer opportunities for deception.

Cheung and Gunby (2022) used a dataset of monthly victimization reports from the New Zealand Police from July 2014 to May 2020 and discovered a correlation between changes in mobility patterns and crime rates. The lockdown in New Zealand began on March 26, 2020, and was lifted on May 27, 2020, and according to the data, during that time property crimes in nonresidential locations decreased by more than half.

In England and Wales, Langton et al. (2021a, 2021b) examined small area variations in crime trajectories during the COVID-19 pandemic. They found that crime declined nationwide in April 2020, when the first full month of lockdowns began. Retail theft had a 60% decline before bouncing back in August 2020 to levels that were still 30% lower than expected. Agrawa et al. (2022) also observed this decrease in crime and analyzed how crime trends evolved during the pandemic. England instituted three national lockdown periods: the first from March 26 to June 15, 2020; the second from November 5 to December 2, 2020; and the third from January 6 to April 12, 2021. Analyzing crime trends before, during, and after each lockdown, Agrawa et al. observed dramatic theft declines in the months when lockdowns were imposed and a return to normal rates in the months when no national lockdown was in place. These findings suggest that theft reduction resulted from significant changes in the population's mobility.

Data from 25 large U.S. cities showed a widespread and immediate drop in crime, with theft decreasing by 28.2% (Abrams, 2021). Ceccato et al. (2022), in their assessment of the effects of stay-at-home orders on crime levels in New York City, found a sharp and consistent drop in crime throughout March, April, and May 2020. The expected theft rate during this time was estimated at 800 counts; however, the reported counts dropped to around 300 immediately following the stay-at-home orders (Ceccato et al., 2022, fig. 4). Another study of crime in New York City found declines in residential burglary, felony assault, grand larceny, rape, and robbery, with increases in nonresidential burglary and motor vehicle theft (Koppel et al., 2023). Meyer et al. (2022) reviewed theft rates in 29 of the largest cities in the United States from January 2018 through December 2020 and found a decrease of 502 thefts per 100,000 people during the spring pandemic lockdown.

As the stay-at-home orders began to be rescinded in May 2020 and social distancing rules loosened, retail theft rates showed mixed results in different parts of the world as populations resumed their regular routines. For example, after lockdown measures were lifted in the United Kingdom, shoplifting rates in England and Wales remained below projections at the end of 2021 (Dixon et al., 2022). In the United States, significant declines were noted in 29 major cities (Meyer et al., 2022). This contrasts with the findings of Borrion et al. (2020), who observed that retail thefts resumed at expected rates in their study conducted in an unnamed city in China.

In the United States, retail theft had seen an increase in certain areas prior to the pandemic; some believed those increases stemmed from changes to laws in some states. For example, in 2014, California raised the dollar threshold for felony theft offenses to $950, reclassifying many thefts from felonies to misdemeanors. Thirty states have increased the dollar threshold for theft offenses since 2005, leading some industry experts to believe that a decrease in enforcement by authorities emboldened thieves to steal without fear of consequences (Corkery & Maheshwari, 2021). By creating lighter punishments for retail thieves, lawmakers created an environment ripe for thefts to occur pre-pandemic as the number of motivated offenders increased (Hong, 2022). As COVID-19 hit the United States, shortages occurred in personnel when fewer people were allowed to work on site. Essential workers such as police, nurses, and grocers were deemed "essential"; however, many Americans had to either work from home or not work at all. This shortage of employees complicates the picture of decreased theft rates as fewer employees were available to prevent thefts. Citing the reduction in arrest rates for shoplifters, the New York Police Department stated, "There was more stealing at stores without security guards who were willing to detain shoplifters" (Hong, 2022). Some retail managers have become disillusioned with the prospect of stopping shoplifters and reporting them to the police altogether, as it is seen as a waste of time and an unnecessary risk (Williamson, 2021).

Researchers analyzing data on retail theft before, during, and after stay-at-home orders were issued have identified lenient theft laws, in addition to labor shortages, as additional variables to consider when studying crime rates. Across the globe, retail theft decreased significantly while these orders were active. As they were loosened or lifted, the results on theft have been mixed in different countries. Some areas have seen a return to average retail theft rates, while others have not. To understand the impact of COVID-19 on retail theft, changes in rates should be considered separately for locales, as opposed to including all retail theft across a large area.

Vehicle Theft and Theft from Vehicles

Vehicles were not immune to theft during the pandemic. As a result of lockdowns and the fear of contracting and spreading the virus, fewer people engaged in activities that required them to drive a vehicle. According to the International Energy Agency (2020), global road transport activity in early 2020 was 50% lower compared to March 2019. Daily vehicle travel decreased by 60% in the United States during the months that lockdowns were imposed (Bureau of Transportation Statistics, 2020). Cheung and Gunby (2022), using Google mobility data in their study on crime and mobility during COVID-19 in New Zealand, observed a sharp decrease in mobility on retail premises and a sharp increase in residential locations, providing fewer opportunities for vehicle theft in unattended parking lots, consistent with routine activity theory's explanation of crime.

According to the National Insurance Crime Bureau (2021b), which tracks insurance claim data, 880,595 vehicles were stolen in the United States in 2020; Colorado, in particular, was hit hard, with a 37% increase in auto theft in 2020 compared with 2019. In Austin and Los Angeles, a significant increase occurred immediately after stay-at-home orders were given (Ashby, 2020), which also happened in Philadelphia (Abrams, 2021); Danbury, Connecticut (Baker, 2022); and New York City (Esposito & King, 2021). Bakersfield, California, had the most recorded auto thefts nationwide in 2020, with California leading all states with 29,162 thefts (National Insurance Crime Bureau, 2021b).

According to Meyer and colleagues (2022), significant increases in auto thefts were reported in a study of 29 major U.S. cities from March to December 2020. The reason may be that car owners who left their vehicles parked and unattended for days were less likely to be effective guardians as complacency set in. Esposito and King (2021), consistent with strain theory, suggested that the psychological stress of a quarantine, increased alcohol consumption, and unemployment resulting from lockdowns increased the proportion of people likely to commit vehicle theft and other crimes. Another explanation for this surge in vehicle thefts may have been higher prices for new and used cars. With the combined conditions of tight supply and heavy post-pandemic demand, used car prices surged as much as 30% from the prior year (Cox, 2021). The president and CEO of the National Insurance Crime Bureau (2021b) indicated that realignments in law enforcement strategies and economic downturn also may have contributed to this increase.

Conversely, decreases in auto theft were observed in different U.S. cities. Chicago and Tucson, for example, saw significant decreases in auto theft (Ashby, 2020), as did Baltimore (Abrams, 2021). Some researchers believe these decreases may have resulted from offenders having less need to steal a vehicle due to the slowdown of productive and social activities (Campedelli et al., 2021). Other explanations for this decrease include fewer car owners driving into populated areas and parking their vehicles in unattended lots, thus leaving would-be thieves with fewer targets.

Thefts from vehicles—or intentionally removing property from a vehicle without the owner's consent—became a lucrative opportunity for car burglars seeking a quick steal during the pandemic. With more vehicles left unattended, thieves had numerous targets to choose from. New York City, for example, experienced an increase of 63% in car burglaries during the pandemic, and Los Angeles saw an increase of 17% (Associated Press, 2020). This low-risk crime produced potential high rewards for thieves who saw many targets left unguarded as their owners remained indoors.

With fewer people driving, owners left their vehicles unattended for days on end, creating an opportunity for thieves. Once again, the change in routine activities altered typical crime patterns. In some areas, the change increased vehicle access, as homeowners did not leave the house and parked their cars outside unattended. In other situations, the reduction in commuting into higher crime areas for work resulted in less theft.

Storage Locker Theft

According to StorageCafe (2022), one in three Americans uses self-storage lockers, with customers' most common reason for renting a locker being a move to another home and a need for temporary space to store property. Likely due to losing a job during the pandemic, to clearing out a garage to make a home gym, or to needing space for a home office, many Americans needed a place other than home to store possessions during the pandemic.

This drove an increase in storage locker rentals. Businesses sometimes rent storage lockers, as well, to store inventory or other items. Regardless of who rents them and why, storage lockers contain valuable items and offer tempting targets for thieves.

Storage companies frequently use antitheft measures such as cameras, bright lights, locked gates, and even security guards. However, a motivated offender can sometimes find ways around these measures with relative ease. Failure to invest in a more sophisticated security system can result in a loss of property for customers and damage to consumers' trust in the storage industry. According to the Janus International Group, most storage locker thefts happen when thieves cut the locks on a unit with a pair of bolt cutters (Morehouse, 2021).

Surprisingly, this type of crime has been neglected in academic literature and is rarely discussed among practitioners. As a result, news accounts provide the only information on storage locker crime during the pandemic. The Arapahoe County Sheriff's Office in Colorado, for instance, reported a spike in storage locker thefts during the pandemic. The sheriff's spokesman said the county saw an 80% increase, with 115 burglaries at 35 different storage facilities (Snowdon, 2021). According to one corporate security expert, the pandemic drove business closures and unemployment, leading to more thefts at facilities with large amounts of goods (Johnson, 2021).

Metal Theft

Metal theft is a growing concern in which thieves steal items such as air conditioners, copper wire and pipes, catalytic converters, bronze plaques, lead roofing, and other items "for the value of their constituent metals" (Whiteacre et al., 2008, p. 3). In other words, thieves steal metal objects, not for their intended use, but to resell them, likely to a scrap yard or recycling center, to earn a profit (Stickle, 2017, 2020b).

Because metal thieves resell their stolen goods to earn a profit, there is a strong connection between the value of metals and the theft rate. Termed the price-theft hypothesis, its validity has been demonstrated by data numerous times (Draca et al., 2015; Posick et al., 2012; Quinn et al., 2023; Sidebottom et al., 2011, 2014). As the market value of metal increases, theft increases in kind. Scrap metal prices are usually driven by two key factors: demand and supply.

The pandemic decreased the supply of metals as mines and refineries closed or slowed production, and the demand for home electronics increased as consumers were in lockdown and working from home. As a result, the value of metals climbed dramatically during the second quarter of 2020 (Yu et al., 2021). While there have been no academic studies of metal theft during COVID-19, there are indications that this crime rose in 2020. For example, the price of copper increased by 90% between January 3, 2020, and March 3, 2022, and the price of rhodium (used in catalytic converters) skyrocketed 1,300% during the first year of the pandemic (London Metal Exchange, 2022).

Because police agencies infrequently track metal theft, it is necessary to turn to other sources. According to the National Insurance Crime Bureau, catalytic converter theft has risen steadily over the last decade. Insurance claims for catalytic converter theft increased from 3,389 in 2019 to 14,433 in 2020, a 325% increase (National Insurance Crime Bureau, 2021a). The bureau has not released data for 2021, but other sources estimate a sharp increase in catalytic converter thefts in 2021. For instance, Been Verified (2021) used Google search data, combined with prior National Insurance Crime Bureau theft reports, to estimate an additional 353% increase in catalytic converter theft during 2021 alone. If these numbers are correct, thefts of catalytic converters may have increased by nearly 700% during the COVID-19 pandemic.

Opportunity is a chief factor in metal theft because thieves mostly steal metal from the built environment (e.g., air conditioners, aluminum doors, gutters, copper wire). Much metal theft occurs at abandoned buildings and construction sites (Stickle, 2017). Pandemic lockdowns closed off many areas where metals abound, such as commercial sites and construction areas. When these sites suspended operations and fewer people were around, guardianship declined and theft became less risky. While academic studies have yet to quantify metal theft during COVID-19, it seems likely that a coalescence of factors—increased market value, greater opportunity, and reduced guardianship—resulted in a significant increase in metal theft.

Package Theft

Package theft, more commonly known by the colloquialism *porch piracy*, is defined as "taking possession of a package or its contents, outside of a residence or business, where it has been commercially delivered or has been left for commercial pick-up, with intent to deprive the rightful owner of the contents" (Hicks et al., 2022, p. 3). Unfortunately, few police agencies track instances of package theft, and retailers and shippers tend not to release their data on package theft. As such, little is known about package theft (Stickle et al., 2020) apart from one crucial source: consumer surveys, which are the basis for this section.

Package theft is emerging as the most common type of crime in America. While it is not a new crime, social media attention, victims' fear (Hicks, 2020), and the financial impact of porch piracy are growing astoundingly. One early study of package theft by August Homes (2016) found that nearly 11 million individuals had been victims of package theft. Less than five years later, a study by Safe Wise estimated that 210 million packages were stolen in 2021 (Carlsen, 2022). Assuming an average value per package of 25 dollars, the impact of porch piracy in 2021 exceeded half a billion dollars. The impact would be even more significant by including expenses for retailers when they replace stolen items, costs associated with reshipping packages, and the loss of consumer trust.

In response to COVID-19, retailers saw a dramatic shift in consumer habits in early 2020. More people than ever before were purchasing items online and having them delivered to their homes. According to a PricewaterhouseCoopers survey in late 2021, the number of persons shopping online was a few percentage points behind traditional physical stores (Torkington, 2021). This dramatic change in buying behavior has shifted crime from retail stores to consumers' homes (Stickle, 2020a), and it presents a new challenge to police, retailers, delivery services, and consumers. The trend toward online shopping has persisted and likely signals a permanent shift in the behavior of consumers, who now buy online and expect products to be delivered conveniently and safely to their home.

Consumer surveys during COVID-19 showed a marked increase in porch piracy. For example, Value Penguin commissioned a survey of retail consumers and found that home delivery orders increased by 40% during the pandemic; 18% of consumers (or nearly one in five) were victims of package theft between March and May of 2020, the height of lockdowns in the United States (Hurst, 2020). A similar study by Security.org in the second quarter of 2020 found that the theft rate continued to hover around 20% (Vigderman, 2020). A rise in package theft was reported at a local level as well. Fox News 31 in Denver found that in the first seven months of the pandemic (March to August 2020), the theft category recorded by police that includes package theft had a rate well above the five-year average (Summers, 2020).

While these numbers come from consumer surveys and not from official police or company reports, they signal that early pandemic predictions were accurate: package theft increased during government-ordered or self-imposed quarantine when consumers ordered more goods online for home delivery (Stickle, 2020a). It seems clear that package theft is another example of a shifting opportunity structure affecting crime types and rates. To address package theft, retailers, lawmakers, shippers, and consumers need to rethink the risk of crime outside the front door and to develop solutions to prevent this crime that spiked during COVID-19 and seems likely to remain high.

Residential Burglary

Residential burglary is the act of entering a dwelling without the owner's consent with the intent to commit a crime. Homeowners commonly try to protect themselves from this risk using different methods (see Stickle, 2015). Consistent with the routine activity perspective, the presence of a guardian at home (homeowner) tends to deter would-be burglars from breaking into the home (Felson et al., 2020). During the pandemic, residential burglaries in the United States decreased early in 2020 as more people complied with stay-at-home orders (Abrams, 2021; Ashby, 2020; Felson et al., 2020; Jackman, 2020). The city of Detroit, for example, experienced a 43% decline in residential burglaries in March 2020 (Felson et al., 2020), affirming the routine activity explanation of crime.

Declines in residential burglaries were not limited to the United States. One study in the United Kingdom revealed that residential burglary rates declined 25% by the first week of the March lockdown in 2020 (Halford et al., 2020). Further, Dixon and Farrell (2021) found significant decreases in residential burglaries in England and Wales from March to June 2020, with rates a third below the expectation in the absence of a pandemic. Other studies using different datasets and lengths of time (but covering March to July 2020) found significant declines in Belgium of 21% (Dewinter et al., 2021); Brazil, 50%, and Sweden, 75% (Ceccato et al., 2022); Mexico, 40% (Estevez-Soto, 2021); and Northern Ireland, 97% (Buil-Gil, Zeng, & Kemp, 2021). Despite some studies indicating no or weak reductions in residential burglaries, most places experienced significant declines during the early stages of the pandemic.

Cities that did not experience a decrease in residential burglaries appear at first glance to be outliers. In a study covering January 20, 2020, to May

7, 2020, Ashby (2020) found that Austin, Louisville, and Minneapolis met their expected burglary rates. Another study examining data from January 1, 2017, to March 28, 2020, showed nonsignificant reductions in burglaries in Los Angeles (Campedelli et al., 2021). Upon further examination, one possible explanation for these conflicting findings is the differences noted earlier in lockdown types and lengths, as the response to the pandemic varied in each state. Stricter lockdown measures likely produced increased strain among residents of these cities, causing their expected burglary rates to be met; previous studies have identified several stressors resulting from quarantines (Brooks et al., 2020). Campedelli et al. (2021) suggest that the combined effect of a partial reduction in situational and opportunistic triggers of crime directly resulting from lockdown and a worsening of the balance between positive and negative psychological stimuli increased the amount of strain in some offenders, leading them to engage in these burglaries even though people were spending more time at home. Consistent with strain theory, Campedelli et al. (2021) conclude that increased strain resulting from quarantine is likely to explain some offending behavior that occurred during the lockdowns.

Soon after the stay-at-home orders were rescinded, residential burglary rates increased to their expected levels throughout the United States (Meyer et al., 2022), and a similar pattern was observed in other countries (Buil-Gil, Zeng, & Kemp, 2021; Ceccato et al., 2022). However, in England and Wales, rates remained well below expected levels (Dixon et al., 2022). Post-lockdown data show mixed results worldwide concerning burglary rates, with some cities returning to expected levels and others remaining lower. Reasons for this variation may come to light as more data become available on burglaries post-lockdown.

Commercial Burglary

Commercial burglaries involve the act of entering a nonresidential building (such as a drugstore or business office) without the owner's consent and with the intent to commit a crime. Businesses typically open to the public but closed during lockdown were targeted by thieves, who took advantage of shuttered establishments with no employees available to act as guardians. Increased commercial burglary in the absence of guardians is consistent with the routine activity perspective, which states, "When guardians are absent, a target is especially subject to the risk of criminal attack" (Felson & Clarke, 1998, p. 4). For example, full-service restaurant traffic dropped by over 88% globally between February 18 and March 17, 2020 (Allen, 2020), leading many restaurants to stop operating and temporarily close. Likely due to these closures, crime at restaurants in Los Angeles and Chicago dropped by 36% during the first five weeks of the pandemic (Pietrawska et al., 2020a). In a similar study, retail crime in Los Angeles during the first four weeks of COVID-19 increased by 64%, with the most significant increases found in vandalism (67%) and burglary (64%) (Pietrawska et al., 2020b).

Many cities worldwide saw an uptick in commercial burglaries during stay-at-home orders. Seattle, Denver, and New York experienced a double-digit increase in commercial burglaries (Jackman, 2020). Felson and coauthors (2020) found a significant increase in commercial burglaries in Detroit for commercial buildings near or adjacent to residential areas. Another study using data from 25 U.S. cities found an increase of 37.8% in nonresidential burglaries during stay-at-home orders (Abrams, 2021). Overwhelmingly, the available data show strong correlations between stay-at-home orders and commercial burglaries in the early months of 2020, affirming the routine activity perspective on crime.

Conclusion

As demonstrated in this chapter, significant changes in property crime occurred during the COVID-19 pandemic. The stay-at-home orders issued by governments worldwide significantly curtailed population mobility, thereby decreasing or increasing opportunities for certain types of theft to occur in particular settings. These changes led to shifts in a broad spectrum of crimes, impacting rates, methods, and places where crime occurred.

Many factors coalesced to impact theft during the pandemic, including disruptions to court operations (Baldwin et al., 2020) and corrections (Abraham et al., 2020), as well as shifting priorities of police (see Jennings & Perez, 2020; Stogner et al., 2020; White & Fradella, 2020). However, routine activities and opportunity changes are among the strongest factors influencing crime, particularly theft. Studies show significant changes in theft rates occurred as interpersonal interactions were severely restricted. The abrupt changes to routine activities brought on by lockdowns may have caused criminals to shift their typical offending patterns. For example, criminals who usually pickpocketed in crowded areas may have switched to stealing packages from porches.

Similarly, as more people stayed at home, residential burglary became riskier, and some offenders may have turned to commercial burglary to avoid this risk. These and other effects resulting from the lockdowns may have lasting impacts on criminals' behaviors. As new opportunities emerge, old opportunities become riskier, and criminals adapt; some criminal behaviors may remain more prominent even post-pandemic.

As a result of the pandemic, criminologists can analyze the nature of theft as never before, likely influencing future crime reduction strategies (see Jossie et al., 2022). The current state of the literature shows a need for more analysis of how stay-at-home orders affected different types of theft, specifically property crime—the most common form of crime—with a focus on storage lockers, package delivery, and metals. With further analysis of how theft rates are affected by restrictions on population mobility, researchers and police will be better equipped to stay abreast of the trends in criminal patterns, opportunities, and behavior.

3. Intimate Partner Violence: Explanations, Trends, and Responses during COVID-19

Shannon Christensen, Taylor Gerry, and McKenna Bennett

Introduction

Public orders put in place to mitigate the COVID-19 pandemic led to more time spent at home, often heightening the intensity and prolonging the length of contact for intimate partners and family. The uncertain duration of the pandemic and its associated policies, increased familial demands of health or childcare, and the navigation of a changing workforce with remote work or even layoff—all introduced new and challenging domestic situations. When stay-at-home orders encouraged people to remain home as much as possible to prevent the spread of COVID-19, unintended effects resulted. Offenders could potentially weaponize the pandemic by dissuading victims from seeking outside social contact for fear of contracting or spreading the virus. Stay-at-home restrictions thus complicated the ability of potential and actual victims to access social services needed to remove themselves from risk and harm. While these orders made sense from a public health perspective, especially given what was understood about the virus's transmission at that time, they also had the potential to create harm.

Many criminologists speculated about the impact of stay-at-home orders on domestic violence because domestic violence incidents are known to increase when families spend more time together (Hansen & Lory, 2020). Domestic violence encompasses intimate partner violence, or IPV, which is a form of abuse or aggression perpetrated by a current or ex-partner, spouse, or dating partner and involves physical, sexual, or psychological abuse (Bradbury-Jones & Isham, 2020; Jetelina et al., 2021; Moreira & Da Costa, 2020). Identifying IPV can be difficult to do when the conditions in a relationship prevent the victim from having a true understanding of the offender's intentions and patterns of behavior. Domestic abuse can include physical, mental, financial, and emotional harm that can be difficult for outsiders and victims to comprehend. For example, victims in an abusive relationship may fall into patterns of self-blame for physical violence they experience while abusers may adeptly use verbal and psychological abuse to control the victim in ways the victim cannot fully grasp. Continued exposure to abusive behaviors can have serious psychophysical impacts on victims. Child abuse and child neglect may be considered elements of domestic violence, since IPV can reverberate throughout the household.

IPV tends to increase during emergencies such as epidemics (Moreira & Da Costa, 2020). This concern was magnified in the COVID-19 pandemic as formal and informal support shifted with the spread of the virus and the isolation measures meant to control it. These shifts included less access to established social services such as family and domestic violence support shelters, a rapidly shrinking housing market that limited residential relocation for victims of domestic crimes, constrained finances, and silo effects in social supports.

This chapter focuses on intimate partner violence, specifically, (1) how the COVID-19 pandemic changed possibilities and opportunities for IPV as understood through various theoretical lenses and explanatory factors, (2) the documented rates and experiences of IPV and the difficulty of tracking this type of crime, and (3) the changed response to intimate partner crimes during the pandemic.

Changed Opportunities, Guardianship, and Stressors

Under any circumstances, IPV is a criminological and policy concern for households. Various theoretical lenses offer insight into this phenomenon, including the intertwined and complex concepts of guardianship, exposure to motivated offenders, economic strain, and changed relationship dynamics. Significant changes to lifestyle, resource availability, and social networks can all affect the prevalence of and response to IPV, and the COVID-19 pandemic altered all of these factors.

Motivated Offenders, Guardianship, and Routine Activities

Routine activity theory posits that crime is more likely to occur when there is a convergence among suitable targets, motivated offenders, and a lack of capable guardianship. The COVID-19 pandemic may have heightened strains on motivated offenders while also disrupting routine activities (including increasing the amount of time spent in contact with potential victims) and reducing chances for capable guardianship such as accessing victim and social services. Among myriad possibilities for increasing IPV events, the pandemic's restructuring of regular household routines, increases in time spent with a partner in isolation from the outside world, and economic hardship may have increased existing relationship stressors that contributed to violence, control, and coercion (Moreira & Da Costa, 2020). Stay-at-home orders and social distancing allowed for abusive tactics, such as surveillance and control, to be implemented more easily by perpetrators, increasing their attempts to exert power and use coercion (Bradbury-Jones & Isham, 2020; Piquero et al., 2021). During the COVID-19 pandemic, victims of IPV spent more time in proximity to their offenders after the closing of nonessential businesses and establishments (Moreira & Da Costa, 2020). COVID-19 made it difficult to publicly address domestic violence and provide resources due to family confinement in the household and the dangers that could pose to victims (Bright et al., 2020). Collectively, these basic changes in lifestyle opened figurative doors for exposure to potential offenders while simultaneously closing figurative doors to guardianship.

Strain and Stressors

COVID-19 changed potential strain and stressors through lockdown measures and altered the nature of work and social relationships. In theoretical terms, once negative stimuli were introduced (e.g., risk of infection), positive stimuli became more difficult to access (e.g., supportive relationships), and additional obstacles emerged to goal achievement (e.g., economic loss) (Bradbury-Jones & Isham, 2020). Experiential documentation by Ravi and colleagues (2022) substantiated this by highlighting how store closings and limited access to supplies created tension between one woman and her partner, provoking fights involving abuse and violence. The immediate financial strains of COVID-19 impacted day-to-day living and added strains to intimate relationships (Moreira & Da Costa, 2020), with financial strain known to be a significant contributor to conditions of IPV (Ravi et al., 2020). In short, the changed dynamics and strains in households introduced the potential likelihood of IPV events and affected the potential ability of victims to escape such circumstances.

Isolation led to increased physical presence within the home for work, social, and familial activities, with less-immediate ties shifting to virtual or more distant spaces. This could significantly strain the benefit or satisfaction of individuals owing to a lack of physical contact with others outside the home. Job loss was an additional strain that significantly impacted conditions related to IPV. Victims who their lost job or experienced a reduction in work hours and pay would have become less able to support themselves and any dependents financially should they want to leave a (potentially) abusive situation (Jetelina et al., 2021). There were additional risks of physical violence experienced by victims through slights and covert expressions of physical behavior, conditioning complacency and acceptance of their perceived risk. These conditions could directly relate to emotional coercive control over victims by perpetrators taking advantage of the fear of financial burden and of contracting or spreading the virus if the victim were to leave (Smyth et al., 2021).

Generally, economic instability can have a disproportionately large impact on IPV and the response to it. The pandemic magnified this. For one, impoverished people often have less reliable access to means of communication such as the internet and cell phone service, making hotlines and crisis centers unreachable and legal aid difficult to access; these circumstances were heightened during the COVID-19 pandemic (Moreira & Da Costa, 2020). Additionally, economic dependence on abusers due to unemployment and the need for childcare could have inhibited those trying to leave a situation of domestic violence (Piquero et al., 2021). Given the tremendous economic impact of the pandemic, those who were already financially marginalized would have been especially susceptible to its financial impact.

Changes in Social Support

Limited access to social support may have influenced IPV events given the isolation of potential victims and their abusers. By staying at home, offenders had increased access to their victims and the ability to cut them off from the world (Smyth et al., 2021). Everyday routines faced tremendous disruption, such as going to the gym, to a place of employment, or socializing with friends. These disruptions put potential victims in greater proximity to offenders while isolating them from social support that might have recognized conditions of abuse and offered assistance to those needing to leave abusive or controlling situations. Informal social support was limited by the absence of contact with friends, family, coworkers, and others who may have previously acted as a support system for victims (Moreira & Da Costa, 2020). With COVID-19 lockdown curfews, limited outside access, and fears of catching the illness, the isolation and restricted abilities to engage with social supports may have changed domestic dynamics and led to the start of or continuation of IPV (Lipp & Johnson, 2023). Some abusers may have weaponized COVID-19 by creating a fear in their victims that coming into physical contact with others could put them at risk. The fear of being exposed to the virus and concerns about transmitting it to others (particularly those in a social support network with compromised health or of advanced age) could be used to coerce and control victims.

Victims were also cut off from previous potential outreach and support centers as access to community health clinics, prenatal health services, day cares, and primary schools was disrupted (Jetelina et al., 2021). The disruption of these connections made victims more reliant onto the isolator, perhaps resulting in disillusionment and forced guardianship over their activities (Smyth et al., 2021). Social isolation can exacerbate the perceived and actual impacts of IPV on victims, especially the removal of support systems and outsiders' opportunities to observe the situation. Often, those around the situation can identify abusive behaviors and provide some element of support to the victim. Guardianship from bystanders allows victims to put and maintain some space between themselves and their living situation, which is important for regulating the behaviors of perpetrators of domestic violence (Nnawulezi & Hacskaylo, 2022).

External Pressures

Perceptions of power and gender structures can be influenced by factors external to the relationship. Changes in the prevalence of IPV globally are often tied to phenomena that are out of the control of offenders and victims. Feminist theories help us understand patterns of domestic violence, which they attribute to dysfunctional masculine attitudes, oppression, and power within relationships and to underlying beliefs about legal and appropriate behavior. Rates of domestic violence increase in times when external stressors challenge perceptions of power from outside the home, including economic pressure (such as the 0.64 per 1,000 rise in IPV cases during the 2008 recession in the United States), environmental change (climate change), and social change (such as the #MeToo movement)

(Caridade et al., 2022; Lucero et al., 2016; Santaularia et al., 2022; Schneider et al., 2016). Theoretically, rises in rates of domestic abuse can be linked to increased stressors in the household or perceived or actual threats to the power that the oppressor feels. Limitations to the control that a perpetrator of domestic violence may hold over the victim could motivate the perpetrator to reassert control and thus lead to additional victimization.

Collective Contributions to Intimate Partner Violence

Collectively, phenomena that can secure the control an offender has over another person are thought to empower offenders to increase their control, guardianship, and suppression of the victim. Often, offenders will seek to limit the contact the victim can have with the outside world, creating a dependence on them. In addition to control as a tactic used by violent partners, isolation can be another. For example, social distancing due to COVID-19 put victims of IPV in potential danger due to the lack of protective factors and the freedom of going to work or school and thus not having access to support and resources from others. In addition, fear of infection and illness could be used by the victim's partner as an excuse for further isolation and control (Moreira & Da Costa, 2020). COVID-19 presented a multifaceted strain on households due to combined financial, environmental, and social changes. The potential for exacerbating previous domestic issues through social isolation was a concern for many officials when making the decision to order lockdown. Most theories and supporting literature suggest that IPV increases during humanitarian emergencies because it aggravates the risk factors that lead to this type of victimization. The next section details whether and how these theoretical likelihoods seemed to translate into behavior.

Documenting Changes in Domestic Violence

In 2019, the Bureau of Justice Statistics estimated that there were 4.2 incidents of IPV per 1,000 persons who were 12 years of age or older (Morgan & Thompson, 2021). These rates dropped to 3.1 victimizations per 1,000 in 2020, with speculation that the reduction was partially a function of reduced reporting and access to resources (Morgan & Thompson, 2021). As the requirements of protecting oneself from the pandemic became stricter beyond residential walls, the pressures within households continued to rise, attributed to fear, increased proximity to perpetrators, and restrictions on movement outside the home. Substantial increases in IPV were reported over the first six weeks of the pandemic, reflected in journalistic reporting and anecdotal stories and in data on service calls to police (Bright et al., 2020). Throughout 2021 and 2022, there were apparent increases in the rates of IPV reported, with rates of 3.3 per 1,000 and 4.9 per 1,000, respectively (Morgan & Thompson, 2021; Thompson & Tapp, 2022). Scholars hypothesized that in the later months of the pandemic, access to resources returned to pre-pandemic levels and allowed for more consistent reporting or use of supportive services that helped to record events. This reflects limitations to the method of measurement or estimation of this type of crime, as there may be discrepancies among surveys, arrest data, call-for-service records, and qualitative investigation (Hansen & Lory, 2020; Thompson & Tapp, 2022).

In general, most scholarship agrees that at the outset of the pandemic (February–April 2020), there were significant increases in reported IPV from community-based organizations as measured by hotline calls and website traffic, as well as police activity data (Hansen & Lory, 2020; Jetelina et al., 2021). Examination of later periods of 2020 appears to show a significant drop in instances of IPV. However, this apparent decline is thought to have resulted from public health policies having reduced or eliminated opportunities for victims to access services. Hanson and Lory (2020) speculate that one reason calls quickly dropped off was increased isolation from friends and social supports, coupled with continued limited opportunities to reach out for assistance. The net results of these changes may have been a reduction in the ability of victims to access social support for leaving a relationship. Hanson and Lory's findings illustrate that victims' calls for help became shorter and quieter due to privacy concerns, while external reports from concerned neighbors and witnesses grew.

Research indicated increases in domestic violence cases through the height of the COVID-19 pandemic (2020–2021) (Demir & Park, 2022; Ertan et al., 2020; Jetelina et al., 2021; Moreira & Da Costa, 2020). Reports of IPV increased both in relationships with prior histories of violent victimization as well as in relationships without such history (Jetelina et al., 2021). However, despite higher reports of IPV through victimization surveys and calls to police for service, arrests for IPV did not increase (Demir & Park, 2022; Jetelina et al., 2021). Bullinger and colleagues (2021) conducted a study that estimated the effects of stay-at-home policies on domestic violence, particularly on calls for police service after the March announcement to stay at home. Their evidence showed a 7.4% increase in domestic-violence-related calls for police service while also showing that the stay-at-home orders decreased police reports of domestic crimes by 6.8% and arrests for domestic violence by 26.4%.

Studies over the period of the pandemic generally found that victims' calls for service and reports of IPV decreased when the strictest stay-at-home orders were lifted (Cook & Taylor, 2023; Demir & Park, 2022; Jetelina et al., 2021; Moreira & Da Costa, 2020), though this varied by location and method of measurement. Some research, however, found little or no decrease in domestic violence trends. Contrary to previous IPV studies, consistent results from multiple cities showed a decrease in police reporting of domestic violence (Bullinger et al., 2021; Leslie & Wilson, 2020). For example, a study conducted by Baidoo and colleagues (2021) assessed police reports of domestic violence from the Chicago Police Department from January to June 2020 and compared them to data on social service availability within Chicago from March and August 2020. These reports spanned 77 neighborhoods in the Chicago area. Compared to the same time frame in 2019, Baidoo and colleagues found a decrease in domestic violence reported by police, of 21.8 crimes per 100,000, after the 2020 stay-at-home orders were implemented. However, they also observed a decrease in the availability of domestic violence service resources, noting this decrease was particularly profound in Black neighborhoods on the south side of the city. Their findings highlight that disruptions to support services were not equal across all places and might have created greater threats for victims residing in communities of color and other disadvantaged areas.

Before the pandemic, IPV was more prevalent in some populations. Certain characteristics elevate the risk for IPV victimization, and some of these increased during the pandemic. In a meta-analysis by McNeil and colleagues (2023), the pre-pandemic correlates of social isolation and unemployment remained stable at a minimum but, in many cases, actually increased in impact during COVID-19. Aligning with strain perspectives, the conditions of the pandemic exacerbated negative stimuli and finance-related stressors. The rise in IPV tended to be concentrated within economically and socially marginalized populations. Those who were unemployed or underemployed, had toddlers, had six or more people living in the home, were pregnant, were trans/nonbinary, and/or were unable to afford rent reported the highest rates of IPV (Jetelina et al., 2021). With identified predictors of IPV being heightened by COVID-19 conditions, certain populations became more vulnerable to domestic violence during the pandemic. Furthermore, protective factors against IPV were heavily disrupted by COVID-19. For example, social support and community cohesion previously provided protection against IPV (McNeil et al., 2023), but COVID-19 stay-at-home orders obstructed victims' ability to reach out to their established social networks that could offer support.

Highlighting the stories of those who experienced IPV during the pandemic, Lyons and Brewer (2021) applied a qualitative thematic analysis to examine convenience data taken from 50 cases of primarily female IPV victims who posted to the Reddit discussion platform. This allowed them to explore the prevalence and perceived correlates of IPV, bridging explanation with empirical evidence. Their data collection consisted of posts made by victims of IPV in forums where they could tell their stories voluntarily and anonymously. These posts made reference to COVID-19 and to general IPV indicators, and the authors presented a connection between the two phenomena. The authors suggest that COVID-19 contributed to and exacerbated previous tension within relationships and was weaponized against the victims as a means of preventing them from leaving the relationship. The authors' general takeaway was that the pandemic was used to harm and restrict victims in ways that went beyond the historical control and coercion strategies used by offenders.

The pandemic had a role in the instigation and continuance of IPV, given the particular context and structure of regulation and strains incurred during this time. Moreira and Da Costa (2020) and others highlight the interplay of social dynamics and institutional responses and recognize that trends in IPV are a multifaceted issue that concerns not only the individuals involved in domestic violence but also the accessibility to and responses by agencies responsible for answering IPV calls for service (Lipp & Johnson, 2023).

Issues of Methods and Measures

The COVID-19 pandemic had an immediate effect on IPV, though various measurement choices can impact how trends are understood. IPV is generally measured by two different methods: official arrest reports through the National Incident-Based Reporting System or other law enforcement agency reporting systems and victims' surveys, such as the National Crime Victimization Survey of households. These two sources capture different aspects of IPV. Arrests necessitate the filing of an official report, an investigation, and the agency's participation in the corresponding reporting system (Morgan & Thompson, 2021). Victimization surveys such as the National Crime Victimization Survey use a nationwide sampling of households and often lend insight into the dark figure of unreported crimes as surveys inquire about victimization experiences directly, seeking to measure victimization experiences even when unreported to law enforcement agencies (Morgan & Thompson, 2021). Historically, the National Crime Victimization Survey and other surveys report higher rates of IPV incidents than the Federal Bureau of Investigation's Uniform Crime Reporting, which is consistent with documented underreporting of IPV and sexual assault (Morgan & Thompson, 2021). Other measurement strategies turn to hotline logs, which document callers seeking help and reporting incidents (Moreira & Da Costa, 2020).

Each of these methods of measure has limitations with respect to accessibility, discretion, willingness to disclose, and human error. Hotlines, while an innovative source of data, may not record incidents that meet the legal definition of IPV, depend on callers having access to phone lines, and may require privacy in reporting (Emezue, 2020). Agency arrest records are subject to the willingness of a victim to report possible IPV and the responding officer to record the event as IPV. This recording depends on discretion, agency practices, and prevailing state laws (i.e., mandated arrest laws). Police departments and other agencies responded to stay-in-place orders by socially distancing their officers and reducing contact with the community (Emezue, 2020; Jennings & Perez, 2020; Nielson et al., 2022). Due to restrictions in police services, apparent decreases in IPV reporting may have come from procedural modifications that limited officers' ability to record such incidents (Demir & Park, 2022).

Victimization surveys are limited by their sampling and response rates, as well as respondents' accuracy in recollection and truthfulness. For these reasons, victimization data from surveys may still underreport events. Further, definitions of IPV have changed over time, in personal understanding and perceived seriousness, which affects whether victims themselves recognize IPV. For example, physical domestic violence was a focus of the media in preventing abuse, with less attention paid to psychological aspects of what makes behaviors abusive (Bright et al., 2020). Many victims may have been unaware of the coercive control wielded by their partners in their state of isolation during the pandemic. In contrast,

Jetelina and colleagues (2020) used an expansive definition of IPV and, through social media surveys, found a much higher rate of victimization than official sources attested, with most victims experiencing heightened insults and screaming. These are components of the definition of IPV but can vary in their interpretation and recording across sources. Because IPV is a behavior difficult to observe behind closed doors, it is a challenge to raise awareness of what counts as IPV and what it means to experience it. Its covert incidence complicates all research and policy efforts to document trends in IPV accurately.

Various research methods have different objectives in examining IPV events and thus provide different insights. Though apparent increases in IPV occurred throughout the pandemic, it is still difficult to measure and operationalize variables that reliably grasp its prevalence. Swells in arrest may be an artifact of a legal change or mandatory reporting policy, whereas increases in hotline calls may result from increased awareness of the resource and more time spent at home near a phone rather than any actual change in the prevalence of IPV. For example, Demir and Park (2022) showed that although calls about IPV to law enforcement agencies increased, arrests did not. This may be an effect of agency policy and recommendations, discretion, or COVID-19 protocols. External factors such as procedural justice issues, jail capacity, and officer safety can all impact law enforcement's response to calls for service, while broader issues such as awareness and obstacles to accessing reporting centers may influence other forms of response and reporting (Emezue, 2020). Using multiple forms of measurement—such as combining victimization surveys and hotline use—may provide more insight into the initial rise in IPV events in relation to COVID-19.

Changing Responses to Intimate Partner Violence

The public health and policy responses to COVID-19 changed conditions that might contribute to an increased likelihood of IPV (e.g., increased economic and relationship stressors, increased contact with offenders, and decreased access to social support systems). These responses also impacted the ability of victims to understand their victimization and risk, to access personal and social support assistance, and to find methods to report their experiences. Social support agencies, the criminal justice system, and the overall accessibility of services were dramatically altered during the rise and duration of the pandemic (Ravi et al., 2022). For example, stay-at-home orders changed procedures used by governing agencies, including the attempt to reduce physical interactions. Hotlines, crisis centers, legal aid, protective services, and law enforcement agencies became limited due to a lack of personnel or funding during this time (Moreira & Da Costa, 2020). In Wisconsin, police officers were encouraged to give more citations or resolve legal infractions in ways that did not involve arrest. While this recommendation was not specific to IPV offenses, the goal was to reduce the rate of physical arrests following a reduction of personnel in order to meet social distancing requirements. It is unclear how crime reporting rates may have been affected and how much identifying and responding to domestic violence was inhibited (Cook & Taylor, 2023).

COVID-19 led to the creation of many barriers to accessing support and resources for IPV victims. For example, mandated closures, social distancing, and travel restrictions limited access to resources and support, specifically affecting domestic violence shelters (Hansen & Lory, 2020; Mantler et al., 2021; Moreira & Da Costa, 2020). Shelters are generally group living facilities, making the restrictions of COVID-19 problematic for their operation. In Ontario, Canada, there was a reduction in occupancy levels at domestic violence shelters because each woman, and potentially her children, could not have her own room and a private bathroom and still maintain regular occupancy. This resulted in a 27% loss of usable space and fewer women residing in the shelters (Mantler et al., 2021). Additionally, access to support and resources can be affected by the location where one lives. For example, law enforcement agencies in rural areas are often smaller, have lower budgets, and have fewer services than urban agencies. Response times in rural areas can take as long as an hour, and access to the means to contact police, such as through a cell phone or the internet, can also be limited (Bradbury-Jones & Isham, 2020; Hansen & Lory, 2020).

Increasing Accessibility

Early and official recognition of the heightened risk of IPV prompted some immediate attention and action. Ertan and colleagues (2020) highlighted potential response plans that emerged as a direct result of stay-at-home orders and other lockdown measures, emphasizing the potential for an increase in risk and the need to have response measures actively in place. Others highlighted strategies such as changing the residential environment and providing hotel rooms instead of shelters, given the high demand, but these strategies also came with their own sets of limitations as long-term and practical solutions (Mantler et al., 2021). Increasing the availability of remote access to service provision was intended to expand access to resources for those who could not remove themselves physically from their abuser or who feared alerting the offender that they were seeking help. Virtual services online could also provide treatment and support to individuals who were sequestered with their abusive partner (Emezue, 2020).

Bright and colleagues (2020) conducted a content analysis to examine the documentation and coverage of domestic violence in the media in the early weeks of COVID-19. Examining 300 news articles on COVID-19 safety measures and responses, they found that media predicted an increase in domestic violence as a result of lockdowns, brought clarity to definitions of IPV, and promoted possible resources for reporting and support, such as shelters or other forms of escape. News articles also drew attention to phone and app-related reporting systems as potentially providing more security and privacy for those facing fears of reporting.

Other research demonstrated the beneficial effects for those who were able to separate from their abuser and indicated that increased isolation was protective rather than limiting. This primarily occurred for victims who were no longer living together with their abuser. At early points in the stay-at-home period, some victims said the isolation caused by mobility restrictions fostered feelings of protection and said they felt relieved that their abuser would not be able to locate them. The stay-at-home orders also provided time to heal, learn, and focus on safety (Ravi et al., 2022). These findings demonstrate the multifaceted effects of some policies.

Changed Systems and Accessibility Issues

Some research found increasing challenges in accessing and providing IPV-related resources, illustrating the complexity of responses. Services such as hotlines, crisis centers, and legal aid suffered from a lack of available personnel and funding, which made many critical services less accessible to victims. At a practical level, limited public transportation impacted victims, as it hindered their ability to reach services that required travel (Ravi et al., 2022), while those in rural areas struggled to access the virtual settings to which many services had transitioned (Nnawulezi & Hacskay lo, 2022). External pressures and events impacted responses to IPV. In tandem with increases in protests in urban areas, access to police was often restricted because agencies had to deploy their limited personnel for order maintenance operations, reducing police resources to respond to and investigate IPV incidents (Bullinger et al., 2021; Dragon & Monk-Turner, 2023). Collectively, access to and delivery of IPV responses faced dramatic shifts and lessened the availability of legal and service resources.

Moreira and Da Costa (2020) stress that domestic violence shelters are generally group-based operations. When shelters for IPV victims restricted occupancy or shut down due to COVID-19, that change minimized support systems for navigating IPV events. Personal reluctance may also have inhibited victims' accessing in-person services such as shelters for fear of potentially exposing themselves to the virus. Other seemingly positive solutions, such as providing hotel stays, presented practical life challenges, such as legal access, counseling provisions, and establishing a daily routine for cooking and errands (Mantler et al., 2021).

Many family courts and justice centers were closed or slowed down procedures, which impeded their ability to serve victims, including serving warrants, holding court proceedings, and processing orders of protection efficiently and effectively. Some court systems largely halted in-person operations, creating long queues of cases requiring judicial attention and processes. During the pandemic, court systems began to implement measures for victims to access legal recourse and began to rely on technological alternatives to in-person processing or to waive in-person requirements of the court (Emezue, 2020). However, such adaptation was not uniformly made, was sometimes quite slow, and, in some jurisdictions, was almost entirely absent.

Reliance on Virtual Services

Service delivery also changed in nature and mode of delivery. For example, a nearly universal pivot to online delivery of social service support challenged principles at the core of social work, particularly for traditional home visits (Holt, Elliffe, et al., 2023). The social worker–client relationship is critical to the support provided by these agencies, and fewer appointments can diminish the building and maintenance of interpersonal connections. Reports documented that face-to-face visits decreased substantially during the pandemic and that technology substituted imperfectly for in-person interactions. Using technology for virtual visits put limits on holistic evaluation, risk assessment, and the creation of an adequate safety plan. Some social workers noted that COVID "made [them] re-evaluate what abuse is and how it manifests in homes" and that it was possible the social worker was "not getting the full picture of what is happening" (Holt et al., 2023, pp. 398, 396). Specifically, limits to reading body language, questioning freely, and providing a holistic assessment were shortcomings of relying on technology in this realm. Other protective measures, such as participating in activities outside the home, contact with others, and access to victims' services, changed.

Using virtual substitutes for social services can present additional problems. For example, security and privacy become worries when using online services for legal counsel (Emezue, 2020) and other social supports (Holt et al., 2023). Technology may allow for unwanted exposure to offenders and greater potential surveillance of victims, and victims may lack access to broadband or the technological acumen to use computer software (Emezue, 2020). Online services remain a reasonable alternative, but having it be the only option presents problems. It can perpetuate inequalities for those who already face structural barriers to accessing services (Koshan, 2020). One of the disparities exacerbated by COVID-19 was economically disadvantaged victims having trouble accessing services. The economic divide caused some victims from marginalized communities to be unable to access the online services many shelters relied on during COVID-19 to deliver services (Koshan, 2020).

Conclusions

COVID-19 policies for social distancing, self-isolation, and lockdown created opportunities for intimate partner violence. Increased exposure to offenders and limited physical mobility, along with disruptions to everyday routines, put victims in proximity to their offenders at higher rates than before the pandemic and removed victims' informal social coping mechanisms (Moreira & Da Costa, 2020). The disruption of regular social routines created an unintended dependency on and exposure to offenders within the household, increasing offenders' ability to employ coercive and abusive tactics (Moreira & Da Costa, 2020). Furthermore, access to IPV services (shelters, hotlines, crisis centers) was compromised, and institutional responses were altered, leaving victims with fewer formal resources. Efforts to increase attention through posting IPV incidents on social media platforms and publicizing IPV trends by news media bolstered awareness and understanding of domestic violence, bringing an oft-hidden type of crime into greater focus. Increased awareness led to the creative deployment of reporting techniques, social media, and app software, which gave victims resources to the social services they may not have accessed previously for reasons of capacity or safety (Emezue, 2020).

Intimate partner violence is a nuanced issue with individualized and subtle techniques, making it extremely difficult for researchers to develop a methodology that can capture the full extent of its occurrence. Privacy concerns with IPV make it difficult to collect data in surveys, and victims' participation in studies may result in retaliation or fear of retaliation. In addition, populations that have experienced IPV may be difficult to reach due to limited awareness, to shame, or to anonymity. Coercive control is a difficult variable to operationalize for research purposes owing to the various means of employing it physically, psychologically, financially, and emotionally. The inability to encapsulate the breadth of IPV with research tools creates issues for researchers attempting to understand these trends. COVID-19, an additional information barrier, has presented various new techniques and issues to be further analyzed by researchers. The pandemic highlights how difficult it is to understand the prevalence of IPV and the policies and resources that most effectively meet the needs of victims. Simultaneously, the pandemic illustrated the many vulnerabilities and gaps that exist in legal and social support networks intended to serve the needs of victims.

4. Labor Trafficking during the COVID-19 Pandemic: Challenges and Services

Erin C. Heil and Andrea J. Nichols

Introduction

In March 2020, the United States was transformed, as many states mandated stay-at-home orders in response to the COVID-19 pandemic. Many jobs were lost after businesses began to close or restrict operations. As communities were experiencing economic hardship, some industries began booming (e.g., construction and the food industry) once certain commodities became essential to sustaining and protecting American lives. Some laborers became susceptible to infection as they worked in positions deemed essential. COVID-19 became a tool to control mobility and instill fear among some workers who were required to continue reporting to work and/or were economically dependent on continuing to report to work. Because of this, COVID-19 became a mechanism of labor trafficking and exploitation. Advocates and experts who monitor labor trafficking began to worry that there would be an increase in identified cases of labor trafficking due to COVID-19. However, because of the lockdowns, it proved difficult to detect situations of suspected labor trafficking. Labor trafficking became more isolated, and the already-existing obstacles to its identification were exacerbated.

This pilot study addresses the challenges in identifying and providing social and legal services to victims of labor trafficking in the United States during the height of the COVID-19 pandemic. The purpose of this chapter is threefold: (1) to outline the issues in identification and service provision to victims of labor trafficking due to COVID-19, (2) to discuss the lack of resources for survivors of labor trafficking because of COVID-19, and (3) to consider the implications of COVID-19 in the context of labor trafficking in the United States.

Issues with Identification of Labor Trafficking

The Trafficking Victims Protection Act defines labor trafficking thus: "The recruitment, harboring, transportation, provision, or obtaining of a person for labor or services, through the use of force, fraud, or coercion for the purpose of subjection to involuntary servitude, peonage, debt bondage, or slavery" (22 U.S.C. § 7102[9]). Sex trafficking, on the other hand, is defined as follows: "The recruitment, harboring, transportation, provision, or obtaining of a person for the purposes of a commercial sex act in which the commercial sex act is induced by force, fraud, or coercion or in which the person induced is under 18" (22 U.S.C. § 7102[9]). Both acts fall under the umbrella term of human trafficking.

Labor trafficking in the United States has historically occurred under the radar, even before the pandemic, as obstacles impeded the identification of its victims. For example, Farrell et al. (2012) found that some of the "challenges inherent to human trafficking cases [include] the hidden nature of the crime and limitations of traditional policing methods, the failure of victims to recognize their own victimization and self-identify to law enforcement, [and] victim fears of reporting" (p. 74). Additionally, exploiters regularly move their workers to another location to escape detection by law enforcement. This movement, alongside labor trafficking commonly being invisible to the general public, creates substantial obstacles to proactive policing efforts (Farrell & Pfeffer, 2014). The layers of isolation created by traffickers have made it difficult, if not impossible, for individuals to self-identify as trafficked victims and to come forward to the police.

Reactive Policing

Because of these obstacles, police are more likely to be reactive in policing this problem. Whereas police can generally rely on proactive strategies to identify cases of sex trafficking, such as monitoring the internet (Heil & Nichols, 2019), they cannot use the same preemptive investigative tools for labor trafficking. Therefore, the police response to labor trafficking is primarily reactive and relies on labor trafficking survivors seeking assistance (Farrell et. al., 2012). A challenge with this passive approach is that labor trafficking victims are not likely to self-identify as victims and are even less likely to come forward to the police. In situations of trafficking undocumented laborers, survivors' fears of detainment and deportation are barriers to their seeking help (Farrell et al., 2019). Survivors may be reluctant to engage with the criminal justice system if they have concerns about violating their worker visas (Egyes, 2017). Furthermore, anti-immigrant sentiments in the United States serve as barriers to service access and utilization (de Vries et al., 2019). In many cases, victims are hidden behind the doors and walls of legitimate businesses. Police are less likely to investigate legitimate businesses without probable cause, thereby keeping potential trafficking situations unidentified.

Lack of Training

Aside from the challenges associated with reactive policing, police face organizational challenges that impede their identification of labor trafficking situations and victims, such as a lack of training. This lack of training compounds a general lack of institutional commitment to, and understanding of, human trafficking. If institutional commitment is lacking, resources become limited, and specialized personnel are unavailable to identify and investigate cases of human trafficking. When police encounter potential cases of labor trafficking or exploitation, they frequently lack the awareness, skills, and resources to properly identify and investigate this crime. For example, "Common mistakes made during interviews [of identified victims] include the use of an untrained or ineffective interviewer, the lack of a translator, the use of a translator who is potentially involved in a case (such as an employer), and lack of cultural sensitivity during interviews" (Farrell et al., 2019, p. 96). The hidden nature of labor trafficking, ineffective policing strategies, and lack of organizational commitment to addressing labor trafficking were all obstacles to identifying cases of labor trafficking before the pandemic.

Vulnerable Status

Obstacles to identifying cases of labor trafficking are closely connected to the vulnerable status of labor-trafficked victims. Many of those individuals trafficked for the purpose of forced labor are undocumented, a status that makes them prime targets for exploitation. Undocumented immigration status is a viable tool that traffickers use to maintain control over workers by leveraging the constant threat of deportation (Desai & Tepfer, 2017). However, the status of being undocumented is not the only immigration issue affecting victims of labor trafficking. Laborers that legally come to the United States on an H-2A visa[1] or H-2B visa are still at risk. Those who recruit workers into situations that end up as labor trafficking will often confiscate the workers' visas so that workers have no proof of documentation (Desai & Tepfer, 2017). This exacerbates the fear of contact with law enforcement, creating a tool of coercion. Additionally, refugees, asylum seekers, and unaccompanied minors face similar vulnerabilities. Immigrant status creates a power imbalance in which the worker becomes dependent on the exploiter.

Of central concern to the trafficked person is the fear of deportation. Farrell and Pfeffer (2014) found that "in roughly one-third of the cases [they] reviewed, at least one victim was detained by immigration authorities before being recognized as a victim" (p. 54). A fear of deportation results in an inherent distrust of law enforcement. Heil (2012) noted that this distrust is critical to the victimization of both documented and undocumented immigrant workers.

Language barriers add to the vulnerability of labor-trafficked persons. Many individuals who enter the United States have limited English proficiency, regardless of their legal status (Office to Monitor and Combat Trafficking in Persons, 2020). As a result, victims might be reluctant to seek assistance from law enforcement, and if they are identified as a potential victim of labor trafficking, the police must often rely on translation services from a third party. Victims who cannot speak English depend on someone else to represent their experiences and status to law enforcement (Farrell et al., 2012). Language barriers prevent victims from reporting their trafficking experience, which leads to greater victimization (Heil, 2012).

The Impact of COVID-19 on Human Trafficking

COVID-19 led to many obstacles that may have increased human trafficking and complicated criminal justice and social service efforts to alleviate this problem. These included increased vulnerability, deteriorated working conditions, decreased auditing by social service providers, new risks, discrimination, economic hardship, and greater isolation (Anti-Slavery International, 2020; Searcy et al., 2022). COVID-19 led to job loss, resulting in many marginalized workers being unable to pay rent and finding themselves homeless. Some landlords began offering housing in exchange for sex on sites such as Craigslist (Council on Foreign Relations, 2020).

Some shelters that were formerly accessed by human trafficking survivors closed as funding streams were reduced or lost (Council on Foreign Relations, 2020). Research has shown that homelessness is a significant risk factor for trafficking among young people (Heil & Nichols, 2019; Todres & Diaz, 2020).

Additionally, COVID-19 affected hospitals. For example, Todres and Diaz (2020) reported that the pandemic impacted identification of trafficking in hospitals, as patients were encouraged to stay home if their symptoms were not severe. Hospitals, especially emergency rooms, that were once a site for identifying victims of trafficking were no longer available as an avenue of support. Overall, COVID-19 caused high levels of financial stress, insecurity, and a lack of outlets for identification, all of which led to increased vulnerabilities associated with both labor and sex trafficking.

Aside from the impact on hospitals and housing, COVID-19 affected the labor force. Farmworkers, construction workers, electricians, plumbers, and food industry workers were among those considered essential workers during the pandemic. These areas of work have been frequently connected to cases of labor trafficking (U.S. Department of State, 2020). Essential work is identified as work being performed that is "necessary to sustain and protect life" (National Conference of State Legislatures, 2020, para. 11.). Workers performing essential work were often more vulnerable to COVID-19 exposure due to work conditions that did not allow for social distancing and other safety measures. At meat processing plants, "workers typically stand elbow-to-elbow to do the low-wage work of cutting, deboning, and packing the chicken and beef that Americans savor" (Jordan & Dickerson, 2020, para. 5). In April 2020, the Smithfield pork factory in Sioux Falls, South Dakota, had more than 640 cases of COVID-19 linked to the plant (Dickerson & Jordan, 2020).

Many of those identified as victims of labor trafficking have traditionally been legal migrants or undocumented workers. Early in the pandemic it was unclear whether even legal migrant workers would be eligible for unemployment benefits or other support under the stimulus packages established by the federal government (Jordan & Dickerson, 2020). Reporters were documenting instances in which migrant workers feared disclosing COVID-19 symptoms in the workplace because they had no health insurance and/or paid sick leave (Jordan, 2020). These workers feared they would be denied work and income, but their attendance at work risked exposing others to the virus. Therefore, despite work conditions conducive to COVID-19 infections, many workers felt they had no choice but to work.

Because of the possibility of temporary closures, some companies took extraordinary measures to ensure that workers remained safe from infection. Agricultural workers were especially vulnerable to infection because they "are often housed in crammed trailers or barrack, sharing rooms, kitchens and bathrooms, and are transported to the fields with up to 40 people on the bus" (Jordan, 2020 para. 13). Lipman Family Farms attempted to alleviate infections by locking down its crews to keep COVID-19 from spreading and jeopardizing the harvest. Workers were ordered to stay within their provided housing or in the fields where they were laboring, with few exceptions allowing them to travel to other spaces. According to Jordan, the farm held some level of control over workers' visas, housing, and wages. Therefore, it was able to enact such restrictions. Interestingly, the Fair Food Program "credits [Lipman Family Farms] with keeping the tomato pickers healthy by restricting them to the farms" (Jordan, 2020, para 25). Unfortunately, lockdowns such as this could potentially lead to a trafficking situation, prevent help-seeking, and limit outreach efforts toward identification, as the mobility of the workers was controlled.

While the vulnerability of essential workers to COVID-19 has been well documented, the relationship of pandemic closures, and the resulting economic and employment vulnerabilities, to labor trafficking is under-examined. Moreover, the research literature identifies vulnerabilities associated with labor and sex trafficking, but the research on COVID-19 and labor trafficking is limited. This pilot study expands on the extant literature to investigate the relationship between COVID-19 and labor trafficking. Specifically, we highlight issues with outreach, identification, and vulnerabilities, as well as additional challenges associated with labor trafficking during the pandemic.

Methods

This pilot study used open-ended interviews with six participants across the United States in December of 2020. Each interview lasted approximately 30 minutes; five were conducted via Zoom meetings and one via phone. Participants worked in various fields, including the federal Occupational Safety and Health Administration, migrant outreach, legal aid, and international assistance. Interviewees were from Virginia (1), Chicago (3), St. Louis (1), and Texas (1). Each interviewee worked directly with victims of labor trafficking. The respondents' sites and the organizational context in which they worked are not reported to protect their confidentiality.[2]

Interviewees were initially identified by their involvement in coalitions against human trafficking in the United States and were contacted via email. We utilized snowball sampling to reach other contacts. During interviews we used a prewritten interview guide (reproduced in the appendix), with allowance for additional follow-up questions and discussion. We stopped after six interviews because, by that point, no further information was revealed (Guest et al., 2006). Five of the interviews were recorded with the permission of the interviewee and transcribed by a professional transcription service. After transcription, the interviews were coded by hand to identify key themes. Further taxonomic analysis uncovered subthemes within the key themes (Spradley, 1979). Following open coding and taxonomic analysis, we merged narrative accounts of each of the key themes.

Results

The findings revealed several key themes in the challenges that the COVID-19 pandemic posed: impeded outreach to potential labor trafficking survivors, workers' increased vulnerability to trafficking, and administrative challenges to resource access and utilization. Pandemic restrictions hampered outreach efforts in places where direct outreach typically takes place, limited the ability to make contact and build trust with potential survivors, and delayed innovative outreach initiatives. Respondents developed strategic practices to address such challenges and continued outreach efforts in new ways, including enhanced community-based response efforts, interagency collaboration, and direct outreach pinpointing spots of likely contact under COVID-19-related restrictions. Respondents described an overall heightened vulnerability to labor trafficking because traffickers were taking advantage of exacerbated economic and employment vulnerabilities and were using COVID-19 restrictions to isolate trafficking survivors and manipulate labor trafficking investigations. Administrative issues included a sociopolitical climate conducive to anti-immigrant sentiments and unnecessary barriers in place for denying or delaying visa applications and other immigration relief, which impeded help-seeking and resource access.

Outreach

Challenges to Outreach and Identification. Generally, respondents noted that outreach practices shifted out of necessity to comply with COVID-19 restrictions and in response to fears of contracting and spreading the virus. Kevin described what typical outreach looked like for him in his organization before COVID-19 and the importance of outreach to building community connections and trust:

> What I like to say is that our number one job is building trust . . . That's what we do. We go visit folks where they live. . . . We connect with church leaders. We connect with folks in Hispanic tiendas [shops]. We meet day laborers that are waiting for work. And what we do is, you know, just establish trust with folks and let them know that not only are we here to connect them to community resources but also just give them a broad overview of the types of things that we specifically do.

Kevin explained that connections in the community were made by sharing experiences, such as where the individual was born, what church they belonged to, and more. Eventually, after many simple conversations, Kevin built trust with members of the community, which allowed him to assist in identifying labor trafficking situations.

Normal outreach practices, however, were stymied for most organizations due to COVID-19. As Kevin indicated,

> it's very difficult for advocates to even be out in the community right now. . . . Because one of the difficult parts of one of the most fulfilling parts of our work, which is connecting with people, but also one of the most difficult parts, is like being out in these rural areas and where our folks are, it's much more difficult to do that in a COVID era.

Kevin explained that connection and outreach had been restricted because of the pandemic.

Evelyn noted that there were shifts in her organization's involvement in proactive outreach in the community, such as through community events and direct outreach to migrant workers, which were no longer being practiced as a result of the pandemic:

> A lot of our outreach in the past has been more to specific grassroots organizations or other service providers. . . . [In the past, there was]

> more direct outreach going on. We have not been doing that since the pandemic started, mostly because a lot of that direct outreach events like health fairs or things like that aren't happening. And we also haven't done direct outreach to migrant workers where we go and leave information for them wherever their contract says that they're living.

Like Kevin, Evelyn highlighted the importance of connection and outreach to assist in identifying victims of labor trafficking. Yet that outreach had been halted during the pandemic.

Multiple respondents indicated that their person-to-person outreach was largely stopped due to the pandemic. Respondents generally explained that their typical outreach efforts were stymied as the pandemic had curtailed their outings in the community and thus their ability to connect and build relationships with people potentially experiencing labor trafficking in spaces vulnerable to labor trafficking. Delia noted that COVID-19 impacted how she typically did outreach, restricting access to usual sites for personal contact. Before COVID-19, there were fewer worker restrictions, but

> now it's very restricted movements, whether we're talking farmworkers or other industries, factories or H2B workers, or landscape workers, just now because of the COVID. . . . . It's something that we know is really underground for now, underground because they really are sheltering in place and there's even more isolation, so there's even less of an ability to connect. And those normal points, access points, some of those traditional access points are now gone, like in-person places of worship or in-person library, you know; those are places that we would, so the things that haven't gone away are those essential services.

Restrictions and confinement affecting workers greatly limited traditional efforts to identify trafficking situations.

In addition to negatively impacting traditional outreach efforts, innovative initiatives were delayed by the pandemic. Nichelle described working with an innovative mapping program intended to guide outreach efforts, but the initiative was delayed because of the pandemic:

> [One of the programs that I was looking forward to implementing] used data from different government databases of labor, of the labor force, specifically in agricultural work, meatpacking plants, and so forth. And what they did is they use that data to map out where

many of these agricultural workers are, which many of them tend to be from immigrant communities. . . . So through that mapping technology that they used, they were able to do really real strategic and pinpointed type of outreach to these agricultural workers . . . so that that type of outreach has been impeded due to the pandemic . . . these types of businesses where we could see a lot of the vulnerable and at-risk communities.

In other words, the pandemic halted or slowed traditional and innovative outreach efforts. Advocates attempted to alleviate the earlier-mentioned obstacles in identifying cases of human trafficking, yet these innovative methods were also blocked by the pandemic.

While respondents described challenges to outreach and identification efforts, they also described ways they were innovating to address these challenges. Commonly used reactive practices, such as working with clients through referrals from other organizations, were still in place. Yet proactive outreach measures were limited; consequently, organizations endeavored to shift how they engaged in worker outreach.

Practices to Address Challenges to Outreach and Identification. Organizations worked to shift their outreach efforts to mediums that would allow some level of contact. Delia described the need to be intentional with outreach efforts under COVID-19 conditions. She noted that previous outreach methods may not be effective based on restricted access to the community. The COVID-19 pandemic had placed barriers to traditional outreach. Still, she worked around these barriers by strategically engaging in outreach where survivors were more likely to be—accessing crisis services, health care, groceries, laundromats, and other essential services still open.

Community-based responses were another method of engaging in outreach focused on interagency collaboration. Delia referred to purposeful engagement with community partners, such as consulates, health care, and crisis services. Other respondents similarly noted relying on and collaborating more with community partners, as Camila explained:

I think we're relying a lot more right now on other partners, like community-based organizations or like the churches. . . . We've had . . . a pretty . . . strong outreach presence, but it's only a couple of people in our team, myself and another colleague. And so, to be able to do that work, it almost amplifies it more easily if we're working through . . . organizations that have a really known presence in the area. And so that's been something that we've been . . . really expanding on now, trying to make those connections with the right folks at different organizations and different agencies to be a point of contact or anything and everything . . . and being a connector.

Overall, respondents indicated that typical ways of engaging in outreach during the pandemic largely involved community-based responses, collaboration, and relying on referrals, as well as continued outreach in areas that were not restricted where potential labor trafficking survivors were likely to go, such as health centers, crisis services, consulates, and other essential services. They noted that these proactive efforts were not ideal, but they were using the methods available to them in strategic ways.

Use of COVID-19 as a Trafficking Tool

When respondents were asked if traffickers were using COVID-19 conditions as a tool of trafficking, their responses focused on increased vulnerability. Such vulnerability included economic dependence, lack of employment options, increased isolation, and lack of social support. For example, Evelyn highlighted the role of COVID-19 in creating further economic vulnerability:

> I just think with financial insecurity and instability, COVID has heightened that for a lot of people, and so [it] can get people into a position where they're desperate and so they're more likely to be exploited or to experience trafficking.

Evelyn elaborated by saying that a labor trafficking situation might be someone's best option due to a lack of other employment opportunities.

Kevin indicated that economic dependency and employment opportunities stretched beyond affecting survivors to impacting recruitment and opportunity in survivors' communities in their home countries:

> we all have these basic human rights of . . . freedom of movement and . . . operating the way that we want to operate in the world. And while we're all subject to certain forms of restriction . . . when folks who are already in vulnerable positions are being told not to do something, oftentimes they obey those orders because they risk broader

consequences, not just of losing their job, but of making labor recruiters [look] bad or disabling folks from recruiting in their hometowns at a later time, which can cut off income streams to very poor, vulnerable communities in Mexico and other areas in Latin America where most of the folks are coming from.

Viewing the present situation as impacting future opportunities might have promoted acquiescence to trafficking situations and prevented help-seeking. Survivors of labor trafficking were put in difficult positions. They opted to stay in the labor trafficking situation so as not to lose employment or potentially limit labor recruitment opportunities for themselves and their communities in the future. In other words, employers would play on laborers' existing economic fears, thereby increasing their control over the laborers.

Camila related that economic vulnerability in the gig economy may have increased trafficking as people took jobs outside legitimate labor. She noted that the economy accelerated some forms of trafficking, with "lots of people relying on jobs . . . that right now they maybe can't enter into traditional economies." Economic constraints on finding legitimate work were worsened by pandemic restrictions. To stay employed and make money, survivors may have taken short-term jobs outside the legitimate labor force. Underground economies make identification of trafficking more difficult and inhibit help-seeking. Isolation exacerbated these conditions, which stymied identification and intervention assistance. Accordingly, traffickers were using COVID-19 to further exploit economic and employment vulnerabilities.

Delia described a case of agricultural labor trafficking in which exploitation and control were intensified under COVID-19 conditions, resulting in lost wages and a lack of recourse:

> because of their incredibly restrictive policies, because of COVID, it ended up being highly restrictive and abusive for the workers where they can't even get their clothes to the laundromat, things like that. And they ended up having to quit and not getting paid for the time that they had worked.

Notably, survivors of labor trafficking were leaving their trafficking situations and simply forgoing the money they were promised, adding an additional layer of exploitation to their situation.

Isolation-Related Vulnerabilities

Isolation was intertwined with trafficking vulnerability and traffickers' use of the situation to their advantage. Nichelle explained that traffickers benefited from the stay-at-home orders or other restrictions on businesses and public spaces because it gave them an excuse to isolate survivors from communities and prevent help-seeking. She pointed out that the general social restrictions implemented because of COVID-19 affected the movement of workers and potential victims.

Camila similarly described pandemic conditions as creating isolation, which traffickers could use as an excuse to control workers' movements:

> I'm thinking like, for example, in a domestic servitude case or domestic work case, I'm using COVID as a means to keep someone even further isolated and saying, you know, because of COVID you can't go out and do this or you can't go out and do that. Using it almost as an excuse.

She further described how isolation was already a challenge before the pandemic but that COVID-19-related conditions had heightened this isolation:

> And I think especially because of the . . . effects of COVID. So, like for agricultural workers, we still had workers coming in this year. But I feel like those workers were even more isolated than normal and down to—you being able to use it as a reason to keep people further isolated or not able to make their own decisions about where to go and when and having not even more for their control.

Respondents were unanimous in affirming that isolation was present before the pandemic but was heightened by the pandemic and its associated public health mitigation strategies. Stay-at-home orders and other mobility restrictions were used as a trafficking tool to isolate workers further, while simultaneously thwarting the identification of trafficking.

Using COVID-19 to Impede Investigations

Delia explained that stay-at-home orders resulted in pushing trafficking farther underground and thus impeding investigation efforts:

> It's so easy to do so, and then it even makes it easier to just hide the crime even more. If we've got folks being trafficked in industries that are impacted by COVID, then those layoffs can happen really easily. That hides the crime in that sense. So, it is in our circles, we do the

same kind of speculation because, again, no hard evidence. But really thinking about this is just the whole situation is really just driving the crime even further underground. So, it's scary. . . . So, when I could tell you this is what we think has happened, just based on what we know and [that traffickers will] use anything to control their folks, so of course, they're going to use coronavirus.

Layoffs were used to hide trafficking by eradicating the trafficked workers—both witnesses and potential complainants. To complicate matters, Delia indicated that labor violations were being examined remotely, which was challenging for investigations of labor violations and the potential identification of labor trafficking.

> What you're seeing as well, it's become more tricky. So, we still definitely do the connection through text, phone, email. But, for instance, investigations for labor violations or for violation of COVID executive orders by the governor. Those investigations are happening remotely. A Perfect Storm of Dual Crises. . . If it comes to a point where the labor investigators need to come in, then maybe there is a way. But how everything has really shifted remotely has made it difficult, I think. And it's just trying to grapple with that reality that makes it frustrating as well.

Patricia indicated there was less on-site investigation because of shelter-in-place orders and concerns about exposing investigators to illness. Because there were fewer on-sight workplace investigations, investigators' ability to monitor and inquire into workplace violations was compromised. She elaborated that, before COVID-19, members of her organization were out on job sites and able to detect and refer cases. During COVID-19, fewer people were on the ground to address trafficking situations. Patricia noted that it now took much longer to do a normal inspection because no one would talk via phone with workers. She noted that employers were handing over bogus lists of workers' names. To access workers, providers relied on electronic and phone communication. Employers were in charge of providing a list of workers' names. In many cases, these names were fraudulent, allowing employers to conceal the workers' identities from the service providers. This concealment let employers skirt the enforcement of labor protocol by rendering workers unidentifiable to service providers. In addition to investigative challenges, some policy and administrative challenges impacted service provision and resource access.

Policy, Visa, and Administrative Challenges under COVID-19 Conditions

Camila described how the lack of support in the Trump administration for immigrants and related anti-immigrant sentiments heightened challenges for people experiencing labor trafficking. The combination of a bad situation (e.g., trafficking) with pandemic circumstances and an administration unsupportive of immigrants created a climate of vulnerability impeding help-seeking.

> But the fact that this is happening during the current administration that we have is only adding to it being more difficult for foreign-born survivors of labor trafficking to come forward. . . . I just feel like the pressure is immense. And you hear so many things about differences in different industries. People, you know, being really threatened if they're talking to anybody, you know, any authority figure, any sort of, you know, even legal aid or things like that. And so, I think that given that there's, again, all of these like, this huge lack of structural support in the administration that we have that is actively vilifying immigrants every day and especially undocumented immigrants who are working here and even folks with temporary work visas. It's just like a recipe for pushing it as far underground as it could possibly be.

Anti-immigrant sentiments and structural challenges negatively impacted survivors' access to key resources. For example, visas became much more challenging to obtain during the pandemic. Regarding what was commonly called the "blank spaces policy," respondents explained that if an application had any blank spaces, even if blank spaces were warranted, it would be declined under changes mandated by the government in 2018. This dynamic was particularly challenging with the heightened need for visas under the circumstances of the pandemic. About the blank spaces policy, Camila said,

> This is a policy that USCIS, which is the U.S. Citizenship and Immigration Services, put out, I think maybe two years ago, maybe 2018. . . . And basically, they said that, you know, these are the immigration forms. You have to submit these forms as part of the application. There's a lot of questions on there that don't necessarily apply to anybody. So, like the example that is probably like one of the most common is if someone doesn't have a middle name, so you leave the middle name

base link, you don't have a middle name. And now under this new policy, that can be enough for either a denial or getting an RFE, which is like a request for further evidence just to delay the process. And so, it's even happening to trafficking survivors who are submitting a visa application. If you leave one space blank, and there's a bunch of other examples that, you know, it would not make sense to fill something out. And if you don't write in and say or if it's a numeric one like zero, you know, it can be denied. And so, it's just adding like—It sounds like a small thing, but on top of all of the other policy changes that have come down the pipeline, it's like just one more thing to make it incredibly difficult for people who like, absolutely without a doubt, deserve it.

Accordingly, applications for T-visas, which protect victims of trafficking, were increasingly denied or delayed.

Nichelle also described increasing challenges to obtaining a visa under COVID-19 conditions:

From some of the things we've heard early on when COVID was around, it was one reason that the administration had to decline visa requests, because of coronavirus, less and less visas were being approved. So, again, that just increases vulnerability of these folks that are already being identified as victims and survivors. So, yeah, I think just the number of visas that have been approved have gone way down.

Nichelle indicated that visa requests were increasingly being declined, with COVID-19 conditions being used as an excuse for doing so. The pandemic was slowing down court proceedings, creating a case backlog at a time when workers needed legal relief. Kevin similarly described that immigration relief was also slowed, with backlogs preventing access to key resources for the survivors he worked with:

A lot of, I would say from the client's perspective, also from my like just stuff has slowed down immeasurably, especially for foreign-born folks. And just trying to like get some type of immigration relief type stuff. A lot of that is just like backlogged even more than it was before.

In sum, respondents indicated that challenges associated with the government were heightened under the COVID-19 pandemic, rendering visas and immigration relief much more difficult to obtain. This was attributed to backlogs, newer policy having made applications more cumbersome, declined applications for minor errors or missing information, and anti-immigrant sentiments displayed by the Trump administration.

Benefits for Work of the COVID-19 Pandemic

To avoid confirmation bias, we were careful to conduct the interviews in ways that would not lead the respondents, so we asked neutrally about the impact of COVID-19 on the respondents' organizational practices. One respondent explained that the COVID-19 pandemic did provide some benefit by drawing media attention to essential workers, including laborers in jobs that were more likely to involve trafficked workers. This heightened awareness might have increased self-reporting in some instances.

Kevin elaborated on this beneficial effect:

> what I can say is that since the start of the pandemic, we have seen workers, even workers who are in vulnerable positions start to speak out a little bit more because in terms of workplace violations publicly, because it was sort of America and the world was a little bit awakened. The folks that are really driving our economy and most particularly the people that we can't live without. Right. In terms of the work that they're doing. And so, I think that when the workers that we represent and work alongside, the vulnerable, low-income workers, were then being required to go in [to work], but then there were not commen-surate protections [COVID-19 protections], right, to be able to keep them safe during a pandemic. And then the data showed that there were these huge breakouts at poultry camps in migrant labor camps, then I think that, you know, workers felt a little bit more empowered, particularly when they have organizations like us to say, whoa, right, we're essential, we're not disposable. We need to be in a position where we have to say something. And this is a moment in time to be able to find something. So, while this has been a tremendously difficult time for everybody, including those workers, I think there's been a sense of empowerment to be able to speak out about things that maybe they didn't feel like they had a platform to do in the past.

Kevin explained that the attention placed on essential workers in the food industry during the pandemic had provided a platform to amplify the voices of labor-trafficked and exploited people.

Yeah, I mean, that's we as advocates, you know, have been trying to use this as a moment of opportunity to say, hey, look, this is the first time where ever in my practice that we affirmatively have folks reaching out to us, whether it be media or other people saying, wow, like what is going on here. And to be able to lift up the worker's voice and to be able to try to use this not just a moment of, you know, immediate change but to use it as a stepping-stone for long-term empowerment and changing certain pieces of the system that are keeping folks impoverished and disenfranchised.

Thus, one potential positive outcome of the COVID-19 pandemic was heightened media attention to essential workers and their working conditions, with the potential for increasing public and political interest in labor trafficking.

Discussion

The academic literature on labor trafficking documents existing barriers to accessing and utilizing key resources (Owens et al., 2014; Schwarz, 2017; Zhang, 2012) and a critical need for social, legal, and health care services (Heil & Nichols, 2019; Preble et al., 2023). The present study indicates that such barriers were heightened at a time when outreach efforts became severely restricted under pandemic conditions. Accessing communities in hot spots for outreach and engaging in person-to-person contact to build relationships, trust, and bridges to future help-seeking were no longer options for all but one organization in this study. Despite such limitations, those engaged in outreach efforts attempted to make contact by focusing on areas still open with fewer restrictions, along with creative outreach endeavors such as gift basket distribution in at-risk communities. Respondents in this study indicated that they could make contact in locations with essential services that survivors would use, such as grocery stores and laundromats, as well as sites of health care services. Respondents suggested innovative community-based responses, such as linking with other social and legal services and consulates, to enhance outreach efforts. Further research should explore additional techniques practitioners use to continue engaging in outreach efforts in times of pandemic-related restrictions, which can be expected to happen again in the future.

Pandemic conditions heightened trafficking vulnerabilities, such as financial need and isolation. Financial need rooted in unemployment makes people vulnerable to a trafficking situation through gig economy work or illegal labor (e.g., panhandling) as well as pay-by-the-job under-the-table work (e.g., a day's work at a construction site) (Murphy, 2016; National Human Trafficking Resource Center, 2018). For those already experiencing labor trafficking, pandemic circumstances heightened coercive control through isolation. Stay-at-home orders or other restrictions prevented labor trafficking survivors from entering their communities and served as a barrier to utilizing community support and resources. Prior research indicates isolation as a trafficking technique and a form of coercion purposely used to prevent help-seeking and exiting the trafficking situation (National Human Trafficking Resource Center, 2018; Owens, 2014; Zhang, 2012). The present study supports this research and indicates that such dynamics are intensified in pandemic circumstances. Local-level law enforcement needs to rely on proactive policing rather than reactive policing. As the respondents explained, survivors were less likely to come forward during the COVID-19 pandemic. Therefore, increased local-level investigations where labor trafficking was likely to take place (e.g., meatpacking plants) were necessary. In addition, this research supports prior work that found anti-immigrant sentiments and policies created barriers to help-seeking (de Vries et al., 2019; Heil & Nichols, 2019). The current study similarly finds that anti-immigrant sentiments deterred help-seeking. Moreover, our findings suggest that policies were put in place to further deny rights to labor trafficking survivors, such those for visa applications.

The results of this study indicate that future research should further explore challenges to obtaining visas, particularly T-visas and U-visas, both in ordinary times and under COVID-19 circumstances. Working to identify such challenges and their impact on trafficking survivors can serve to identify needed legislative action and administrative intervention. For example, changes in 2018 requiring further documentation to obtain a visa, often in ways that did not make sense or were not possible, should be further explored and revised. Respondents indicated that visa applications were being denied during the pandemic because of blank space policies and an overload of cases. For example, applications required that applicants provide a middle name, which fails to acknowledge that middle names are uncommon in some nations and cultures. Applications could be rejected for failing to identify a middle name, with no clear remedy or instruction for how applicants without a lawful middle name should complete this basic element of the application. The research literature indicates that while protections for trafficking survivors are part of federal legislation, the protections are implemented in discretionary ways, particularly for visa applications (Egyes, 2017; Polaris, 2020). The current study shows how COVID-19 conditions exacerbated this dynamic by delaying applications and increasing application denials associated with blank space rules. For labor trafficking survivors to self-report their victimization, support services that are supposed to be provided according to the Trafficking Victims Protection Act should be fulfilled without increased barriers. These barriers served to revictimize workers by denying their basic rights as trafficking victims in ways that are antithetical to federal law.

The benefits of COVID-19 conditions were not identified as particularly prevalent. However, continued media exposure of the necessity of migrant labor in our society can potentially assist in highlighting the experiences of labor-trafficked people, amplifying their voices and experiences with labor trafficking and reframing the narrative of anti-immigrant xenophobia for essential workers. It is well documented that labor trafficking is not a social issue that has garnered much public and political attention, particularly compared with sex trafficking (Heil & Nichols, 2019; Owens et al., 2014; Preble et al., 2023). Further media exposure may work to draw added attention to the needs of labor-trafficked and exploited people.

Limitations

Although the findings of this study illustrate the new obstacles that legal professionals and advocates faced in identifying and protecting victims of labor trafficking during the COVID-19 pandemic, there are limitations to the study. First, because of the pandemic, we could interview only six individuals. Geographically, the sample was not as representative as we would have liked. Through snowball sampling, we identified interviewees from the Midwest, the East Coast, and the South of the United States; ideally, we would have had representatives of other areas. Despite these geographic and numeric limitations, our respondents all gave similar answers, and we believe that recruiting additional participants from other areas of the United States would have yielded similar results.

We found that interviewing via Zoom meetings (and one phone call) did not allow for the same personal experience as in-person interviews.

Had we talked to interviewees in person, we could have observed them in their environment and engaged in day-to-day activities in their roles as advocates and legal professionals. Generally, in-person interviews elicit more in-depth data that we could not get via Zoom. Still, with each interview, there was a personal connection, and it was possible to follow up with the interviewees if we or they had additional questions.

A last limitation to this study was its time frame, given that the data were collected one year into the pandemic. At the time of this writing, we learned that dynamics related to the pandemic involved ongoing changes. Consequently, we saw shifts in how advocates and legal professionals assisted victims of labor trafficking. If another pandemic develops, we suggest that researchers continue to monitor the effects of the pandemic and policy responses over time to determine how patterns change regarding the identification and protection of victims of labor trafficking in the United States.

Conclusion

The current study uncovered the challenges under COVID-19 circumstances experienced by organizations that provide services to labor trafficking survivors. Its findings can guide further research and inform potential policy and practice recommendations in the case of another pandemic. The findings suggest a need for strategically shifting outreach efforts to places where making contact is still likely and for enhancing community-based response efforts to hone outreach and identification efforts. Traffickers seemed to take advantage of economic and employment-related vulnerabilities and used COVID-19-related restrictions to isolate survivors further, which highlights the importance of continued outreach through available means. Identified limitations to online investigations indicate that in-person investigations of suspected labor trafficking should continue in pandemic circumstances, with enhanced provisions of personal protective equipment for investigators. Furthermore, policies such as the blank spaces rule, which seems designed to deny visas and immigration relief, should be rescinded to be consistent with the protections for labor trafficking survivors in the U.S. Trafficking Victims Protection Act. Further research should continue exploring these areas using a larger sample, inclusive of more geographic regions, to account for possible regional nuances and potentially to uncover further challenges and responses for addressing labor trafficking during the COVID-19 pandemic.

Appendix

Please tell me about which agency you work with and your role at that agency.

How long have you been with them?

How many cases do you believe that your agency, in terms of labor tracking, that you have identified?

Can you describe to me some of the proactive strategies that you use in identification?

Since COVID, have you seen any sort of impact on how labor trafficking may have changed?

Do you believe traffickers are using the fear of COVID as a tool of isolation?

Do you believe the dynamics of labor trafficking changed in this new era of a pandemic?

How do you believe COVID has affected survivors' self-identification of labor trafficking?

What do you think would help the general public better identify situations of labor trafficking?

Did your agency receive any of the CARES Act funding?

Do you think there is a relationship between what we're experiencing with the pandemic and labor trafficking today?

Notes

1. Temporary visa that allows non–U.S. citizens to work in the agricultural industry in the United States.

2. *Disclosure of potential conflicts of interest*: No potential conflicts of interest were identified in this study. *Research involving human participants and/or animals*: Research was limited to nonintrusive interviews with participants aged 18 and older. *Informed consent*: Because of COVID-19 restrictions, interviewees gave oral informed consent, which was recorded in their Zoom interview.

5. Policing Perceptions: Campus Officers' Job Commitment, Fit, Satisfaction, and Self-Legitimacy amid COVID-19

David R. White and Andrew Hartung

Introduction

When considering the overall impacts of the COVID-19 global pandemic on law enforcement, the experiences of campus police officers must be taken into account. Approximately 15,000 sworn police officers and 11,000 non-sworn security staff serve an estimated 900 public and private four-year colleges and universities in the United States, with a combined student population of about 12 million (Reaves, 2015). While campus officers are similar in some ways to their full-service law enforcement counterparts, they work within the organizational framework of higher education and face challenges particular to that environment. Because COVID-19 has had unprecedented impacts on higher education, it is important to evaluate how the pandemic conditions created new strains for campus officers. In this chapter, we examine how COVID-19 affected campus officers' perceptions of job commitment, job fit, and job satisfaction as well as the confidence they have in their authority—something commonly referred to as *self-legitimacy* (see, generally, Bottoms & Tankebe, 2012).

By late March of 2020, colleges and universities across the country abruptly closed their campuses and rapidly shifted students to online learning to comply with stay-at-home, stay-safe orders (Johnson, 2020). These sudden closures were difficult at best, and related difficulties continued into the following academic year (2020–2021), which saw a mixture of online, hybrid, and face-to-face learning in ways never done before. These abrupt shifts led to serious questions about the logistical and budgetary impacts the pandemic would have on many aspects of campus life and the learning environment. Undergraduate enrollment shrunk by 20%, accounting for $19 billion in lost revenue from tuition, room-and-board contracts, and other campus fees (Kim et al., 2020). Financial concerns also included losses in state funding, endowments, and donations (Blankenberger & Williams, 2020). This led to the layoff of an estimated 51,000 campus employees nationwide by July 2020, mainly nonacademic staff, as well as other cost-saving measures (Hess, 2020; see also Burke, 2020). Meanwhile, logistical issues regarding compliance with public health mandates to keep students and staff safe made the administration of university operations challenging and more costly.

Along with the rest of the country, campus communities experienced increased infections through the fall of 2020 (Centers for Disease Control and Prevention, 2020; Flaherty, 2020; Walke et al., 2020). College students' propensity to socialize placed them at greater risk of infection (Flaherty, 2020) and made them a focus of public concern (e.g., Johnson, 2020). To combat this concern, campuses implemented a variety of mitigation efforts and, in many cases, took aggressive steps to reduce risks, hoping to avoid making the situation worse. Despite the efforts, by May of 2021, there had been more than 700,000 confirmed COVID-19 cases and 100-plus deaths of either students, faculty, or staff on America's college campuses (Hodge et al., 2022).

From a policing standpoint, all police officers, not just campus officers, faced increased risk of exposure to COVID-19, due to the essential nature of their work and the potential to encounter someone infected with the virus (Lange & Terry, 2020). This risk is reflected in the fact that, by September of 2020, COVID-19-related fatalities had exceeded all other causes of death among police officers for calendar year 2020 (Ingraham, 2020). By May 2022, there were more than 600 verified police officer deaths related to COVID-19 nationwide (Officer Down Memorial Page, 2022), including at least six campus police and security officers (International Association of Campus Law Enforcement Administrators, 2022). In addition to other stressors associated with policing, fears related to COVID-19 had the potential to affect officers' physical and psychological well-being as they confronted the fact that they might become infected at work and could bring the virus home to their loved ones (Frenkel et al., 2021; Weinstein, 2020).

In addition to the risk of exposure to COVID-19, police officers assumed the responsibility for enforcing the evolving COVID-19 public health mandates, such as mask orders and social distancing, which grew increasingly unpopular among the public, including college students. This duty added to officers' job stress (Stogner et al., 2020) and may have damaged officers' legitimacy with the public (Jones, 2020). In campus contexts, officers enforce not only state and local health mandates but also campus policies. As campus policies may be more restrictive than other local mandates, their enforcement may be more difficult and may lead to frequent questions from students and other stakeholders. Importantly, campus police officers have long faced additional struggles not encountered by their full-service counterparts when it comes to maintaining their legitimacy as "real" law enforcement officers (Jacobsen, 2015; Wilson & Wilson, 2011). As a result, there are reasons to suspect that the additional COVID-19 strictures may have placed more strain on the relationship between campus officers and their communities. As this occurred, the impact of such strain could have affected campus officers' job satisfaction, affective commitment, sense of suitability for the job, and self-confidence in their own authority (see White et al., 2020).

In this chapter, we explore how COVID-19 concerns affected campus police officers on two levels. First, we evaluate officers' personal fears about COVID-19 exposure and their perceived ability to police during the pandemic—something we contextualize as the officers' *individual concerns*. Second, we assess the officers' perceptions of how well their employing campus was managing the crisis and how confident they were in their school's ability to ensure everyone's safety. We operationalize this as the *organizational response*. We assess the relationships between these two COVID-19 concerns and four outcomes: *job satisfaction, affective commitment, job fit,* and *self-legitimacy*. Although conducting research was difficult during the pandemic, we were able to use an online survey to reach out to campus police and security officers in Michigan (N = 93) in June and July of 2020.[1] While the results of a small convenience sample should be interpreted cautiously, our findings offer insights into how COVID-19 affected campus police officers' attitudes relative to the four outcomes. We end our discussion by describing some potential policy implications as well as directions for future research relative to campus policing.

Policing in a Campus Context

Campus police are an understudied group relative to their law enforcement peers in other jurisdictions (Patten et al., 2016). Originating as watchmen, campus officers were often retirees from occupations other than policing until around the 1950s, when retirees from municipal police organizations began to fill the ranks (Sloan, 1992). These watchmen performed mainly custodial duties in protecting the campus from fire, water, or other damage (Sloan, 1992). These watchmen eventually took on the responsibility of enforcing campus rules and regulations, moving them away from their maintenance role and toward a more police-oriented function. Modern campus police officers were not widely employed until the late 1960s or early 1970s (Sloan, 1992), and even today, their role requires a balance between working within campus structures and fulfilling police-oriented functions.

Much of the call volume on campuses pertains to issues associated with a college-aged population (Fisher, 1995; Henson & Stone, 1999), and campus officers' duties are generally oriented more toward parenting or acting as a role model than toward policing in the traditional sense (Sloan, 1992; Sloan et al., 2000; Willis, 2015). Despite this, these officers are typically granted the same authority as their municipal counterparts. This is evidenced by the fact that 92% of campus officers serving public institutions and 38% serving private ones have sworn arrest powers (Reaves, 2015). However, many campus stakeholders see these officers as less legitimate than their full-service counterparts (Jacobsen, 2015; Patten et al., 2016; Wada et al., 2010). This questioned legitimacy owes, in part, to the fine line that campus officers walk in working for colleges and universities with their distinctive administrative capacities while also being legally and fully empowered as law enforcement officers.

Ideally, campus police officers should be comfortable with this dual role and with taking a community- and service-oriented approach to their duties (Sloan et al., 2000; Jacobsen, 2015). However, officers who enjoy engaging in traditional crime-fighting may experience more role conflict than their colleagues (Howe, 2015). Younger officers, especially, may be dissatisfied with service-oriented tasks such as unlocking doors and making security checks of buildings (Howe, 2015). In the face of the COVID-19 pandemic, the additional responsibilities associated with virus mitigation efforts (e.g., enforcing mask mandates and limitations on social gatherings) may have further undermined some campus officers' sense of legitimacy.

How, then, did COVID-19 affect campus police officers' job satisfaction, commitment, fit, and self-legitimacy? We offer several factors to consider. First, as with full-service police personnel, campus officers' personal fears about their exposure to COVID-19 on the job and about their ability to carry out their duties amid pandemic conditions were well-founded concerns. Second, significant budget reductions, angst among college and university administrators over the pandemic's financial implications, and early cost-saving moves such as layoffs led many campus police and security officers to worry about their job security. As many campuses shut down on-site operations in the spring of 2020, sending students home and faculty and staff into remote working conditions, campus officers might have viewed their job security as increasingly vulnerable.[2] Finally, although campus officers were involved in their institution's response to COVID-19, they may have wondered about the larger picture: Do I believe campus leaders made the right decisions during the crisis? How confident am I that they were looking out for everyone's best interest? How much do I trust them to handle this ongoing crisis or future crises?

We would be negligent if we did not also recognize that the COVID-19 crisis coincided with a social movement that brought heightened public scrutiny to police and the justice system over racial injustice. The deaths of George Floyd and Breonna Taylor touched off widespread civil unrest during this time. As a result, concerns about police officers' job satisfaction, commitment, fit, and self-legitimacy were not limited to COVID-19 factors; these attitudes were likely affected in negative ways by the broader sociopolitical climate as well. Similar concerns were widely discussed following the death of Michael Brown in Ferguson, Missouri, in 2014 (e.g., Wolfe & Nix, 2017).

Elements of Campus Police Officers' Attitudes

Job Satisfaction

Job satisfaction is generally recognized as an emotional response to "the perception that one's job fulfills or allows the fulfillment of one's important job values" (Locke, 1976, p. 1307). Assessments of job satisfaction often evaluate the impact of the job's characteristics, environmental conditions, and individual-level correlates (Johnson, 2012). In most cases, individual factors—such as sex, age, education, and tenure—produce mainly weak or nonsignificant results (Cantarelli et al., 2016; White, Kyle, & Schafer, 2022), whereas job characteristics—such as variety, autonomy, or task identity—tend to have more empirical support (e.g., Humphrey et al., 2007). Although environmental factors can conceptually cover many things, role ambiguity, which is defined by an uncertainty about how to carry out a work role, has been a consistent (negative) predictor of job satisfaction (Abramis, 1994), as has role conflict, which is defined, in part, by competing organizational demands or differences among several roles filled by the same person (Rizzo et al., 1970, p. 155; see also Schuler et al., 1977). Additionally, the research includes job stress and strain, which are defined as the "tension, anxiety, worry, emotional exhaustion, and distress" caused by work (Lambert & Paoline, 2008, p. 548) and the "internal tension the employee feels when required to do work tasks the employee dislikes or feels ill equipped to perform" (Johnson, 2012, p. 160). Job stress is negatively related to job satisfaction; furthermore, a meta-analysis demonstrated that mental health (e.g., anxiety, depression) is related to job satisfaction (Cass et al., 2003). Although studies of job satisfaction among police officers are less common than studies of other populations, the evidence generally suggests similar outcomes. Relative to our study, officers' personal stress over potential COVID-19 exposure may have compounded with some degree of role confusion, ambiguity, or conflict in having to enforce evolving COVID-19 mitigation policies.

Perceived organizational support is another factor that has consistently demonstrated a relationship with job satisfaction (Eisenberger et al., 1986). Organizational support is defined as the belief that employers care about the contribution and well-being of employees (Riggle et al., 2009). Organizational support consistently predicts about 38% of the variance in job satisfaction (Riggle et al., 2009, p. 1029), and some recent research demonstrated that organizational responses to COVID-19 represented one aspect of organizational support (Daniels et al., 2022). Perceived organizational support is often an important predictor of job satisfaction among police officers, including perceived supervisory support and issues of fit between an officer's own outlook on the job compared with those of the officer's supervisors (see, e.g., Ingram & Lee, 2015; Johnson, 2012; Paoline & Gau, 2020; White et al., 2021). As the worst of the pandemic is still fresh in memory and studies exploring its impact are limited, our study adds value to such exploration by assessing the effects of COVID-19 on individuals' attitudes toward work.

The available research on police job satisfaction provides conclusions similar to those of the broader literature, reporting that job character-istics and environmental factors exert the strongest influences on job satisfaction, while individual-level factors tend to produce weak or non-significant associations (see Ingram et al., 2021; Zhao et al., 1999). This work highlights that officers with high levels of work stress and strain tend to be more dissatisfied at work (Ingram & Lee, 2015; Johnson, 2012; Paoline & Gau, 2020). When there is an incongruence between officers' expectations or values relative to those of the leadership team, this lack of fit results in reduced job satisfaction (e.g., Ingram & Lee, 2015; White et al., 2021). White et al. (2021) even indicate that, independent of fit and other individual factors, officers' self-legitimacy—the confidence they have in their own authority—is significantly related to job satisfaction. Despite the interconnectedness of these factors with job satisfaction and the likely impacts of COVID-19-related strains, scant research thus far has addressed the impacts of COVID-19 concerns on police officers' job satisfaction.

Affective Organizational Commitment

Organizational commitment is frequently related to job satisfaction (e.g., Meyer et al., 2002). Many of the same issues affecting job satisfaction also affect organizational commitment, including job characteristics and environmental factors (Mathieu & Zajac, 1990). Affective commitment, perhaps the most-studied form of commitment, is defined by an emotional attachment to an organization (Kuo, 2015, p. 32). Importantly, police officers' perceptions of organizational support are associated with more organizational commitment (Johnson, 2015). This finding is consistent with a meta-analysis of broader organizational research, which demonstrated that perceived organizational support was the strongest positive predictor of affective commitment (Ahmed et al., 2015; Meyer et al., 2002; Riggle et al., 2009). Relative to the current study, officers' perceptions of their organizations' responses to COVID-19 could serve to either increase or decrease their commitment.

There is also evidence that high job stress is associated with low organizational commitment (Griffin et al., 2010; Lambert & Paoline, 2008). It is worth noting that job stress is also strongly correlated with emotional exhaustion, and while it is analytically distinct from the concept of burnout, long-term job stress is seen as "the end results of prolonged exposure to job stress" (Griffin et al., 2010, p. 242). Among a sample of police officers, Johnson (2015) acknowledged that, while there is evidence in the literature showing that job stress and organizational commitment are related, he found no such relationship in his secondary analysis of data from 11 police agencies in the Phoenix metropolitan area. This led him to conclude that "perhaps the individuals volunteering for service as law enforcement officers enter the field anticipating high levels of stress" (p. 1171). Regardless of these mixed findings, it is evident that COVID-19 added stress to campus police officers' jobs and that such pressure may have manifested both in concern over personal safety and well-being and in perceptions of organizational support.

Job Fit

The theoretical framework of person–environment interactions examines how individuals "fit in" at work, and empirical research consistently reveals that a good fit tends to produce positive outcomes for both the employer and employee. Kristof-Brown et al. (2005) contend that "theories of person–environment interactions have been prevalent in the management literature for almost 100 years" (p. 281). Fit is frequently defined as a level of congruence between individuals and their work environment based on a variety of conceptualizations, including the congruence of values, personality, knowledge, skills, and abilities (Ostroff & Schulte, 2007). Researchers have categorized the various aspects of how someone fits in at work, which includes aspects of person–organization, person–supervisor, person–group, and person–job fit (Ostroff & Schulte, 2007). A meta-analysis demonstrated that fit is strongly related to job satisfaction and organizational commitment, among other similar outcomes (Kristof-Brown et al., 2005).

Research on person–environment fit among police officers is relatively sparse, though there have been a few studies in the past decade (e.g., Ingram, 2013; Ingram & Lee, 2015; Rief & Clinkinbeard, 2020; White et al., 2020; White, Kyle, & Schafer, 2022). These studies have focused primarily on person–supervisor fit (Ingram, 2013; Ingram & Lee, 2015), person–group fit (Ingram et al., 2021), or on combinations of person–organization fit, person–supervisor fit, and person–group fit (Rief & Clinkinbeard, 2020; White et al., 2020; White et al., 2021; White, Kyle, & Schafer, 2022). Only one of these studies included job fit (Rief & Clinkinbeard, 2020). Among the general findings of these studies, a satisfactory fit with top managers (organizational fit) has been related to increased job satisfaction (White, Kyle, & Schafer, 2022). Some mixed evidence has shown that person–supervisor fit is related to job satisfaction (Ingram & Lee, 2015; White, Kyle, & Schafer, 2022), and further evidence has been found that group fit is linked to job satisfaction, though this appears more nuanced (Ingram et al., 2021). Supervisor fit is also related to reduced role ambiguity (Ingram, 2013). Finally, hierarchical models of fit that include congruence with top managers, supervisors, and coworkers are a strong positive predictor of police officers' self-legitimacy (White et al., 2020).

Self-Legitimacy

Police legitimacy has been the focus of much discussion, but Bottoms and Tankebe (2012) point out that this emphasis has been placed almost exclusively on citizens' perceptions of police rather than on police officers' perceptions of their own authority. The legitimate exercise of governmental power, such as that used by police, requires a dialogue between the citizen and the power holder. Bottoms and Tankebe assert that the power holder's perception of their own legitimate authority importantly shapes how and when a power holder may assert certain claims to power. In simple terms, self-legitimacy defines the "power-holders' recognition of, or confidence in, their own individual entitlement to power" (Tankebe, 2014, p. 3).

Researchers have demonstrated that police officers' self-legitimacy is, in fact, positively related to embracing more democratic modes of policing (Bradford & Quinton, 2014; Tankebe, 2019; Trinkner et al., 2016; White et al., 2021), which includes less willingness to resort to threats of physical force (Tankebe & Meško, 2015). Others have indicated that improved self-legitimacy is related to greater engagement with community members (Wolfe & Nix, 2016) and better perceptions of moral alignment with the community (White et al., 2021).

The antecedents of self-legitimacy are in the organizational environment, which includes assessments of organizational justice, revealing that officers who have positive working relationships with supervisors and coworkers generally report better self-legitimacy, while individual-level factors have generally resulted in weak or nonsignificant findings (see White et al., 2020). Relative to our study, research has demonstrated that self-legitimacy is correlated with trust in the organization (Wolfe & Nix, 2017) and with better perceptions of person–environment fit (White et al., 2020; White et al., 2021). However, no studies have addressed how COVID-19 has affected police officers' self-legitimacy, and no published studies have directly explored campus officers' perceptions of self-legitimacy.

Methodology

Our study focuses on campus police officers' perceptions of *job satisfaction, affective* (organizational) *commitment, job fit,* and *self-legitimacy* during the COVID-19 pandemic. Specifically, we assessed officers' COVID-19-related job perceptions on two levels. First, we assessed their *individual concerns* over exposure to the virus and their ability to do the job during this crisis.

Second, we assessed their perceptions of their school's *organizational response* to the pandemic, which we believe demonstrate a form of organizational support in this unprecedented event. We hypothesized that less personal worry over COVID-19 (individual concerns) and better perceptions of organizational response would both relate positively to all four outcomes. Simply put, officers who worry less about their exposure to COVID-19 and the ability to do their job effectively amid pandemic conditions, as well as those who believe their organization was effective in managing the initial crisis, will report statistically better job satisfaction, affective commitment, job fit, and self-legitimacy—the four outcome variables.

To test these predictions, we used data from responses to an online survey of campus police officers ($N = 93$) administered during June and July of 2020. Working with the president of the Michigan Association of Campus Law Enforcement Administrators, we distributed our survey request to campus public safety directors and administrators at colleges and universities throughout Michigan, and we asked them to forward the request to their respective staff. At the time, there were 616 certified campus police officers at 12 colleges and 14 universities across the state.[3] Although some non-sworn security staff members were included in our sample, approximately 87% reported that they were certified, sworn officers.

To measure COVID-19-related concerns, we asked officers about their *individual concerns* relative to exposure to the virus and their perceived abilities to do their job amid the pandemic, and we asked them for their perceptions of their school's *organizational response* to the crisis. We measured *individual concerns* by asking officers the extent to which they agree with the following statements: "I personally worry a lot about being exposed to COVID-19 while on duty" (reverse coded); "I feel prepared to do my job the way it should be done, despite the challenges of the COVID-19 crisis"; and "I personally do not think the COVID-19 crisis will change the way I go about my daily job." These questions, and all dependent and independent variables in the survey, were measured on a five-point scale of agreement from "strongly disagree" to "strongly agree." The responses to the three items were summed in a scale where higher scores represented less individual concern relative to COVID-19.[4] On a scale ranging from 3 to 15, the mean score for *individual concerns* was 10.07 (standard deviation = 2.58).

We similarly measured officers' perceptions of their campus's response to the COVID-19 crisis as the *organizational response* with three statements: "I think my college/university did a good job managing the mid-semester shutdown this past spring (2020)"; "I think my college/university will be better prepared to manage similar pandemic crises in the future"; and "I feel confident that my college/university will work hard to ensure students, faculty, and staff are all as safe as possible when returning this fall (2020)." We summed the responses in a single scale where higher scores represented officers' greater confidence in their organization to manage the COVID-19 crisis.[5] On a scale ranging from 3 to 15, the mean score for *organizational response* was 11.53 (standard deviation = 2.82).[6]

Relative to our outcome variables, we measured *job satisfaction* with five items from Johnson (2012). These included such statements as "I find work stimulating and challenging" and "I enjoy all the things I do on my job very much." The items were measured on a similar five-point scale of agreement, from "strongly disagree" to "strongly agree." The responses were summed in a scale ranging from 5 to 25, with higher scores representing greater job satisfaction. Despite the potential stressors of COVID-19 and general concerns over legitimacy, officers in this study reported being generally satisfied with their jobs, with a mean score of 18.07 (standard deviation = 4.63).[7]

Affective commitment was measured using three statements modified from Kuo (2015): "I have told my friends that campus public safety work is a worthy profession"; "It does not matter how people may criticize public safety on campus; I am willing to serve as a public safety officer"; and "I am proud to tell people that I am a campus public safety officer." Responses to the items were summed so that higher scores represented greater commitment. As with our finding for job satisfaction, officers seemed strongly committed to their roles, with the mean score for *affective commitment* being 11.95 (standard deviation = 2.76) on a scale ranging from 3 to 15.[8]

Four statements were modified from Saks and Ashforth (1997) to measure *job fit*: "My current job enables me to do the kind of work I want to do"; "My current job is a good match for me"; "My knowledge, skills, and abilities match the requirements of my current job very well"; and "My job fulfills my needs for what I look for at work." Responses to the items were summed in a scale from 4 to 20, with higher scores representing better perceptions of job fit. As with some of the other outcomes, officers generally reported high perceptions of job fit, with the mean score being 15.58 (standard deviation = 4.07).[9]

We used five statements modified from White (2019) to measure our final outcome variable, *self-legitimacy*: "I am confident in the authority vested in me as a campus safety officer"; "I am confident I have enough authority to do my job well"; "I believe my public safety department can provide security for all members of the campus community"; "I feel my job positively impacts the members of my campus community"; and "I do not hesitate to use my authority when I believe it is necessary to intervene in a situation." These items were summed in a single scale ranging from 5 to 25, with higher scores representing greater self-legitimacy. Overall, officers reported very high self-legitimacy, with the mean score of 21.47 (standard deviation = 3.41).[10]

In addition to the four outcome variables, we included sets of individual and organizational factors. Our individual factors were *gender, race, rank, education, military service, tenure* (collected categorically), *age* (collected categorically), *certified* law enforcement officer versus non-certified officer, and *previous* law enforcement experience outside higher education. For organizational factors, we included college or university *school type* as two-year school versus four-year school. We then asked the officers if they were covered by *collective bargaining*, and we quantified their school's *student population* in three categories: less than 10,000, 10,000–14,999, and 15,000 or more.

Results

As a small convenience sample, our results come with clear limitations that cannot be understated and are addressed in our discussion. Nonetheless, the descriptive data demonstrate that our sample is not that different from national census data for campus police officers. Our final sample ($N = 93$) represents about 13% of the total population of certified campus police officers in the State of Michigan. The full descriptive data for the sample are provided in Table 5.1.

Bivariate correlations are presented in Table 5.2. At this level of assessment, several of the outcomes—*affective commitment, job fit, job satisfaction*, and *self-legitimacy*—are strongly correlated with one another. The first three are all similar concepts, while self-legitimacy differs slightly. It is noteworthy that self-legitimacy is strongly correlated with these other perceptions. This supports the notion that all the concepts are interrelated. Why these four factors converge in this way in our sample is outside the scope of what we address in this chapter; instead, we focus on how each of these factors relates to the officers' COVID-19 concerns and to individual and organizational factors.

Table 5.1 Descriptive Statistics for the Sample

Variables	Percentage
Gender (% male)	90.5%
Race (% White)	81.7%
Rank	
Patrolman / Security officer	50.5%
Supervisor / Command staff	49.5%
Bachelor's degree or higher	62.4%
Military service	12.8%
Tenure	
0–10 years	52.3%
10–19 years	27.9%
20 or more years	19.8%
Age (% 40 years or older)	69.9%
Certified law enforcement officer	87.1%
Prior work in law enforcement outside higher ed	74.4%
Serve at a 4-year college/university	58.1%
Collective bargaining (% yes)	70.8%
Student population	
Less than 10,000	23.6%
10,000 to 14,999	22.5%
15,000 or more	53.9%

Among the individual-level factors, White respondents had significantly better *affective commitment, job fit, job satisfaction,* and *self-legitimacy*; however, given the small sample size, this finding should be interpreted cautiously. Similarly, respondents age 40 and older also reported better *affective commitment, job fit,* and *job satisfaction*. What's more, certified campus officers reported greater *self-legitimacy* than non-certified security officers. None of the other individual factors was significantly correlated with the outcome variables.

As it relates to COVID-19 *individual concerns* and *organizational response*, race (as White or non-White) was significantly correlated with perceptions of *organizational response*, with White respondents having better perceptions, as was *age*, with older respondents reporting better perceptions. *Individual concerns* were not strongly linked with any of the control variables but were closely associated with perceptions of *organizational response*. This relationship was in the expected direction. Respondents who expressed less individual concern over COVID-19 were also significantly more likely to think that their organization did a satisfactory job in response to COVID-19.

At this bivariate level, the two COVID-19 variables, both *individual concerns* and *organizational response*, were significantly correlated with all four outcome variables. These are reported in Table 5.2. All the relationships were in the expected direction. Less individual concern over COVID-19 and better perceptions of organizational response were positively correlated with better *job satisfaction, affective commitment, job fit,* and *self-legitimacy*.

Moving beyond the bivariate correlations to a multivariate analysis, we used several ordinary least squares regression models to explore the relationships between COVID-19 concerns and the four outcome variables. The full results of these models are found in Table 5.3 and in the notes at chapter's end. Our results are somewhat mixed. First, as it relates to *affective commitment*, the only significant predictor variables were *organizational response* and *rank*. Officers who believed their organization performed better in its organizational response to COVID-19 exhibited higher affective commitment. Meanwhile, the officers' *individual concerns* over COVID-19 did not significantly relate to their *affective commitment*, nor did any of the other individual or school factors included in the control variables, aside from *rank*. Overall, the significant factors predicted a little over one-third of the total variation in *affective commitment* (36%).

In the multivariate test of *job fit*, *organizational response* was significant again, and *age* and *gender* were also significant, with older and male respondents reporting better *job fit*. As expected, those who reported higher *organizational response* scores also reported significantly better perceptions of *job fit*. Forty percent of the variance in *job fit* was explained by the included variables. The results for *job satisfaction* similarly revealed that *organizational response* was a strong predictor; additionally, *rank* emerged as significant, with supervisors and commanders reporting more *job satisfaction* than frontline officers. Consistent with the test of *job fit*, the explained variance in *job satisfaction* was about 41%. *Individual concerns* were not a significant predictor of *job fit* or *job satisfaction*.

Table 5.2. Bivariate Correlations

Variable	1	2	3	4	5	6	7	8	9	10	11	12	13	14	15	16	17	18
1. Gender	1																	
2. Race	.112	1																
3. Rank	-.113	.089	1															
4. Education	.143	.264*	-.014	1														
5. Military	-.126	-.078	.069	-.105	1													
6. Tenure	.204	.081	-.289**	.186	-.196	1												
7. Age	.000	.296**	.007	.071	.056	.247*	1											
8. Certified officer	.098	.399**	.068	.164	-.141	.093	.097	1										
9. Prior police work	-.187	.037	.055	-.180	.145	-.311**	.349**	-.077	1									
10. School type	-.039	.049	-.231*	.149	-.019	.298**	-.415**	.128	-.402**	1								
11. Collective bargaining	.031	.166	.103	-.181	-.223*	.153	-.095	.277**	-.137	.115	1							
12. Student population	.133	.075	.020	-.074	-.141	.044	-.114	.258*	-.076	.097	.281**	1						
13. Individual concerns	.039	.112	-.048	.030	.012	-.132	.110	.152	.050	.009	-.061	.097	1					
14. Organizational response	.175	.266*	.005	.030	-.134	-.012	.255*	.122	-.025	-.133	.034	-.116	.351**	1				
15. Affective commitment	.049	.242*	-.143	.118	.125	.025	.301**	.175	-.053	-.029	-.065	-.133	.336**	.574**	1			
16. Job fit	-.146	.215*	-.013	-.024	-.031	.008	.420**	.069	.106	-.159	.001	-.089	.331**	.575**	.747**	1		
17. Job satisfaction	-.078	.261*	-.144	.113	-.020	.053	.347**	.134	.070	-.059	-.022	-.166	.358**	.619**	.811**	.852**	1	
18. Self-legitimacy	.130	.297**	-.131	.192	-.039	.106	.204	.268**	.003	.105	-.014	-.144	.497**	.605**	.704**	.623**	.705**	1

Statistical significance: * $p < 0.05$; ** $p < 0.01$

Finally, *self-legitimacy* was predicted not only by *organizational response* but also by *individual concerns* over COVID-19. Only one control variable, *student population size*, emerged as significant, with officers at smaller schools reporting greater perceptions of self-legitimacy. In this test, these three factors explained about 42% of the variance in self-legitimacy. As observed in the bivariate relationships, those who expressed less individual concern over COVID-19 likewise expressed significantly better self-legitimacy.

Discussion

This study was carried out in June and July 2020, that is, between spring semester 2020, when in-person classes and campus life were disrupted in March, and the following fall semester, August through December. During this time period, schools were forced to devise longer-term solutions to the pandemic. Because the pandemic and its mitigation strategies were still evolving, this state of flux may limit, or at least should situate, our findings. Still, the results provide at least two clear conclusions.

First, respondents who were more confident in their organization's response to the crisis were statistically more likely to report better job commitment, fit, and satisfaction as well as self-legitimacy. For all four of these models, the explained variance was between 36% and 42%, which demonstrates the importance of leadership and organizational response to crisis in framing these perceptions. Akin to other forms of organizational support, the response of organizations to the COVID-19 crisis, or to any traumatic experience, matters to employees.

Perceived organizational support includes the sense that an organization cares about the well-being of its employees, and prior research has consistently demonstrated that this perception positively relates to organizational commitment, satisfaction, and fit (Ahmed et al., 2015; Dawley et al., 2010; Riggle et al., 2009). COVID-19 forced organizational leaders to make swift and high-stakes decisions. While researchers have only begun to evaluate the pandemic's impacts on the workplace, it is already clear that the support provided by leaders during and after the pandemic has clear implications for employees' perceptions (Daniels et al., 2022). Our study adds to that evidence and makes clear that, in policing contexts, this impact extends to perceptions of campus officers' self-legitimacy—the confidence they have in doing their jobs. This finding has implications beyond campus policing and likely extends to full-service law enforcement officers as well.

Table 5.3 Ordinary Least Squares Regression Results

Variable	Affective commitment			Job fit			Job satisfaction			Self-legitimacy		
	b	SE	β	b	SE	β	b	SE	β	b	SE	β
Gender	−0.283	0.814	−0.037	−2.973	1.263	−0.247*	−2.500	1.395	−0.186	0.625	0.990	0.064
Race	−0.609	0.788	−0.084	0.623	1.216	0.054	−0.059	1.349	−0.005	0.478	0.959	0.052
Rank	0.848	0.278	0.334**	0.489	0.437	0.120	0.966	0.485	0.215*	0.510	0.339	0.157
Education	−0.290	0.525	−0.060	−0.998	0.816	−0.131	−0.001	0.904	0.000	−0.269	0.639	−0.044
Military	1.091	0.709	0.164	−0.567	1.096	−0.054	0.105	1.219	0.009	−0.294	0.863	−0.035
Tenure	−0.290	0.382	−0.071	−0.331	0.594	−0.071	−0.054	0.655	−0.010	0.107	0.465	0.028
Age	0.699	0.738	0.135	2.300	1.148	0.280*	1.394	1.278	0.152	−0.324	0.898	−0.049
Certified officer	1.081	0.886	0.134	0.258	1.372	0.020	1.598	1.518	0.112	1.512	1.078	0.146
Prior police work	−0.705	0.632	−0.136	−0.698	0.976	−0.085	0.134	1.087	0.015	0.635	0.768	0.096
School type	−0.023	0.628	−0.005	−0.613	0.989	−0.084	0.028	1.091	0.003	0.810	0.763	0.139
Collective bargaining	−0.256	0.579	−0.052	−0.274	0.905	−0.035	−0.011	0.998	−0.001	−0.715	0.705	−0.112
Student population	−0.185	0.293	−0.068	−0.112	0.459	−0.026	−0.520	0.513	−0.106	−0.748	0.357	−0.213*
Individual concerns	0.049	0.103	0.050	0.071	0.159	0.045	0.196	0.176	0.113	0.305	0.125	0.242*
Organizational response	0.354	0.100	0.395**	0.551	0.156	0.386**	0.729	0.172	0.462***	0.441	0.122	0.385***
R^2	0.364			0.403			0.410			0.426		
F-test	2.742**			3.184**			3.271***			3.559***		
Intercept	9.24***	2.229		11.368***	3.198		7.768*	3.538		11.649***	2.514	

Statistical significance: * $p < 0.05$; ** $p < 0.01$; *** $p < 0.001$

Second, in this sample, officers' individual concerns about exposure to the virus and their ability to do the job during the ongoing pandemic significantly affected their perceptions of job commitment, fit, and satisfaction in the bivariate test, but this did not hold true in the multivariate analysis. Even in a regression model that excluded organizational response, which might condition the relationship of individual concerns to the outcome variables, individual concerns were nonsignificant.[11] This suggests that fears about safety or the stress over possible exposure to COVID-19 was not as relevant to individual officers as was their organization's response to the pandemic. While this is not a direct comparison with other research, this finding aligns with evidence indicating that stress is not a consistent predictor of police officers' job satisfaction. Specifically, Johnson (2015) claimed that perhaps those in policing expect exposure to higher levels of stress, and our finding may be an extension of that mentality to the COVID-19 context. As an aside, it was interesting to find that these individual concerns were not correlated with age, given that age increases the potential health risks of COVID-19.

Although the officers' individual concerns were not related to other job perceptions, these attitudes were significantly related to perceptions of self-legitimacy. This finding suggests that—though officers did not allow the stress of COVID-19 to affect their job commitment, fit, and satisfaction—it still had some bearing on how confident they felt in fulfilling their responsibilities at work. Specifically, officers who worried less about COVID-19 exposure and their ability to do the job amid the pandemic reported better self-legitimacy. In a recent study by Kyprianides and colleagues (2022), which examined police officers in the United Kingdom during the COVID-19 crisis, the authors indicated "that officers' confidence in their own authority to police COVID-19 [i.e., self-legitimacy] *hindered* their well-being" (p. 516, emphasis in original). In other words, they found that officers with greater self-legitimacy likewise reported more problems with their personal health and well-being, including worry over their elevated risk of contracting the COVID-19 virus. This seems inconsistent with our findings, but research on this topic is relatively sparse. Kyprianides and colleagues also reported that positive organizational climate amid the COVID-19 crisis was positively and significantly correlated with greater self-legitimacy. At least anecdotally, this finding—and much of the previous work on self-legitimacy—seems to resonate with our results on organizational support during crisis. The extant research highlights that officers who express greater self-legitimacy are more likely to embrace democratic modes of policing, including being less cynical and more supportive of restrictions on the use of force (Bradford & Quinton, 2014; Tankebe, 2019; Trinkner et al., 2016; White et al., 2021), and may be more willing to engage with community members (Wolfe & Nix, 2016). If individual COVID-19 concerns affected officers' self-legitimacy, then managing these concerns could have consequences for how officers interact with members of the public.

Our study is not without some limitations. Its reliance on a small convenience sample creates clear limitations to the generalizability of our findings. The pandemic conditions generally made research efforts more challenging, limiting the extent to which researchers were able to assess various conditions in the middle of the crisis. For that reason, we are glad that our study provides some provisional insights into conditions at that point in time. The time-bound nature of a cross-sectional study such as this one represents a second limitation. Attitudes and perceptions about the COVID-19 pandemic were not static, and they may have changed along with the dynamics of the evolving crisis. If questioned today, these respondents may voice perceptions different from what they did when conditions were more uncertain. All the same, the response of leadership in crisis situations is relevant, as evidenced by our results. Finally, while our study offers some insights into campus police officers' experiences, it underscores how little we know about campus policing, campus police officers and security personnel, and the conditions in which they operate. We encourage others to advance research that helps us better understand how campus police fit into the landscape of American law enforcement.

Conclusion

The response of organizational leaders to crisis influences employees' perceptions. These perceptions concern whether or not the employer cares about them, supports them, and, ultimately, lives up to the shared values that bond employees to the organization. The COVID-19 pandemic created unprecedented pressures on institutions of higher education, thereby placing additional strains on campus police officers. As essential frontline employees who are asked to help maintain public order and ensure safety on their campus, these officers reported, in response to our online survey, that the supportiveness and responsiveness of their organization to the needs of those affected by the pandemic importantly shaped their job satisfaction, commitment, fit, and self-legitimacy. This should serve as a reminder to organizational leaders that it is paramount to recognize their employees' emotional and psychological needs, particularly when employees might be experiencing heightened stress.

Notes

1. This project was approved by Ferris State University's Institutional Review Board.

2. Similar fears might have understandably been felt by campus employees working in food service, in custodial operations, and in other roles that were less clearly essential and that could not be carried out remotely in the face of institutional fiscal crisis.

3. Certified campus police officer numbers were made available from the Michigan Commission on Law Enforcement Standards.

4. Cronbach's alpha = 0.706.

5. Cronbach's alpha = 0.900.

6. We combined all six COVID-19 questions into an exploratory factor analysis using principal axis factoring with varimax rotation. The items loaded as expected as two unique factors (eigenvalues > 1): Kaiser-Meyer-Olkin = 0.747; Bartlett's test of sphericity = <0.001; explained variance = 76.74%; factor loadings = >0.530.

7. Cronbach's alpha = 0.892; skewness = −0.812, standard error = 0.253; kurtosis = 0.524, standard error = 0.500.

8. Cronbach's alpha = 0.786; skewness = −1.16, standard error = 0.251; kurtosis = 1.26, standard error = 0.498.

9. Cronbach's alpha = 0.918; skewness = −1.13, standard error = 0.253; kurtosis = 0.946, standard error = 0.500.

10. Cronbach's alpha = 0.870; skewness = −1.38, standard error = 0.258; kurtosis = 2.15, standard error = 0.511.

11. This model was not shown in the tables ($\beta = 0.054$; $p = 0.604$).

6. A Perfect Storm of Dual Crises: Understanding Officer Perceptions during the COVID-19 Pandemic and Defund the Police Movement

Janne E. Gaub and Marthinus C. Koen

Introduction

As COVID-19 emerged as a global threat in the spring of 2020, police officers in the United States and elsewhere quickly came to be viewed as heroic frontline workers in a deadly pandemic. Then, on May 25, 2020, Minneapolis police officer Derek Chauvin knelt on the neck of George Floyd for more than nine minutes, suffocating him to death, while horrified onlookers pleaded for the officers to stop. Video footage captured and distributed by onlookers caught Floyd's repeated pleas of "I can't breathe!"

People across the United States—and indeed, around the world—took to the streets with signs painted with the words "I can't breathe!" to protest police brutality, a lack of police accountability and transparency, and general racial inequality. Some protests got violent or destructive. Protests in Minneapolis, where the incident occurred, resulted in property damages of over \$350 million, with neighboring St. Paul suffering over \$80 million in damage (Bakst, 2021).

Overnight, police transformed in the public eye from being heroic first responders fighting on the front lines of an invisible threat to the subject of national protests, anger, and frustration. The contrast between how the public viewed and treated police—and how police viewed themselves and their job—at the beginning of the COVID-19 pandemic versus after the death of George Floyd was stark, and police were unprepared for the backlash.

In this chapter, we situate policing within the context of the "dual crises" of the COVID-19 pandemic and the George Floyd protests to shed light on how police officers viewed this transformation. We interviewed frontline police officers and sergeants in the United States and Canada, discussing what these experiences mean for policing as they weathered the "perfect storm" of pandemic and protest.

Government Response to the COVID-19 Pandemic

To contain the spread of the virus that causes COVID-19, both the United States and Canada took similar, top-down policy approaches whereby local and state/provincial governments were responsible for battling the pandemic, while receiving funding, strategic guidance, and other resources from their respective federal governments (Detsky & Bogoch, 2020; Haffajee & Mello, 2020). Both nations implemented lockdowns, physical distancing mandates, quarantining of the infected and potentially infected, travel restrictions, and temporary border closures. These measures ebbed and flowed across place and time as waves of the virus (and subsequent mutations) impacted the two countries.

Despite taking similar approaches to pandemic response, the two countries differed in their execution of them. For example, with a handful of exceptions, Canadian society experienced a pandemic discourse that was largely congruent across local, provincial, and federal government officials. Despite Canadian officials not always strictly following what public health experts recommended, how Canada executed its response to the pandemic was relatively effective in mitigating the impact on public health (Gaub et al., 2022).

In the United States, the initial federal response to the pandemic was lackluster. As cases of COVID-19 began to break out in the United States, President Trump was focused on the fallout of his first impeachment and downplayed the seriousness of the pandemic, despite being briefed on the potential magnitude of what was to come. Moreover, the president decided to double down by claiming that the pandemic was not serious and would "disappear" by April 2020 (Wolfe & Dale, 2020). Mixed messages reverberating through different levels of government about the nature and spread of the virus and how to combat it caused much confusion for the public and forced some local and state governments to take matters into their own hands. A lack of coordination from the federal government made initial response efforts virtually futile (Haffajee & Mello, 2020).

At the same time, some public figures undermined the recommendations of those in the scientific community by promoting audacious conspiracy theories, supporting pseudoscience, and breaking federal guidelines and recommendations (Carter & May, 2020). For example, Senator Rand Paul (a Republican from Kentucky) on many occasions quarreled with Dr. Anthony Fauci about the veracity and legitimacy of COVID-19 vaccines during congressional sessions. Moreover, Senator Paul promoted the drug hydroxychloroquine as a potential cure for COVID-19, even though multiple randomized controlled trials had failed to back those claims. Unsurprisingly, it turned out that the senator's wife owned shares in a company that made a medicine used to treat COVID-19 complications (Baxter, 2021). Similarly, Representative Nancy Pelosi (a Democrat from California), who was a vocal proponent of lockdowns and mask mandates, was caught on camera getting a haircut in a salon in San Francisco without wearing a mask during the first peak of the pandemic (Gregorian, 2020).

Despite containment efforts by the U.S. and Canadian governments, the consequences of the pandemic reverberated across myriad aspects of society beyond public health outcomes. The pandemic had serious impacts on both the U.S. and Canadian economies (Galea & Abdalla, 2020), educational systems (Stanistreet et al., 2021), political discourse, and social relations (Bernauer & Slowey, 2020; Carter & May, 2020). Making matters worse, in May of 2020—when people began to realize the pandemic would not be short lived—frustrations boiled over as the world learned the circumstances around the deaths of Ahmaud Arbery, Breonna Taylor, and George Floyd.

Policing during a Pandemic

Research on policing in the pandemic, while still growing, currently falls into three predominant camps: organizational environment factors, officer-level concerns, and police operations. The literature on the policing environment has mostly considered public expectations and crime rates (Ashby, 2020; Ghaemmaghami et al., 2021; Malpede & Shayegh, 2022; Nix, Ivanov, & Pickett, 2021; Nouri & Kochel, 2022). One study found that the public supported precautionary policing but did so by a slim margin. Public opinion split over whether the police should engage in social distancing enforcement; for example, only 55% supported shutting down large gatherings, and 52% supported the enforcement of social distancing ordinances (Nix, Ivanov, & Pickett, 2021)

Many police agencies ceased proactive and community-oriented policing efforts, fielded some calls remotely, or tried to limit their public interactions as much as was feasible (Gaub et al., 2022). This caused some anxiety among segments of the public. The public felt less safe as the police were less visible and disengaged from order maintenance efforts (Ghaemmaghami et al., 2021; Nouri & Kochel, 2022).

Some research has considered the initial consequences of pandemic lockdowns and stay-at-home orders on crime rates. One study, focused on San Francisco and Oakland, found significant reductions in crime after stay-at-home orders were implemented (Malpede & Shayegh, 2022). Others considered types of crime across various jurisdictions and found similar crime reductions; there were, however, some categories of crime that remained constant or even increased over time, most notably intimate partner violence (Ashby, 2020; Nix & Richards, 2021; Stickle & Felson, 2020).

Another vein of literature considered how the pandemic could affect police officers' mental health. Some have drawn parallels between the COVID-19 pandemic and other global and national catastrophes (e.g., the HIV epidemic or Hurricane Katrina) in discussing the potential for the COVID-19 pandemic to cause occupational stress for officers (Drew & Martin, 2020, 2021; Jennings & Perez, 2020; Newiss et al., 2021; Papazoglou et al., 2020; Stogner et al., 2020) Given that police officers often consider their departments to lack adequate resources for day-to-day police functions, a global pandemic might add significant strain on officers and their organizations alike, resulting in increased levels of officers' stress and burnout (Papazoglou et al., 2020; Stogner et al., 2020; White & Fradella, 2020).

Some research has confirmed that officers are likely to report increased levels of vexation and less job satisfaction after encountering bodily fluids, such as arrestee saliva, when weaponized during an encounter (Jennings & Perez, 2020; Papazoglou et al., 2020): for example, when a citizen knows they are infectious and deliberately spits on an officer as an act of contempt, defiance, or assault. Not only are officers concerned that they may contract a disease (like COVID-19), but they are also concerned that they may infect people with whom they live or for whom they care (Drew & Martin, 2020, 2021; Papazoglou et al., 2020). This was especially the case among frontline officers responding to calls for service in the early phases of the pandemic (Newiss et al., 2021).

One study addressed these questions organizationally, finding that early and sustained messaging positively affected police vaccination rates (Mourtgos & Adams, 2021). Similarly, a survey of officers in California found that when agencies implemented strategies that would result in fewer average police-citizen contacts, officer perceptions of safety increased, while stress decreased (Shjarback & Magny, 2022). Officers also seemed to be more buoyant when their department took safety measures such as providing adequate personal protective equipment and enforcing physical distancing and mask mandates (Gaub et al., 2022).

The literature on the pandemic's impacts on police operations is a robust line of inquiry as several studies have investigated these operations using different methodologies. Agency size and the rate of infection in a particular jurisdiction seemed to affect the extent to which police organizations pivoted in response to the pandemic (Mrozla, 2022). A common response to the pandemic was implementing some form of written policy to guide officer actions. Such policies would outline how officers should respond to calls, including reducing arrests for minor offenses, limiting proactive stops, and paring back community-oriented policing efforts (Maskály et al., 2022). Lum et al. (2020) found that during the early phases of the pandemic, about 90% of responding agencies had implemented some form of written policy to guide patrol actions, which later spread to specialized units as well. In some police agencies, however, the presence of policies limiting intraorganizational contact among officers appeared not to change the way officers behaved (Gaub et al., 2022; Maskály et al., 2021).

At the same time, agencies began to pivot to using telecommunication technologies or applications to communicate with the public and/or respond to calls (Lum et al., 2020; Maskály et al., 2022; Mrozla, 2022; Gaub et al., 2022). For example, police agencies began to rely more on social media or other digital platforms to maintain communication with the public (Farmer & Copenhaver, 2022; Hu et al., 2022). Such communication typically contained information about COVID-19, changes to services, and reminders of pandemic-related policies and restrictions (e.g., lockdowns; Farmer & Copenhaver, 2022). Moreover, some agencies used remote strategies to deal with petty offenses and misdemeanor calls for service (Lum et al., 2020; Maskály et al., 2022). While there seemed to be an overall reduction in reactive policing (Lum et al., 2020), some agencies saw larger reductions than others (Maskály et al., 2022). The same was true for proactive policing strategies such as community-oriented policing and problem-oriented policing (Lum et al., 2020; Maskály et al., 2022). Interestingly, at some police agencies, officers engaged in sustained or even increased levels of directed patrols (Maskály et al., 2022), which makes sense because simply patrolling hot spots does not require that officers interact with the public.

Training was also impacted by the pandemic as agencies had to reallocate resources or rethink existing strategies. For example, the classroom portions of in-service training were able to occur remotely, and officers seemed to warm up over time to remote learning (Gaub et al., 2022). At the same time, certain forms of training, such as field training, scenario-based in-service training, and pre-service academy training, posed more difficulties for the police (Gaub et al., 2022). Training academies seemed to be particularly hampered by the pandemic, with single-agency academies experiencing the most disruption compared with those who served multiple agencies. Academies were faced with canceling classes, suspending instruction for weeks at a time, and/or relying more heavily on online instruction (White, Schafer, & Kyle, 2022).

Ahmaud Arbery, Breonna Taylor, and George Floyd

As the first wave of the pandemic was peaking in the United States, three separate stories of Black people being killed under dubious circumstances erupted in public discourse. These were the deaths of Ahmaud Arbery in Georgia, Breonna Taylor in Kentucky, and George Floyd in Minnesota.

Ahmaud Arbery: Jogging while Black

Ahmaud Arbery was killed in late February 2020. News of his murder did not become well known until early April 2020 when (ironically) one of the suspects in the case, Gregory McMichael, asked his lawyer to share the video of the killing with a local television station (Kennedy & Diaz, 2021; Kornfield, 2021). The video, which showed Travis McMichael shoot and kill Arbery with a shotgun after a quick confrontation, went viral within hours. Details emerged that Arbery was going for a jog when he was chased down by the McMichaels in their pickup truck before being killed. The McMichaels mistakenly assumed Arbery was involved in a string of thefts that had happened in their neighborhood, which prompted the encounter.

When the video was released, the public was outraged that no charges had been filed against either the McMichaels or Roddie Bryan, who had filmed the encounter, two months later. Making matters worse, it turned out that the prosecutor who initially had jurisdiction over the case asked the police not to pursue the investigation. Greg McMichael had previously worked in law enforcement, leading to speculation that he had received preferential treatment (Kennedy & Diaz, 2021; Kornfield, 2021). After the video's release, the Georgia Bureau of Investigation took over the case. Two months later, all three men were arrested and charged with malice murder, felony murder, and other crimes. Almost two years after Arbery's murder, the three men were found guilty of most of the charges brought against them, with Travis McMichael being convicted of malice murder.

While Arbery was not murdered by police officers, the McMichaels' connection to law enforcement, the hesitation by the prosecutor to file charges, and the dubious circumstances of his death exemplified systemic racism and perceived corruption in how non-whites are treated by the criminal justice system (Nguyen et al., 2021). The public criticized how the case was handled from start to finish. Many remarked that McMichael's confidence in having done no wrong was what prompted him to request that the video be made public. It was one more example of Black people being unable to participate in everyday activities (like jogging) without concern for their well-being.

Breonna Taylor: Sleeping while Black
Around the time Arbery's murder became known to the public, news of Breonna Taylor's death began to circulate. She was a 26-year-old Black woman who was killed by Louisville Metro Police officers while they executed a no-knock warrant at her apartment (Lovelace, 2021; Vadala, 2021). The police had suspected Taylor's ex-boyfriend, Jamarcus Glover, of keeping drugs and/or money at her apartment. They had evidence that a car registered to Taylor had been parked at a known drug house not far from her apartment. The police also claimed that Glover had received packages sent to Taylor's address that potentially contained drugs (Vadala, 2021). The warrant said that they had worked with a U.S. postal inspector to determine that drugs were indeed sent to Taylor's house, a fact heavily disputed by the postal inspector in Louisville, who claimed never to have been included in the investigation (Oppel et al., 2021).

When the police executed the warrant on March 13, 2020, three plain-clothes officers forced their way into Taylor's apartment. Taylor and her current boyfriend, Kenneth Walker, were in her apartment at the time. Details of the sequence of events and what exactly was said are murky, as there are discrepancies in the accounts of witnesses, Walker, and the police. However, the evidence suggests that the police might have knocked once and announced their presence before forcing their way into the apartment (Oppel et al., 2021; Vadala, 2021). Walker, who did not hear the police announce themselves, fired his 9-millimeter pistol in self-defense (thinking that someone was entering the home illegally). This bullet was likely the one that struck one of the officers (Oppel et al., 2021). The officers then fired 32 rounds into the apartment, killing Taylor but leaving Walker unhurt. After the shooting, the police never searched her home for drugs or money. Like Arbery's case, the news of Taylor's death did not emerge in public discourse until months after she was killed.

A grand jury was convened in September 2022 to investigate the officers' actions in the case and ultimately failed to indict the officers on any charges related to her death. The only indictment was for a single officer's wanton endangerment of the occupants in the neighboring apartment (Legal Defense Fund, 2020). A grand juror later filed a motion seeking the release of the grand jury's proceedings, which was granted in the form of audio recordings. Among others, the NAACP Legal Defense Fund reviewed the recordings and concluded that Kentucky's attorney general, Daniel Cameron, substantially deviated from standard grand jury procedure in presenting the case. Most importantly, the review found that, contrary to Cameron's public statements, he did not present the charge of homicide or the explanation of self-defense. In other words, the grand jury was not even presented with the *opportunity* to indict the officers on the charge of homicide, nor was it presented with evidence that Walker may have been acting in self-defense. It was not until August 4, 2022, that the U.S. Department of Justice (2022) filed federal charges, including civil rights violations, against four current and former Louisville police officers for the events that led to Breonna Taylor's death.

George Floyd: "I Can't Breathe"

On Monday, May 25, 2020, George Floyd, a 46-year-old black man, was murdered by Officer Derek Chauvin in Minneapolis, Minnesota (Oriola & Knight, 2020; Weine et al., 2020). After being arrested for using a counterfeit 20-dollar bill to buy cigarettes (which prosecutors believed warranted a citation, rather than a custodial arrest), Floyd expressed that he was feeling claustrophobic, recovering from COVID-19, and was having difficulty breathing after a brief struggle between Floyd and one of the arresting officers (Taylor, 2021). While Floyd was handcuffed, some of the arresting officers asked Floyd if he was on drugs, which he denied, again stating that he was anxious and having difficulty breathing. When officers attempted to put Floyd in the patrol car, another small struggle ensued with Chauvin assuming command and taking Floyd to the ground, resting his knee on the back of Floyd's neck (Oriola & Knight, 2020; Taylor, 2021; Weine et al., 2020). Bystanders and Floyd pleaded with Chauvin to remove his knee from Floyd's neck as he was no longer resisting, was handcuffed, and was clearly having difficulty breathing. After a few minutes, bystander video shows Floyd dying with Chauvin casually leaning on his neck before making feeble attempts at reviving him (Taylor, 2021). Video of the murder deeply vexed viewers as it vividly depicts Floyd's agonizing last moments in detail. As a result of the video, Derek Chauvin was arrested for second-degree murder on May 29, 2020. In March and April 2021, Chauvin was tried and ultimately convicted of unintentional second-degree murder, third-degree murder, and second-degree manslaughter and sentenced to 22.5 years in prison (Xiong et al., 2021).

Public Outcry and Calls for Police Reform

All three deaths were the latest in a long line of high-profile police-related deaths of Black men and women in the United States, but they served as a flash point that renewed calls for police reform. The three murders became emblematic of systemic racism and oppression that still pervades the United States and the rest of the world. Consequently, demonstrations in protest of the three deaths took place around the country and in other countries, despite a raging pandemic (Gaub et al., 2022; Lovelace, 2021; Lum et al., 2021; Nguyen et al., 2021).

The public response to the deaths of Arbery, Taylor, and Floyd reinvigorated the Black Lives Matter and #SayHerName campaigns (African American Policy Forum, 2022), while simultaneously giving rise to the Defund the Police movement. "Defunding" the police called for demilitarizing the police and diverting resources to other entities to handle certain police-citizen interactions (Lum et al., 2021; Vermeer et al., 2020). While the vast majority of protests were peaceful (Armed Conflict and Location Data Project, 2021), some instances turned into riots as the public felt they were being placated and nothing was being done. For example, in Minneapolis, Atlanta, and Louisville, what began as peaceful protests turned into brutal clashes with the police. Making matters worse, people died or were severely injured during some of these protests, either at the hands of the police or by "anti-protestors" (Jeong et al., 2021). Property damage from protests across the country totaled nearly $2 billion, far surpassing the previous record held by riots in Los Angeles following the death of Rodney King in 1992 (Kingson, 2020).

Public figures and organizations that had before been quiet about police brutality and systemic racism began to speak out, demanding accountability and justice. For example, the National Football League—which had all but blacklisted Colin Kaepernick for kneeling in support of the Black Lives Matter movement during the national anthem at football games—came to show support for players doing it (Levenson, 2021). Furthermore, the league even prompted the football team in Washington, D.C., to change its name from the Redskins to the Commanders (Belson & Draper, 2020). Sir Lewis Hamilton, a Black Formula 1 driver, urged his team (Mercedes) to race in all-black car liveries for the 2020 and 2021 seasons and compelled the organizers of Formula 1 to devote time before each race to promote equality and inclusion (Smith, 2020). After winning the Tuscan Grand Prix, Lewis Hamilton stood on the podium wearing a shirt with Breonna Taylor's picture on the back under the text "Say Her Name," with the front of the shirt reading, "Arrest the Cops Who Killed Breonna Taylor."

Political figures in the United States also seemed to pick sides, adding to the sociopolitical chasm forming in the American polity. Republican Senator Mitt Romney marched with a group of protesters in Washington, D.C., in support of Black Lives Matter on June 7, 2020, mere weeks after the video of George Floyd's death proliferated across social media (Coppins, 2020). Muriel Bowser, the mayor of D.C., commissioned a section of northwest Washington to be named "Black Lives Matter Plaza," with the words "Black Lives Matter" written in massive yellow letters across the pedestrian section of 16th Street NW (Weil, 2021). Others were less supportive, such as President Donald Trump (Beer, 2021; Coppins, 2020). He criticized Mitt Romney for his support of Black Lives Matter, referring to BLM protestors and demonstrators as "thugs," "terrorists," and "anarchists." In Canada, the response to systematic oppression and racism had been more unified. For example, Prime Minister Justin Trudeau made a surprise appearance at a "No Justice = No Peace" rally in Ottawa, showing his support for the movement (Bronskill et al., 2020).

This quick transition in public sentiment proved too much for some police representatives. For example, Mike O'Meara, the president of the

New York Police Benevolent Association, stood in front of a group of police union representatives and addressed the public response to police brutality, venting his frustrations with the public for framing all officers as brutal and castigating the media for "vilifying" officers (Moreno, 2020). Though he denounced Derek Chauvin's actions, O'Meara, in what could best be described as a toddler-like meltdown, puffed his chest, balled his fists, and screamed that he was tired of the police being treated like "thugs" and "animals." This sentiment was shared by many police unions, which saw the death of Floyd as an isolated incident and stood in opposition to systemic police reform (Moreno, 2020).

The Perfect Storm

The COVID-19 pandemic and calls for police reform collided, both for policing as a profession and for the general public. Indeed, a massive divide opened in American society as opposing views were entertained by news media, promulgated by public figures, and spread through social media. On one side, those calling for sweeping police reform (to the point of de-funding or abolishing the police, in some cases) also obeyed stay-at-home orders and other COVID-19 mandates. In fact, most Black Lives Matter protests were a sea of mask-wearing, peaceful marchers. Conversely, the other side vehemently "backed the blue" and called for law and order, with some embracing QAnon conspiracies and casting doubt on the effectiveness of COVID-19 vaccines and other related public health initiatives. While the summer and fall of 2020 were marked by George Floyd protests, there were also numerous armed protests of mask mandates and stay-at-home orders during that time (Armed Conflict and Location Data Project, 2021; Censky, 2020).

Through it all, stark differences were observed in how police managed and responded to each type of protest. Aggressive containment tactics, such as "kettling" (Grantham-Philips et al., 2020), were generally reserved for peaceful Black Lives Matter protests, whereas police remained stoically passive when confronted with aggressive, angry anti-mask protesters (Armed Conflict and Location Data Project, 2021). Data showed that police were three times as likely to use force against left-wing protests (e.g., Black Lives Matter) than right-wing protests (e.g., pandemic-related protests or early "Stop the Steal" protests following the November 2020 presidential election) (Armed Conflict and Location Data Project, 2021).

For police, this turmoil meant reckoning with difficult truths. In a short period of time (beginning in spring 2020 and continuing through summer and into fall), they had gone from experiencing an outpouring of appreciation to calls for their dismantling. Though the common turn of phrase claims that police "protect and serve," it was becoming painfully obvious that not all police met that expectation while too many were doing the exact opposite for communities of color. In fact, the police have no duty to protect the public at all, according to the U.S. Supreme Court precedent set by *Castle Rock v. Gonzales* (2005) (Cyrus, 2022). How police managed this internal and external strife would determine their trajectory moving forward, yet little is known of what police officers themselves thought about these issues and how these issues were manifesting in their departments. The data we present here take advantage of the "natural experiment" afforded by the pandemic and George Floyd protests to disentangle police perceptions of themselves, the public, and the role and job of policing.

Methodology

Our data come from a qualitative study of line-level police officers in the United States and Canada. Semi-structured interviews and focus groups were conducted with 20 officers and frontline supervisors in the beginning months of the pandemic (April–June 2020; phase 1, or P1). After May 25, 2020, these conversations organically took on a very different tone, with a palpable shift in perspective. As such, follow-up interviews were conducted with 10 of these officers and supervisors approximately 18 months later (January–February 2022; phase 2, or P2). The initial conversations focused on changes to policing due to the pandemic, including the prevalent use of personal protective equipment, modifications to internal policies or procedures, and the impact the pandemic had on public perceptions of police and on officers' perceptions of their job. In follow-up interviews, the same questions were asked again to gauge the persistence of pandemic changes to policing, while also including questions that focused on the perceived impact of the "dual crises" of the pandemic and the Black Lives Matter and George Floyd protests in the summer and fall of 2020 and the continued societal shift in attitudes about the police. Interviews and focus groups generally lasted 45–60 minutes and were recorded via Zoom. The recordings were then transcribed for analysis. We used both deductive and inductive thematic coding (Boyatzis, 1998; Braun & Clarke, 2006), which is appropriate as the events of the pandemic were still unfolding and there was no baseline for reference (Gaub et al., 2022).

Findings

In our conversations with frontline officers and supervisors, both before and after the death of George Floyd, it was clear that policing had reached something of a turning point during 2020. The ways in which officers—and departments—viewed and responded to that turning point led us to three generalizations. First, it was clear that a two-front (internal and external) culture war was ongoing. Police as an institution faced resistance from the outside, whereas individual officers faced resistance from within. Guyot (1979) once likened attempts to change or reform policing to "bending granite," and this became apparent during this experience. Second, our respondents described initial changes to police practice and procedure early in the pandemic in ways that were, ironically, predictive of the very suggestions that would later be made by reform advocates. And yet once reformers began making those demands, police chiefs and others argued that those changes were only temporary and were not indicative of the "real job" of policing. In some cases, police responded to what they viewed as insulting demands by withdrawing or even flat-out leaving the profession. Finally, our respondents consistently asserted that police departments should be learning organizations—yet after the death of George Floyd, those assertions became sharper and more refined in their tone.

The Culture War within Policing

One of the key topics our respondents discussed was the two-front culture war at play within policing during the pandemic. Policing as a profession and institution experienced both external and internal strife. Externally, the Defund the Police and Black Lives Matter movements forced an "outside-in" approach to reform, as noted by this participant:

> I don't know that the change is taking place, in a significant way. Because a lot of the changes that we're seeing, a lot of the progressiveness that we're seeing, it is not coming from the inside out, it's forced on an organization. (Officer 2531, P2)

The external pressure to reform had led to substantial declines in police morale (Mourtgos et al., 2022; Shjarback & Magny, 2022). Frustrated with the changing tides in public views of the police—and a perception of public ungratefulness for all they do—many police officers believed the effort was not worth the reward of low pay and terrible hours. Like many other industries, policing suffered a "Great Resignation" in the latter months of the COVID-19 pandemic (Mourtgos et al., 2022), as evidenced by these comments from participants:

> [In Seattle] you've got a mass exodus of officers because of low morale, and you got low morale in Minneapolis, or some of these other cities, and people are just like, I'd rather just get out of the business and not deal with it for whatever reasons, because it's [cumulative]. (Officer 2531, P2)

> Recruiting has been tough, we're trying new things to get people to come to the department. Then keeping them—you know, retention. We're just losing people, 10 or 12 a month. [. . .] We're getting a lot of just straight-up resignations from folks that, I would say, have 10 years and less service time. Lot of resignations. I don't know for sure, but the people I've talked to seem 50–50. Some are leaving policing and some are going to other departments that are either paying better [. . .] which there aren't too many [nearby] that pay more than us. But there are a lot that are comparable pay, a lot less [. . .] stress. (Officer 1885, P2)

> Now all of a sudden, everybody's on board with doing different things, with changing their policies to allow headgear, or beards, or longer hair for different cultures and religions, tattoos, things like that. And all of a sudden, the door's wide open, everyone wants to try stuff. And I'm like, "Well, where was the willingness to try all this before?" The whole point of diversifying is to represent your community as much as possible, but nobody wanted to do that. But now they're being forced to. And so I think that it's less that the culture has changed, and it's more out of necessity, which is okay. [. . .] I think that before we could, we could simply attract Millennials with, "Hey, look, we have a decent paying job. And it's safe and secure." Now we're grappling with the Great Resignation, people are resigning because they want something better. How can we make our agency, our culture, the job more attractive to them? (Officer 1403, P2)

At the same time, internally, officers also experienced resistance from their own peers. In many cases, officers who acknowledged the need for reform or change were viewed almost as traitors to the profession and excluded from the internal work group. Rather than adjust the culture to accommodate necessary reform, the culture doubled down on itself, forcing those who disagreed to leave.

> And so those who want to do the right things, the right things from the inside out, those are the ones who were ostracized, and they're never put in a position where they can make those things happen. [. . .] And we know that in the culture of policing, if you speak up and speak out, you become the black sheep, and next thing you know, you can't be put into specialty units or you can't get promoted because you know "the system" will do what they can to put you in a corner so that you don't get out and influence the masses. Because [. . .] what is the number one role of government? [T]he government's number one role is to preserve itself. And so whether you're talking about a pandemic, a health crisis, a public health crisis, whether you're talking about civil unrest, the government's role is to always make sure it exists. (Officer 2531, P2)

> It was a miserable time to be a police officer, and everyone felt it in their own way. It started becoming nasty among each other at work based on how it was. And if you didn't toe the party line and you weren't a "cop's cop" here—shielding, blue line, protecting us from the public that doesn't understand us, etc.—you were an outcast. [. . .] I saw both sides. I understand why the public is in unrest and I understand that it's not our department that did it, but we are all wearing blue; and if you see that played over and over in the news, how are you not going to be upset and have questions? And if our reaction is just "They don't understand and they need to understand use of force science, human behavior science, and how all this comes down," [. . .] I go, "You need to understand them. You work for them to a degree." And that just didn't fly. It really was, like, this is groupthink right now. This is our echo chamber, this is our silo. You're either in it with us, saying the chants and the mantras, or you're out. You could not be critical of the profession from inside during this. If you were critical inside the department as this was going on, you're an enemy. (Officer 1616, P2)

Ebb and Flow: Predicting and Retreating from Reform Demands

Additionally, we found that the initial adjustments to police procedures during the pandemic nearly predicted the demands of reformers only months later. For example, police departments undertook more social service roles, like handing out food to the elderly or delivering school lunches to students in need. Additionally, police learned they did not need to respond to every call with "boots on the ground"; rather, they handled many calls via telephone or internet-reporting mechanisms. Many of our respondents believed this would be a fruitful option to keep beyond the pandemic, though some believed small-town residents would still expect a greater level of customer service from their police department.

> The school shut down, so the [school resource officers] weren't working in the schools, community events shut down, so we weren't doing those. A lot of stuff that we did—big public outreach, public gatherings, that sort of stuff—we stopped doing. So, I think the goal stayed the same, but we had to be nimble and try to reinvent how we did certain things. We have a big senior population, we've done a lot of work around interacting with seniors. So we had to shift instead of going to retirement homes and do in-person stuff, we started looking to see where we could help with their vulnerabilities. We worked on food delivery projects, and those sorts of stuff that helped out the community, but was not stuff that we've done before, for sure. (Officer 1833, P1)

> And I think we need to reevaluate what calls we actually respond to. And I think what COVID[-19] did was also pointed out to our superiors that, you know what, the city was fine when PD didn't respond. They really were, you know, one or two citizens might have been upset but they're upset at us anyway. [. . .] So, I think from a certain perspective, it changed the mission in that, yeah, we want to provide good customer service, community service. But that doesn't mean you need two cops at your doorstep when there are other calls for service that are of a higher priority. (Officer 2135, P1)

> We initially scaled back and enforcement almost nothing. Initially, we started to build back up our enforcement a little bit, but essentially, officers that are doing enforcement are waiting for the egregious stuff. (Officer 1885, P1)

Yet in the throes of calls for reform, many police withdrew from public interaction altogether, known as "de-policing" (Wallace et al., 2018). They reduced their response to calls for service even further, virtually eliminating proactive activities and any discretionary response.

> With George Floyd, everyone did that classic police culture thing where collectively everybody was hurt—everybody went home, turned on the news, felt as if their social self-identity was in question because they identify as a police officer. It's a part of who we are. And police officers are on the news as racists and beating people. So with all that going on, that's where I really see some of the pullback. It was "You don't want us, fine. Call a felon when you need help." But really just not engaging in any sort of proactive patrol. I think they might reason that "Hey, the reason we aren't stopping cars is because of the pandemic," but a lot of the younger officers love going out and being proactive. That's their jam. The real reason they aren't doing that is because it's just, kind of, a collective pullback. (Officer 1616, P2)

The controversy prompted an exodus of police personnel from the profession (Mourtgos et al., 2022), which further exacerbated difficulties in responding to calls as departments encountered substantial understaffing. All of this—along with other factors known and unknown—contributed to the staggering rise in crime experienced in 2020 and 2021, as the full force of these actions began to be felt (Cheng & Long, 2022; Mourtgos et al., 2022; Nix, Adams, & Mourtgos, 2021).

Learning from the Perfect Storm

Finally, we asked our respondents what could be learned from the "dual crises" of the pandemic and calls for police reform. Most respondents believed police departments should be learning organizations, continually adjusting to the needs and norms of the public they serve. Several participants noted these changes were necessary because "public safety" takes many forms.

> [COVID-19 has] made us think a little bit about how much of what we've been doing we can do without, or changing the way that we respond to certain crimes or calls for service. I could see some of the changes being permanent in terms of doing more reports over the phone, instead of spending the time sending officers to, you know, lost property calls and that sort of thing. I think it could change some of those operations permanently. But I think in terms of mission, and it's even more difficult to do in this time, I think we've become more community-oriented, doing those kinds of community activities instead of the enforcement activities. (Officer 1885, P1)

I think that law enforcement is a component of public safety. But I think what people, at times, don't realize is that a cop walking down the street, going to grab a coffee, is also public safety. And if that cop does nothing but chat with some people, drink the coffee, answer a question, then that's just as important as them going to deal with someone that stole a bag of chips for 50 cents or one dollar or whatever. So yeah, I think that people see law enforcement and public safety as one and the same. [. . .] Enforcing the laws is a component of policing, but for the most part, it's got nothing to do with that. I mean, really, it's just dealing with people and disagreements. (Officer 1833, P2)

When initially asked if they believed police agencies should—or even would—learn from the pandemic, many of our respondents voiced hope that they would.

I think that for us, like as a smaller agency, it's given us a good opportunity to really dig down into what our core services are and how do we deliver that core service in a variety of ways. (Officer 1833, P1)

We can learn that we can do service delivery. It's forced innovation, it's forced us to be creative where it was never on the radar before the pandemic forced it. So if we're fighting budget cuts [. . .] my sergeant wonders what are we going to be doing for next budget cycle, it's going to be hard to really advocate for us to keep the resources that we have coming when we've proven and stats have shown that service delivery and they're able to provide alternative methods. (Officer 2266, P1)

It does seem that we're forced to really triage and prioritize what we're going to spend our time on and what things we are going to enforce. For all those factors, the logistics of our own attention, the logistics of the courts, really having to be a little surgical in how we operate, which I think is a good thing. And it's kind of cut down on a lot of things we do just because we do them. So, the excessive traffic stops, a low-level drug offense, a lot of the stuff that, you know, in the past we thought maybe would help increase quality of life. (Officer 1616, P1)

But following the death of George Floyd, many of our participants recentered their focus on the culture of policing, wondering whether policing as an institution—and departments individually—could adjust alongside calls for reform.

So because of necessity, hopefully, we're getting a different type of—many different types of officers. We get different types of officers that will change the culture. And hopefully with that change in culture, it sort of perpetuates itself. (Officer 1403, P2)

I think everything we do is 20 years behind the private sector but yes. All the change slowly diffuses to us and next thing you know "Oh, yes, we have body cameras now and here's how we use them and how we review them." Whether or not we want it to happen, it slowly permeates the profession. [. . .] I love all the ideas and the background we have. It's just so hard to implement in a department. The stars have to align. You need a progressive chief, you need people around them in city hall / town hall that support that and are pushing that, too. Really it just takes every right person on every seat of the bus. (Officer 1616, P2)

So at some point, you're either going to change or the change is gonna come to you. And you're not even gonna have a seat at the table to determine where, why, or how. (Officer 2531, P2)

Additionally, our participants noted the historically short memories of police departments, and of policing as a whole, and worried that would inhibit the ability of departments to adapt in advance of the next crisis.

We do a decent job at initial crisis response. I don't think we do a very good job of managing a long-term crisis. We do after-actions and those types of things, but I think we have a short memory. You know, we had the pandemic, George Floyd, the protests we've had through the summer. Our initial responses to all those things I think were pretty decent. But then there's that follow-up to make sure we're even better the next time. And some of it's even small stuff—a couple weeks ago we kind of got surprised by nine inches of snow. (Officer 1885, P2)

I see opportunities for change. But I don't see our department taking advantage of those changes right now. I really don't. I feel like we went through George Floyd, and as soon as the rioting stopped, we're like, "All right, we're good." We're willing to do the community outreach. And the way you defuse a riot, I think, is not 10 minutes before, it's probably 10 years before it happens. And so everyone is kind of sitting around the department with all these changes that are happening, saying, "We're gonna coast on what we've built." But we'll coast for about four or five years, and then everything is going to come crumbling down, because we have not maintained that infrastructure or those relationships, those community partnerships. So there are opportunities to build out, but I just don't see our department taking advantage of them right now. I don't. It's like we have forgotten about George Floyd. It's like we've forgotten that whenever police kill a person of color, and it's clearly egregious, our memories are so short about it. We forget about our history with people of color in this country, our profession's history with people of color, and the role that we've played. And we were like, "Well, that happened, it's over, everybody's fine." And we forget about building out. (Officer 1403, P2)

I'm hopeful, I know I'm being proactive about being a part of the change, I'm not waiting for somebody to do something, I'm going out there and doing it myself. [. . .] It's not gonna just happen on a dime, it's gonna be slow, albeit deliberate, it's still gonna be slow. And we all want to see change happen tomorrow or tonight. And we know that when it comes to systemic change, or systematic change, that is a long, complex endeavor that does not take one or two weeks, it's gonna take some time, especially when you're trying to change a culture. (Officer 2531, P2)

I mean, it's hard to be that kind of very authoritarian, military culture. Especially when you have these students coming out of our policing and criminal justice classes where we are telling them all that's wrong in policing and they're bringing that with them to some extent. I'm optimistic and I do see some changes coming. I think that the broader inclination of policing is to kind of protect itself and use its little ways to increase its power, so to speak, is definitely at play. I think that's the hardest problem you have currently in policing. (Officer 1616, P2)

As Officer 1403 clearly describes, policing has a history with communities and people of color, and that cannot be forgotten. Rather than withdrawing into themselves and becoming insular, police departments should reach out, "build out" as the officer describes, and strive to do better in the long run.

Conclusion

The timing of the COVID-19 pandemic and the social upheaval following the death of George Floyd created a perfect storm of dual crises and served as a significant stress test for a mélange of police functions. Initially the pandemic forced police to adjust their responses in the face of a public health crisis unmatched in a century. Yet in a matter of two months— while the disease of COVID-19 was still raging through the United States and elsewhere and most areas were still under stay-at-home or similar orders—public outcry over the highly publicized deaths of Ahmaud Arbery, Breonna Taylor, and George Floyd reached a boiling point. Large-scale protests across the country demanded reform and accountability. Some protesters spoke of defunding or altogether abolishing the police.

From a scholarly perspective, a valuable aspect of this study stems from the "natural experiment" afforded by the timing of the data collection. By sheer chance, our research on the effects of the COVID-19 pandemic was conducted both before and after the death of George Floyd, which let us capture evident shifts of perception from our participants. The follow-up interviews permitted a more nuanced understanding of the long-term effects of the pandemic, police reforms, and responses to both from policing as a profession.

That said, our study is qualitative and, as such, has a small sample size. As with all qualitative research, the experiences of our participants are not necessarily generalizable to all police officers in the United States and Canada. Yet ours is the first qualitative study to explore the dynamics of these two events as they happened in real time. Thus, the results of our exploratory study can inform future qualitative and quantitative research into these confounding events. Specifically, future research might consider retrospective avenues for determining and understanding shifts in perceptions that might have occurred among police officers in different organizational contexts as the pandemic played out. It is imperative that data collection efforts persist to eventually produce a nuanced narrative of policing in the era of the COVID-19 pandemic.

The findings of this study have implications for both research and practice. Our findings can serve as a warning to police agencies to be learning organizations and not wistfully return to the pre-pandemic ways of doing things because "that's how it's always been done." We urge department leadership to critically assess their department's relationship with all aspects of their community and to take stock of policies and practices that may be inefficient, ineffective, or both. The police need to see themselves as leaders in innovation as opposed to guardians of tradition, which requires a cultural shift from top to bottom, across individual organizations and the entire police institution. The police response to the pandemic has shown the public that police can make swift and drastic changes. What remains to be seen is whether the police can do this proactively. It is the responsibility of criminal justice scholars to build relationships with their local police agencies as opposed to criticizing them in academic journals that leaders of those agencies hardly read. Such a relationship could promote a productive communication of police craft and science that stands to lead the police toward become leaders in innovation.

7. Plea Bargaining Later in the Pandemic: COVID-19 Mitigation Strategies and False Guilty Pleas

*Jacob W. Forston, Shi Yan, Miko M. Wilford,
and Rachele J. DiFava*

Introduction

The Sixth Amendment of the United States Constitution offers several protections to defendants in criminal cases, including the right to a speedy trial, the right to a trial by jury, and the right to know the charges and evidence supporting the allegations brought against them. Despite the constitutional emphasis on the trial process, the overwhelming majority of criminal defendants waive these rights by entering a guilty plea. As of 2018, the most common form of case disposition in the federal criminal justice system was a guilty plea (90%), followed by charge dismissal (8%). Only 2% of federal criminal cases were resolved by jury trial (Gramlich, 2019). This shift away from trials was best illustrated in *Lafler v. Cooper* (2012) when Justice Anthony Kennedy stated, "criminal justice today is, for the most part, a system of pleas, not a system of trials" (p. 11).

Plea bargaining has undoubtedly changed how the criminal justice system processes cases. While some scholars have applauded plea bargaining because of the efficiency and flexibility it brings (Easterbrook, 1992; Scott & Stuntz, 1992), others have voiced concerns over the informal nature of the process and the potentially coercive properties contained within negotiated pleas (Bibas, 2004; Hessick, 2021; Newman, 2023; Schulhofer, 1992; Wilford & Redlich, 2018). The coercive nature of negotiated pleas largely centers around the differences in sentence outcomes depending on the method of case disposition. Cases resolved by trial often result in longer sentences as well as more punitive forms of punishment (Ulmer & Bradley, 2006), which can make a plea bargain appear less risky. This coercive effect can be amplified by the release status of the defendant. If the prosecutor offers a sentence that does not involve jail time, defendants housed in pretrial detention may choose the immediate gratification of getting to leave jail, even though the guilty plea comes with the long-term consequences associated with a conviction, regardless of the defendant's guilt status (Edkins & Dervan, 2018).

Before March 2020, defendants awaiting trial in jails already had clear incentives for wanting to end their stay in pretrial detention. Detained defendants have to put their freedom on hold for an undetermined amount of time as they await their trial (Kellough & Wortley, 2002; Sacks & Ackerman, 2012). The start of the novel coronavirus pandemic (COVID-19) in March 2020 became the newest factor that defendants had to consider when deciding whether to accept a negotiated plea or go to trial. The early stages of the pandemic placed strains on the court system and added new health risks to carceral spaces (Piquero, 2021; Watson et al., 2020). However, later stages of the pandemic brought forth a sense of normalcy, especially as COVID-19 mitigation efforts were introduced to communities. This study examines how varying levels of COVID-19 mitigation efforts in a jail setting, such as vaccine distribution, mask requirements, symptom screening and testing, and social distancing, influenced plea decision-making.

Literature Review

Theoretical Basis of Plea Bargaining

Theoretically, the salient mechanism driving plea bargains for both the prosecutor and the defendant is the probable outcome of the trial, a supposition known as the shadow-of-the-trial theory (Bibas, 2004). The shadow-of-the-trial theory posits that the decisions made in plea negotiations are rooted in the perceived potential outcome of the trial (Scott & Stuntz, 1992). According to the theory, a critical component impacting both parties is alleviating risk. Put differently, negotiations can reduce the costs associated with a more formal legal process and can reduce the risk of uncertain and unpleasant outcomes for both parties.

Innocence and the Shadow-of-the-Trial Theory. A major concern about plea bargaining involves the number of tools available for prosecutors to maximize the chance of plea acceptance (Hessick, 2021). During the negotiation process, prosecutors have the discretion to drop or reduce charges, sometimes meaning the difference between a felony and a misdemeanor.

Prosecutors are given the creative flexibility to bring forth charges that maximize the possibility of pleading guilty, even if that means offering pleas too good for even innocent defendants to pass up (Wilford & Khairalla, 2019).

Aside from charge bargaining, prosecutors can also leverage the length of the sentence within the sentencing range of the indictable charges, with those found guilty at trial facing longer sentences (Ulmer & Bradley, 2006). Innocent defendants offered sizable plea discounts to the sentence have a strong incentive for entering a guilty plea, especially when the alternative is the maximum allowable sentence length if convicted at trial (Schneider & Zottoli, 2019). The difference in outcomes can be difficult to measure when plea offers have alternative sanctions, but the largest sentence reductions can range upwards of 60% of the length of the original sentence (Yan & Bushway, 2018).

The premise of the shadow-of-the-trial theory holds up well empirically, especially the notion that individuals respond differently when plea conditions vary (Bushway et al., 2014). For example, Petersen and colleagues (2022) found that the shadow-of-the-trial theory may even underestimate how sensitive defendants are to the risk of going to trial, meaning that the baseline of guilty pleas may be higher than anticipated under the model. This suggests that, overall, defendants are more likely to plead guilty than originally predicted by the shadow-of-the-trial theory.

Pretrial Detention and Guilty Pleas. Another source of pressure that may increase the likelihood of innocent defendants pleading guilty is their release status. Defendants housed in pretrial detention forfeit their freedom until their trial date, and the effects of this are amplified when considering the unpleasant conditions of jails (Lerman et al., 2022; Toman et al., 2018). For example, Kellough and Wortley (2002) found that interviewed defendants in detention were over two times more likely to enter a guilty plea compared with their released counterparts. Edkins and Dervan (2018) used a vignette to manipulate release status. They found that innocent defendants housed in pretrial detention were over twice as likely to enter a guilty plea than were innocent defendants in the community. One glaring concern, especially relating to false guilty pleas, is that being detained pretrial is not synonymous with guilt. The above research demonstrates, however, that the influence of pretrial detention can still invoke additional pressures to plead, for both innocent and guilty defendants.

COVID-19 and the Criminal Justice System

In the first months of 2020, COVID-19 began ravaging the United States and the rest of the world, signaling the start of a viral pandemic unlike anything seen before. To make matters worse, it became clear that the United States, in particular, was not well positioned to handle a pandemic (Barrett & Yaffe, 2020). The initial response to COVID-19 in the United States was fragmented and chaotic. As time went on and the pandemic continued to rage, some states were able to reduce rates of transmission and fatalities through various initiatives such as mask policies, capacity restrictions, and, ultimately, vaccine rollouts in the spring of 2021 (Hallas et al., 2022). However, these eventual COVID-19 mitigation efforts were distributed unequally, meaning that the effects and experiences of COVID-19 varied depending on the jurisdiction (Wong & Balzer, 2022).

The early stages of the pandemic also created stressors for the criminal justice system, including the court system and carceral facilities (Piquero, 2021). Many courts began to halt nonessential operations, such as jury trials, and to prioritize more time-sensitive court proceedings such as first appearances (Baldwin et al., 2020). Retrospectively, available case-processing data from federal courts provides evidence of judicial strain during the early stages of the pandemic. Specifically, federal courts filed 29% fewer cases involving criminal defendants, likely to decrease workload at a time of constrained resources (Germano et al., 2022). Beyond the shift of prioritizing certain types of court proceedings, most courts had to adapt their day-to-day practices to a virtual setting. This created its own set of challenges and setbacks, with Nir and Musial (2022) observing that issues with technology in a virtual court setting contributed in some capacity to the delays in court processing during the pandemic. These impacts trickled down to individual courtroom actors. In a survey of criminal defense attorneys, a majority cited hardships in being able to consult with clients effectively. Many reported concerns about prosecutors wielding greater sentence reductions to avoid adding to the growing number of pending jury trials (Daftary-Kapur et al., 2021). With virtual proceedings, many of the more informal opportunities to communicate such as in courthouse hallways are not available, which can add some additional uncertainty to the entire process (Johnson, 2024).

Pretrial detention was made even more onerous during the pandemic. In addition to its already unpleasant aspects, defendants now had to factor in the likelihood of exposure to a potentially life-altering disease. Thus, more defendants may have pleaded guilty to get out of pretrial detention as soon as possible (Cannon, 2020). Using an animated simulation of legal procedures, Wilford, Zimmerman, et al. (2021) found that participant-defendants who were made aware of the potential consequences of the pandemic by their defense attorney were more willing to plead guilty. Moreover, innocent participant-defendants ranked concerns related to COVID-19 higher than did guilty participant-defendants in their plea decision considerations.

Carceral facilities have been disproportionately affected by COVID-19 compared with the general population (Charles et al., 2022; LeMasters et al., 2022; Plummer et al., 2023; Watson et al., 2020). Additionally, COVID-19 and other infectious diseases may pose a stronger threat to jails compared to prison (Franco-Parades et al., 2020). Prisons have a relatively stable population, whereas jails have a constant flux of individuals entering and leaving the facility (Chan et al., 2021; Freudenberg, 2001). This makes understanding the nature of COVID-19 in jails crucial from a viral standpoint; the "revolving door" of jails increases the risk of disease spread both inside the facility and out into the community. This is particularly relevant given the various mitigation strategies jails could implement at multiple points during the pandemic.

COVID-19 Mitigation Efforts in the Criminal Justice System. The development of the COVID-19 vaccination was touted as the best way to gain herd immunity without jeopardizing lives (Pandolfi & Chirumbolo, 2022). However, the distribution of vaccinations within jails varied from state to state, and research suggests that incarcerated individuals and correctional staff may have been hesitant to take vaccines (Tyagi & Manson, 2021). Additionally, Wallace and colleagues (2021) found that correctional staff were the main drivers of COVID-19 transmission within facilities by introducing the virus into the institutional setting. Only 10 states prioritized all incarcerated individuals during the first vaccination phase, with the remaining states either including incarcerated individuals in a later phase or failing to include this population in the plan altogether (Quandt, 2020).

Mask usage was crucial at peak stages of the pandemic. This was a source of variation from state to state, with just over half of states requiring masks to be worn by correctional staff and less than a third of states extending this requirement to incarcerated individuals (Widra & Herring, 2020).

Later in the pandemic, some facilities began to drop mask mandates once a certain vaccination threshold was achieved within a facility (Marks, 2021). Some jails implemented screening procedures to identify COVID-19-positive individuals in order to isolate them from the general population. This depended on jail policy and the availability of and commitment to testing protocols; again, implementation varied greatly by jurisdiction. A handful of states were able to offer comprehensive testing throughout their facilities, but many states were unable to fully adopt testing protocols, or their screening process existed on the books but not in practice (Widra & Hayre, 2020). Social distancing was attempted in facilities but was arguably the most difficult strategy to implement in a setting of mass incarceration (a long-recognized concern; Dolovich, 2020).

While many of the underlying structures that led to mass incarceration are still in place, COVID-19 was the impetus for showing that correctional practices can change under the right circumstances. Specifically for jails, the Bureau of Justice Statistics reported that just over 200,000 individuals had an expedited release due to the COVID-19 pandemic (Minton et al., 2021). However, the jail population steadily increased after the initial steep decline as the pandemic continued to evolve (Sawyer, 2022). Decarceration efforts were not distributed equally. For example, Texas saw only a one percentage point drop in the number of incarcerated individuals, whereas Washington saw a 33% reduction in the total number of incarcerated individuals (Widra, 2022). California reduced its jail population rather rapidly at the initial stage of the pandemic, going from 68,000 individuals in custody in February of 2020 to roughly 48,000 individuals in custody in May of 2020 (Kubrin & Bartos, 2023). Overall, estimates suggest that pandemic-related jail decarceration efforts resulted in a net decrease of 7% (Sawyer, 2022).

By the time that data collection for this study occurred, much of the country had moved into post-pandemic operations, with the lifting of mask mandates at the state level and new guidance from the Centers for Disease Control and Prevention (Hersher, 2022; Mandavilli, 2022). Within the criminal justice system, mitigation efforts had allowed for operations to return to a semblance of normalcy. As the worst of the pandemic appeared to have passed, some states had either decreased the frequency of COVID-19 reporting for carceral facilities or stopped tracking and reporting COVID-19 information altogether (Behne, 2021).

Current Study

This study uses a two-group between-subjects design. One of the key findings of Wilford, Zimmerman, et al. (2021) was that the pandemic was considered more influential in the decision to plead guilty for innocent participant-defendants. This suggests that factually innocent participant-defendants may view the possibility of catching COVID-19 in pretrial detention as more of a factor given their innocence. To better understand how the pandemic influenced plea decision-making for innocent defendants specifically, all participants in this study were presented with an experimental scenario in which they were formally charged with larceny but were factually innocent.

Hypothesis 1: Participant-defendants assigned to the higher COVID-19-mitigation scenario will have a lower guilty plea acceptance rate.

Hypothesis 2: When asked to assess their willingness to accept a plea on a numeric scale after learning of the jail's mitigation efforts, participant-defendants assigned to the higher COVID-19-mitigation scenario will be less willing to enter a guilty plea.

Methodology

Plea Simulation

The simulation depicts the participant's avatar being falsely accused of stealing a pair of sunglasses and subsequently charged with larceny in court (see Forston [2022] for more about the scenario). The defense attorney in the simulation provided the participant-avatar with information about the negotiated plea offer, as well as the jail's high or low COVID-19 mitigation efforts. The sentencing outcome was not manipulated, meaning that all participants were offered the same plea deal of six months of probation, if they accepted the guilty plea, or nine months of county jail time, if found guilty at trial. Before being directed back to the survey, participants chose either to accept or reject the presented plea offer (see Wilford, Sutherland, et al. [2021] for more information and illustrations of the simulation).

Four mitigation efforts were manipulated based on the above discussion of the criminal justice system's response to the pandemic. These were (1) within-facility vaccination rate; (2) mask usage and enforcement; (3) screening procedures; and (4) social distancing within the facility.

Mitigation Effort 1: Vaccination Rate. In the high-mitigation scenario, participant-defendants were told that the vaccination rate for the jail's incarcerated individuals and correctional staff was well above the state average. In the low-mitigation scenario, participant-defendants were told that the vaccination rate was well below the state average for incarcerated individuals and correctional officers.

Mitigation Effort 2: Mask Availability and Usage. In the high-mitigation scenario, participants-defendants were told that the jail provided and required masks. Alternatively, participants-defendants in the low-mitigation scenario were told that the jail did not require or provide masks.

Mitigation Effort 3: COVID-19 Screening Procedures. Participant-defendants in the high-mitigation scenario were told that the jail had a screening process to detect and isolate individuals displaying symptoms of COVID-19. In the low-mitigation scenario, participant-defendants were told that the jail did not have a screening process to detect and isolate symptomatic individuals.

Mitigation Effort 4: Social Distancing. Participant-defendants in the high-mitigation scenario were told that the jail had reduced capacity, so it was unlikely that they would have to share a cell with another individual. Participant-defendants in the low-mitigation scenario were told that the jail had not reduced capacity, so it was likely that they would have to share a cell with another individual.

Survey and Variables

Participants were asked a battery of demographic questions as well as questions assessing their legal decision-making (see Forston [2022] for a discussion of all survey questions). Three primary dependent variables were obtained from the survey and simulation. The first dependent variable is a binary measure of whether the participant accepted (1) or rejected (0) the plea deal after viewing the entire simulation. To expand beyond the binary variable of accepting or rejecting the plea, the next dependent variable is the participant's post-COVID-19-condition willingness to accept a plea (WTAP), measured on a scale between 0 (completely unwilling) and 100 (completely willing). In the simulation, participants were asked to provide their WTAP score before and after the defense attorney discussed the jail's COVID-19 mitigation efforts. This allowed for measuring how their WTAP changed in response to the COVID-19 mitigation information. As such, the final dependent variable is the difference in WTAP, which is the post-mitigation-info WTAP minus the pre-mitigation-info WTAP. This score ranged from −100 to 100, with negative scores indicating a decrease in WTAP score after the participant-defendants learned of the mitigation measures and positive scores indicating an increase in WTAP score after learning of the mitigation measures. A pre-test/post-test variable allowed for understanding the baseline likelihood of pleading guilty regardless of the experimental condition. The independent variable of interest is the experimental condition to which the participant was randomly assigned. As discussed below and in the chapter's notes, COVID-19 vaccination status was included as a control variable. This was coded as a binary variable, with individuals who received one or more doses of the COVID-19 vaccine being assigned a value of 1 and individuals who had not received any doses of the COVID-19 vaccine being assigned a value of 0.

Procedure

The sampling frame for this study included 200- and 300-level criminal justice students enrolled in on-campus or online courses. Once they entered the online survey, participants were randomly assigned to an experimental condition (either the low or high COVID-19 mitigation effort scenario) and were directed to the simulation. The survey was active from January 26, 2022, through March 1, 2022. The survey was visible to 1,821 students and received a total of 241 responses, yielding a response rate of 13.23%.

Sample

Both experimental groups were confirmed to be demographically similar.[1] The main portion of the analysis consists of comparisons between the two groups and the dependent outcome variables while also testing for statistical significance.[2] To be included in the final sample, participants had to correctly answer a series of questions to ensure they paid attention to the survey and the manipulations.[3] In total, 48 participants were removed for not answering the dependent variable questions or failing the manipulation and attention checks, resulting in a final analytical sample of 193 participants.

Results

Descriptive Statistics

Table 7.1 presents demographic information for the full sample, as well as the balance test results within each condition. Importantly, both groups were similar for all variables except vaccination status.[4] For the full sample, the average age was 22.55 years old. For gender identity, 72.54% of the sample identified as female, 26.42% as male, and 1.04% as nonbinary or other. For race and ethnicity, 45.55% of the sample identified as White, 6.81% as Black or African American, 0.52% as Indigenous or Native American, 3.14% as Asian, none as Native Hawaiian or Pacific Islander, 32.46% as Hispanic, 9.52% as multiracial, and 2.0% as other.

Turning to COVID-19-related information, 77.96% of participants indicated they were vaccinated for COVID-19, and 22.04% indicated they had not been vaccinated. Lastly, descriptive statistics were calculated for the three dependent variables. For the full sample, 52.85% of participant-defendants entered a guilty plea, the average post-WTAP score following the simulation was 58.39, and the average difference between the pre- and post-condition WTAP scores was 6.30, suggesting a slight increase for the average participant-defendant's willingness to plead guilty.

Main Analysis

Table 7.2 presents the results for the dependent variables, with Figure 7.1 providing additional visual clarity. Participants in the low-mitigation condition entered a guilty plea 56.88% of the time, and participants in the high-mitigation condition entered a guilty plea 47.61% of the time. In other words, defendants given information about the lack of COVID-19 mitigation strategies in jail had a higher plea acceptance rate by 9.27 percentage points. However, the chi-squared test did not show statistical significance at the $p < 0.05$ level, with an associated p-value of 0.201.

The next test was a t-test for the relationship between the post-WTAP score and the experimental condition. Defendants in the low-mitigation condition had an average post-WTAP score of 60.56, and defendants in the high-mitigation condition had an average post-WTAP score of 55.58. This shows a marginal difference in the WTAP score for those in the low-mitigation effort condition by 4.98 points; however, this difference was not statistically significant, with a p-value of 0.313.

The final t-test expanded the analysis by considering the difference between the pre- and post-condition WTAP scores. Defendants in the low-mitigation condition had an average WTAP score change of 8.17, and participants in the high-mitigation condition had an average change of 3.86. The WTAP score for both groups increased following exposure to the mitigation information, but the difference between WTAP scores is greater for those in the low-mitigation group by 4.32 points, meaning that

Table 7.1 Descriptive Statistics and Balance Tests

Variable	Full sample			Low mitigation			High mitigation		
	Mean	Median	SD	Mean	Median	SD	Mean	Median	SD
Age	22.55	20	6.81	22.28	20	5.51	22.90	20	8.20
Level of conservatism	45.05	50	22.97	44.70	50	23.46	45.49	50	22.45
Plea knowledge	3.50	3	0.92	3.40	3	0.88	3.64	4	0.96
Trial knowledge	3.50	3	0.80	3.44	3	0.79	3.57	4	0.81
Mandate effectiveness	38.18	40	24.33	36.97	35	23.46	39.74	40	25.48
Female identifying	0.73	—	0.44	0.73	—	0.45	0.73	—	0.44
White	0.46	—	0.5	0.42	—	0.50	0.49	—	0.5
Black	0.07	—	0.25	0.04	—	0.19	0.11	—	0.31
Indigenous	0.01	—	0.07	0	—	0	0.01	—	0.11
Asian	0.03	—	0.17	0.05	—	0.21	0.01	—	0.11
Hispanic	0.32	—	0.47	0.38	—	0.49	0.25	—	0.44
Mixed race	0.10	—	0.32	0.11	—	0.32	0.12	—	0.33
Prior legal system experience	0.23	—	0.42	0.24	—	0.43	0.23	—	0.42
Mask usage	0.86	—	0.35	0.84	—	0.36	0.87	—	0.34
Immunocompromised	0.10	—	0.30	0.08	—	0.27	0.13	—	0.33
Vaccinated	0.78	—	0.42	0.85**	—	0.35	0.68**	—	0.47
Plea acceptance	0.53	—	0.5	—	—	—	—	—	—
Post-condition WTAP	58.39	65	33.88	—	—	—	—	—	—
Difference in WTAP	6.30	1	22.65	—	—	—	—	—	—
Observations	(n = 193)			(n = 109)			(n = 84)		

Note: ** $p < 0.01$ between low- and high-mitigation conditions. SD = standard deviation

Table 7.2 Main Analysis Results

Dependent variable	Low condition Mean	SD	High condition Mean	SD	Difference	SE	p-value
Decision	0.57	0.50	0.48	0.50	0.09	0.07	0.201[1]
WTAP post-condition	60.56	32.76	55.58	35.27	4.98	4.91	0.313[2]
Difference in WTAP	8.17	23.64	3.86	21.21	4.32	3.28	0.190[2]

Note: *SD* = standard deviation; *SE* = standard error
[1]Chi-squared test
[2]Student's *t*-test

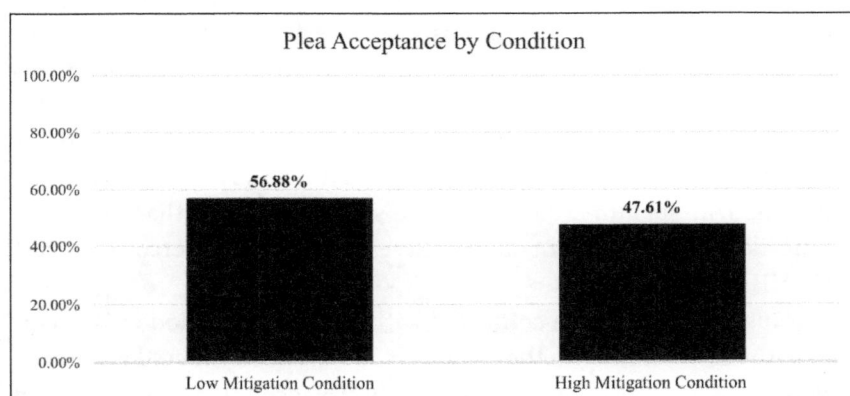

Figure 7.1. Overall Plea Acceptance by Condition

disclosure of the level of COVID-19 mitigation strategies led to a larger increase in the WTAP score for the low-mitigation condition. However, this was not a significant difference between groups, with a *p*-value of 0.190.

Main Effects Diagnostics

One important consideration relating to these results is the time period in which the data were collected. Given the ever-changing nature of the COVID-19 pandemic, it is necessary to contextualize both the threat posed by the pandemic and the status of government regulations and reports by the media. Throughout the data collection period, the Omicron variant was largely retreating, with news outlets reporting that the daily rate of new COVID-19 cases had fallen below the peak of the Delta variant (Cheng et al., 2022; Shammas et al., 2022). These changes resulted in a move to end COVID-19-related restrictions nationwide, with many of these changes coming on the heels of the Omicron variant (Hersher, 2022). This also resulted in the Centers for Disease Control and Prevention announcing new recommendations for masks relative to the level of COVID-19 transmissibility (Mandavilli, 2022).

In addition to the formal mitigation efforts, another consideration involves how the public responded to and perceived these mitigation efforts throughout the pandemic. Newer variants, such as Omicron, were more transmissible but not necessarily as lethal compared with earlier pandemic stages (Lorenzo-Redondo & Hultquist, 2022). This is crucial to consider, given the role that risk perceptions play in the support of COVID-19 mitigation efforts. More specifically, when higher risks are associated with a COVID-19 diagnosis, such as death or severe long-term side effects, the support for adopting and implementing mitigation efforts is greater (Graso, 2022). This effect is undercut by pandemic fatigue, which can cause individuals to lose motivation to adhere to mitigation efforts (Delussu et al., 2022). Data collection occurred two years into the COVID-19 pandemic with its numerous waves and surges, meaning that pandemic fatigue likely played a role in our results, especially as the perceived threat of COVID-19 lowered.

Because data collection coincided with this erratic period of the pandemic, the tests relating to the main effects were reconsidered according to when participants completed the study. To account for the timing of COVID-19 restrictions lifting, the change in guidelines from the Centers for Disease Control and Prevention, trends of COVID-19 cases nationwide, and the approximate halfway point during data collection, February 15th was used to split the data into two different time groups (i.e., Time 1 and Time 2). Data collected on this cutoff date was included with the Time 2 group. This split allowed us to determine whether timing impacted any dependent variables of interest.

The first reanalysis involved the decision to accept or reject the plea by COVID-19 mitigation condition for Time 1 and Time 2 (Table 7.3). For individuals in Time 1, the average plea acceptance rate for individuals in the low-mitigation condition was 55.26% and was 42.37% in the high-mitigation condition. Individuals in Time 2 had an average plea acceptance rate of 60.60% for individuals in the low-mitigation condition and 60.00% for individuals in the high-mitigation condition. The difference between the means for Time 1 was 12.89 percentage points, and the difference between means for Time 2 was 0.60 percentage points (Figure 7.2). These results indicate that the magnitude of the COVID-19 mitigation effect on plea decision-making shrank later into the pandemic, as its impact lessened.

The same trend was apparent when examining the difference between the pre- and post-WTAP scores (Table 7.3). The average Time 1 difference in WTAP scores was 8.62 for those in the low-mitigation condition and 3.59 for those in the high-mitigation condition. For Time 2, the WTAP score change for those in the low-mitigation condition was 7.15 and for those in the high-mitigation condition was 4.48. When looking at the two time periods, the WTAP score change between conditions was 5.03 in Time 1 and 2.67 for Time 2 (Figure 7.3). Again, this demonstrates a reduction in

Table 7.3 Main Effect Diagnostics

Outcomes by time period	Low condition	High condition	Difference
	Mean	*Mean*	*Difference*
Plea acceptance before 2/15/2022	0.55	0.42	0.13
Plea acceptance on or after 2/15/2022	0.61	0.60	0.01
Post-condition WTAP before 2/15/2022	60.11	54.17	5.94
Post-condition WTAP on or after 2/15/2022	61.61	58.92	2.69
WTAP difference before 2/15/2022	8.62	3.59	5.03
WTAP difference on or after 2/15/2022	7.15	4.48	2.67
COVID-19 influence level (guilty plea) before 2/15/2022	2.83	2.35	0.48
COVID-19 influence level (guilty plea) on or after 2/15/2022	2.35	2.29	0.06

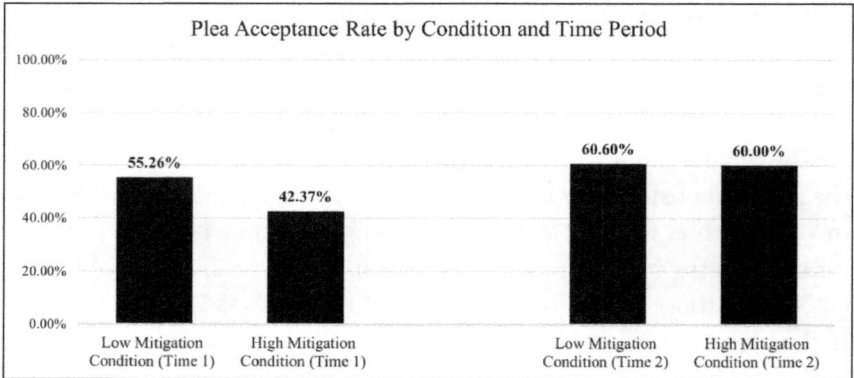

Figure 7.2. Plea Acceptance by Condition and Time Period

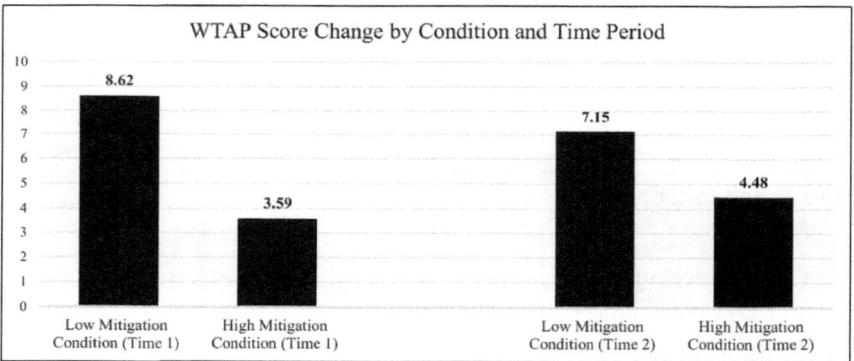

Figure 7.3. WTAP Score Change by Condition and Time Period

the magnitude of the manipulation's effect based on the time period of participation. This may help to explain why the main effects did not reach statistical significance.

Finally, defendants who accepted the plea offer were asked to rank five factors, indicating how each of the factors influenced their decision to enter a guilty plea. These factors included the strength of the evidence against the participant, avoiding a potential jail sentence, avoiding pretrial detention altogether, and COVID-19-related risks. Participants could also write in their own factor. Higher scores indicate that a factor was more influential. Participant-defendants who pleaded guilty during Time 1 had an average COVID-19 ranking of 2.65; and during Time 2, the average ranking for COVID-19 was 2.32. In other words, after February 15th, COVID-19 became less influential in the participant-defendant's decision to plead guilty, regardless of experimental condition. In fact, COVID-19 as a factor had the largest change between the two time periods compared with the other four factors. These changes in the magnitude of our manipulation's effect based on the time of participation likely reflect changes in the pandemic itself. The emergence of the widespread (but more minor) Omicron variant, followed by a decrease in COVID-19 cases and subsequent policy changes, occurred during the data collection period. As a result, people's perceptions of the risk posed by COVID-19 changed in kind.

Discussion

This experimental study examined the effects of COVID-19 mitigation efforts on plea decision-making in a jail setting simulation. We hypothesized that individuals in the low COVID-19 mitigation condition would be more likely to enter a guilty plea and would increase their willingness to accept a guilty plea (relative to those in a high COVID-19 mitigation condition). Findings indicate that COVID-19 mitigation efforts alone were not enough to significantly impact plea decision-making (at least not at this stage in the pandemic). While the primary hypotheses did not reach statistical significance, the results still offer several implications and possible explanations to better understand plea decision-making and how it can be affected by a fluctuating pandemic.

Although COVID-19 mitigation efforts did not have a statistically significant impact on plea decision-making, it is still worth noting the trends in decision-making following exposure to either COVID-19 mitigation level. First, the difference in the WTAP score before and after exposure to the COVID-19 mitigation condition indicated that both groups increased their WTAP. Thus, just the reminder of COVID-19's potential presence, even in the high-mitigation condition, increased the WTAP score. This overall increase for both groups could have contributed to the nonsignificant impact of the mitigation manipulation on change in WTAP. The unbalanced nature of the vaccination status variable offers insights into plea decision-making later in the pandemic. There were more vaccinated individuals in the low-mitigation condition (see note 4). When vaccination status was controlled for, the WTAP score change coefficient was reduced. This suggests that vaccinated individuals may be less sensitive to the risk of being exposed to COVID-19, which may be explained by the perceived immunity given by the vaccine.

Previous research has illustrated that jail has a reputation for being unpleasant (Toman et al., 2018) and that many defendants see entering a guilty plea as a way to escape the immediate unpleasantness of jail (Edkins & Dervan; 2018; Sacks & Ackerman, 2012). Regardless of the mitigation level described by the defense attorney, COVID-19 may amplify an already unpleasant environment. This finding echoes the findings of Wilford, Zimmerman, et al. (2021), who discovered that presenting information relating to the pandemic to participant-defendants made it significantly more likely they would accept the plea offer.

Since the COVID-19 pandemic began, both epidemiologists and policymakers have cautioned of its ever-changing nature, especially with the potential for new variants and surges (Lonas, 2022; Sun, 2020). The Omicron variant, which was much more contagious yet seemingly less severe, led to changes in COVID-19 mitigation strategies and in the behaviors and perceptions of the general public (Lonas, 2022). For example, medical experts recommended that individuals upgrade to KN-95 or N-95 masks because cloth masks would not protect them from the Omicron variant (Rogers, 2021) and because of the possibility of breakthrough cases for vaccinated individuals (Le Page, 2022). To put the effects of the Omicron variant into perspective, data from the Centers for Disease Control and Prevention (2022b) showed that the highest daily case count before the Omicron variant was in January 2021 with 293,325 reported cases. The daily case count for the peak of the Omicron variant was 1,259,946 reported cases. Following the peak, cases began to decline rapidly, signaling that the worst of Omicron had passed. At the time of our data collection (between late January and early March 2022), the pandemic was becoming less of a concern, and the majority of states were lifting COVID-19 restrictions (Mandavilli, 2022; Shammas et al., 2022).

Although purely exploratory, splitting the data into two periods supports the explanation that COVID-19 was perceived as less of a concern as the Omicron variant continued to wane. The pandemic was incredibly dynamic, meaning that the influence of COVID-19 on an individual's decision-making may have fluctuated. Many Americans expressed the desire in 2022 to return to normal, with data suggesting that people were feeling more comfortable resuming normal activities such as going to a grocery store, dining at a restaurant, and attending an indoor concert—all activities that would have been considered high risk at earlier stages of the pandemic (Gramlich, 2022).

Another consideration involves what the response to COVID-19 in correctional facilities looked like during Omicron. For example, in response to the combined effects of the Omicron variant and the return to pre-pandemic carceral capacities, many facilities resorted to periods of lockdown to reduce the possibility of COVID-19 spreading (Schwartzapfel & Blankinger, 2021). While not the best indicator of jail practices, the Federal Bureau of Prisons (2022) has taken a tiered approach to decide what COVID-19 preventive measures are still needed depending on the vaccination rate of the facility, the rate of incarcerated individuals in medical isolation, as well as the level of community spread. While most federal facilities have resumed near-normal operations, at the time of writing, masks are still required indoors regardless of COVID-19 risk level. Looking beyond the Omicron variant, this could be the closest the pandemic jail experience will be to the jail experience before the pandemic.

This does not suggest that COVID-19 mitigation efforts should not be implemented or are no longer helpful. Detention facilities have a duty to keep individuals relatively safe and healthy. The findings of this study indicate that jail is still perceived as an experience worth avoiding by way of making a guilty plea, regardless of what COVID-19 measures are in place. Recall that, in this study, all the participant-defendants were factually innocent, yet plea acceptance rates were still around 50%. This is unsurprising given the previous literature highlighting the effect that pretrial detention has on plea decision-making. Ultimately, this study underscores the importance for practitioners to recognize that decisions made about who will be held in pretrial detention can affect case outcomes, especially regarding how the case will be resolved.

Several limitations to the study are worth discussing. The first limitation involves the sample itself. This sample consisted of Arizona State University college students, so the findings should be considered with that population in mind. Notably, university policies relating to COVID-19 may have influenced how the students perceived COVID-19 and COVID-19 mitigation efforts. Another concern relating to a college student sample is the possibility that the sample may not have the same risk tolerance levels compared to a defendant sample, although the rates of our participants with prior legal system experience help to alleviate this concern.

Beyond the sample characteristics, there are also concerns relating to the sample size. While similar studies had more experimental manipulations, making a larger sample size necessary, the most comparable study to the present one is Wilford, Zimmerman, et al. (2021), which had a final sample of 704 individuals for their 2 × 2 factorial design. Using this previous study as a benchmark, even with only one manipulation, a sample size closer to 300 would have been ideal. A larger sample may have provided more statistical power to detect a significant difference in COVID-19 mitigation efforts if a difference existed.

There is also a limitation relating to the timing of data collection. Although collecting data as the Omicron variant became less prevalent was purely coincidental, there are concerns over how this affected the findings. Issues relating to the manipulations themselves may have also contributed to the lack of statistically significant findings. The mitigation efforts we included were informed by various sources and jurisdictions regarding strategies to reduce COVID-19 in carceral spaces; however, they might not fully reflect the actual day-to-day operations within a jail setting. Additionally, future research assessing mitigation efforts should include a measure of how influential each mitigation effort was to the participant-defendant to understand better how well the manipulation was implemented.

Conclusion

Plea bargaining continues to be the backbone of the criminal justice system, even though it has been criticized for many of its associated prosecutorial practices and due process shortcuts (Hessick, 2021). Although innocent individuals would ideally not accept a guilty plea, the current plea-bargaining system puts a great deal of pressure on individuals to accept a guilty plea in lieu of a trial. COVID-19 is an additional factor that defendants now have to consider when making a plea decision. The criminal justice system was deeply affected by the hardships relating to the pandemic. This experimental study investigated the intersection of plea bargaining, pretrial detention, and COVID-19 mitigation strategies in the later stage of the pandemic. Although the strategies used to curb the spread of COVID-19 in the jail setting simulation did not statistically impact plea decision-making, the more general effects of COVID-19 were present in the results.

The pandemic put defendants housed in pretrial detention in a position where they had to choose between the harmful consequences of potentially contracting COVID-19 or the harmful consequences of a guilty plea. Although COVID-19 appears to be becoming less of a health threat, the residual effects of having experienced a pandemic may still shape how individuals view high-risk environments such as jail. The pandemic thrust many glaring issues in criminal justice and plea bargaining into the spotlight. It took a pandemic for public leaders to reckon with the fact that jails and other correctional spaces pose a risk to the health and safety of those inside, especially when operating at or above capacity (Widra, 2022). Many prosecutors showed more leniency when negotiating pleas during the pandemic, which inadvertently increased the pressure to plead guilty when a defendant otherwise may have considered trial (Daftary-Kapur et al., 2021). COVID-19 pressured the criminal justice system to change how it operates relatively quickly. Now that the criminal justice system has demonstrated that it can change to address acute issues, it is time to address the chronic issues related to the combination of plea bargaining and the implementation of pretrial detention.

Acknowledgments

We want to thank the entire team at the Plea Justice Project for making the interactive simulation and this research possible. We would also like to thank Ojmarrh Mitchell for providing feedback and guidance on an earlier version of this study. Lastly, we thank the editors of the Perspectives on Crime and Justice series for providing a platform for our work to be shared.

Notes

1. Balance tests were done by comparing the median score for continuous demographic variables using the Wilcoxon rank-sum test. For dichotomous demographic variables, Pearson's chi-squared test evaluated the similarity between both groups.

2. The main portion of the analysis used a chi-squared test between the experimental condition and the dichotomous decision dependent variable. Additionally, t-tests were done between the experimental condition and the two dependent variables relating to the WTAP score.

3. In total, six manipulation checks were administered, and participants needed to successfully complete four in order to remain in the analytical sample. In addition to correctly responding to four out of the six manipulation checks, participants also had to answer the survey questions relating to all three

dependent variables to remain in the sample. Lastly, two attention checks were given to ensure participants took the time to read each of the questions.

4. Vaccination status was the only variable that was unbalanced, with an associated p-value of 0.003. There were more vaccinated individuals in the low-mitigation condition compared to the high-mitigation condition. Given the unbalanced nature of vaccination status, regression analyses controlled for vaccination status and tested the robustness of the main findings. The WTAP score change variable was the only variable to be significantly impacted by vaccination status ($p = 0.041$). When vaccination was controlled for, the change in WTAP decreased.

8. COVID-19 in Corrections: Analysis of Protocols and Trends

Matthew Vanden Bosch

Introduction

The COVID-19 pandemic has exposed glaring flaws in the correctional system in the United States and has brought renewed mainstream attention to the issue of infectious diseases in correctional settings. However, it is not the first disease to expose our systems' challenges as we attempted to curb its spread and negative consequences. While the pandemic has affected all aspects of the correctional system, this chapter focuses on prisons, as the relatively stable population of prisons allows for a more accessible examination, presentation, and understanding of rates and case numbers, as well as the longer-lasting impacts, of COVID-19 in corrections.

This chapter first explores the effects of COVID-19 on the correctional system, including spread and response, and discusses how this differs from the pandemic's effects on the public. It then considers a parallel discussion of other institutionally prevalent diseases and their impact on the correctional system, and it uses these understandings to inform our contemporary understanding of COVID-19 and how correctional institutions can and have responded. The chapter concludes with a summary of how careful consideration of illnesses can help us understand the prevalence and spread of disease in correctional facilities and how best to address it moving forward for future pandemics or epidemics and general disease management and health care.

During the early stages of the pandemic, advice regarding COVID-19 management strategies was vague and variable for the public and correctional facilities. The lack of clear and actionable advice may help to explain why, during the early pandemic, 9 of the 10 largest outbreaks occurred in or originated from prisons (Maxmen, 2020). Key aspects of these instances demonstrated how good intentions led to harshly adverse outcomes. In one case, an outbreak in a California prison prompted the transfer of roughly 120 high-risk individuals to San Quentin Prison from the California Institution for Men. These individuals were transferred out of a concern for their health, moving vulnerable individuals away from an active COVID-19 outbreak, as the California Institution for Men was one of the first prisons in the state to experience an outbreak of COVID-19 (Wesley & Beyer, 2021). However, these individuals were not tested for COVID-19 nor properly isolated upon arrival in San Quentin. The resulting outbreak in San Quentin infected over half of the staff. Many individuals who were incarcerated there also subsequently tested positive for COVID-19 (Maxmen, 2020).

Public and institutional understanding and response to COVID-19 evolved in the first months of the pandemic. Early phases of the pandemic were defined by high levels of cases with no available vaccine, such as in the fall of 2020, when COVID-19 had been active for months but before vaccines were widely available. At this stage, research provided some reliable information on the spread of COVID-19, offering a more comprehensive understanding of management strategies. Notably, the Centers for Disease Control and Prevention was given more latitude to retool the advice for the general public and correctional facilities.

As of December 2023, the time of writing, the attention to and the severity of the pandemic is lessening, in large part due to the role of vaccines being made publicly available as well as some natural immunities for those infected and the generally weaker variants of COVID-19 that have emerged and taken over as the primary infections. However, COVID-19 remains ongoing and illustrates a significant example that may inform us about the weaknesses of our systems in prisons and beyond. In fact, in October of 2023, there was an average of 16,115 new COVID-19 admissions to hospitals each week, more than half the rate of COVID-19 admissions to hospitals each week in August of 2020 (the earliest date for which this information is available from the CDC's COVID Data Tracker). Much literature on COVID-19 (and many other diseases) in the correctional system comes from medical research rather than strictly criminological research. Still, the findings provided by medical research can help us identify weak spots in correctional systems and their trends in dealing with COVID-19. Most related criminological research focuses on the existence and quality of prison health care rather than disease rates or the intersections of public health and correctional research (Lambert et al., 2020).

Motivations for Understanding
Health Care in Corrections

There are three distinct reasons we should care about the health of incarcerated individuals, particularly in a preventive and moral sense. Overall, by focusing on prevention, we can avoid significant long-term and short-term adverse effects on individuals, their communities, and our society. As the old saying goes, "An ounce of prevention is worth a pound of cure." This outlook guides the best responses to diseases that threaten individuals incarcerated in our nation's prisons.

First, we have an individual and public moral responsibility to ensure the well-being of incarcerated individuals. We are confining these individuals in close quarters and have a duty to keep them free of disease and in relative human comfort. Courts have accepted the arguments for why we need to provide an uncrowded prison for incarcerated persons (Abraham et al., 2020; Pyrooz et al., 2020). These arguments have frequently relied on general concerns over accessibility to mental and physical health care in prisons (Forrester et al., 2014). Because many prisons lack intensive care units (Sivashanker et al., 2020), prisoners who become particularly sick must be taken to outside hospitals, possibly straining those external resources. If we can prevent these individuals from becoming sick in the first place, we can avoid not just individual adverse outcomes but also help to minimize the spread of illness.

A second reason to care about the health of persons who are incarcerated is that we have a clear financial incentive to protect the health of our nation's inmates, even more so than other individuals. Simply put, we pay the bill for any health issues that they have. While incarcerated individuals are often responsible for some amount of money as a co-pay (Grodensky et al., 2018), the rest of the cost is covered by taxpayers. Prevention is almost always cheaper than treating or curing a disease, and analyses have shown substantial costs saved because of widespread COVID-19 vaccinations, even before accounting for the preservation of human life (Wang et al., 2021).

Third, the vast majority of those incarcerated in correctional facilities, including prisons, will at some point be released back into their communities (Jacobi, 2005). If returning citizens have recently been exposed to or infected with a communicable disease, this disease could be passed to families and communities. Other high-prevalence diseases, such as sexually transmitted infections or tuberculosis, can lay dormant for some time and emerge later in life—even potentially after the individual has been fully reintegrated. The returning population provides a clear transmission vector through which diseases spreading through portions of our correctional system can move into the broader public. If we reduce the number of people being pushed into and removed from our correctional institutions, we can break a recurring cycle that allows for the exposure of incarcerated populations to diseases beyond the bounds of their facility. Additionally, this would reduce the likelihood of diseases being exported to the public from a facility experiencing an outbreak.

However, even if no incarcerated persons were being released to society, the basic functions of a correctional institution require daily travel between the prison and the community, as staff, vendors, and service providers arrive to work at the prison and return home each day. Any infectious disease transmitted to them at any time threatens to jump into the community (Nowotny et al., 2021), whereas an incarcerated individual would need to be infected near in time to their release or be infected with a disease that has an incubation period. Therefore, the breaking of the constant cycle of incarceration and release would not necessarily prevent prisons from experiencing major outbreaks of any number of diseases.

The Public, the Prison, and the Pandemic

At the time of writing, there have been over 103 million confirmed cases of COVID-19 in the United States, representing about 30% of the total U.S. population, and over 1.1 million individuals have died. Notably, due to a lack of widespread testing, both figures likely understate the true extent of COVID-19, though this is a more significant concern for case counts than deaths. Individuals who do not present symptoms but have the disease, known as asymptomatic infections, are much less likely to be tested. Given that anywhere between 25% and 95% of COVID-19 cases are asymptomatic (Kronbichler et al., 2020; Marcum, 2020), known COVID-19 cases could dramatically undercount the prevalence of the disease.

COVID-19 Rates and Fatalities in Incarcerated Individuals

The rate of COVID-19 infections is even higher among those who are incarcerated in our nation's prisons, though this may be partially due to more testing. While not every prison conducted mass testing on inmates, testing revealed many previously unknown or asymptomatic cases in some places where it was done. In a sample of 16 correctional facilities holding 16,400 individuals, the known case rate before mass testing was 642 (3.9% of the combined sample) (Hagan, 2020). After mass testing, the known case rate was over 8,200 individuals, representing roughly 50% of the combined sample, and one tested facility had a total known case rate of almost 83% after testing. In more focused studies, San Quentin Prison in California had an outbreak infecting more than 60% of inmates, Avenal State Prison (also in California) had over 80% of inmates infected with COVID-19 (Parsons & Worden, 2021), and still other facilities had over 75% of their prisoners infected (Marcum, 2020). The lack of repeated mass testing throughout the correctional system risks dramatically undercounting the true prevalence of COVID-19 in our prisons, furthering its spread and risking COVID-19 becoming a cyclical disease in correctional settings.

Though likely undercounting the true rates of COVID-19 infections, testing estimates remain the best information available. At the end of 2019, just before COVID-19 began to impact the United States seriously, there were a total of 1,464,400 individuals incarcerated in prisons (Carson, 2020). By September 12, 2022, there had been almost 650,000 confirmed cases of COVID-19 among individuals incarcerated in prisons in the United States. The roughly 650,000 positive cases would represent over a third of the prison population and likely undercounted positive cases. With an estimated one in three persons who were incarcerated having tested positive for COVID-19, incarcerated individuals were at a heightened risk of exposure and to the long-term consequences of infection.

The number of deaths from COVID-19 for inmates from 2020 to 2023 was 2,933. While small, this represents a death rate for confirmed cases of COVID-19 of just under 0.47%. This is less than half of the roughly 1% death rate for confirmed cases of COVID-19 among the public. This lower figure may be explained by two things: the younger average age of inmates and a higher amount of testing in correctional facilities. Put differently, the official death rate from COVID-19 in the public is likely inflated in real terms by the prevalence of elderly individuals in our communities and artificially by the lack of mass testing.

The data for the number of prison cases are more likely to be accurate than the data for the number of COVID-19 cases in the public. Members of the public are likely to get tested for COVID-19 only when they or someone close to them is showing symptoms. By contrast, in some prisons, if one individual tests positive for COVID-19, this can lead to testing everyone in the facility (Hagan, 2020). Thus, the statistics for COVID-19 in prisons are likely more accurate than those for the general population. While the characteristics of a prison (overcrowding, shared spaces, weak health care) all increase the likelihood of spreading diseases, the ability to conduct mass tests is much better. It is entirely possible that if we could have conducted mass testing in the public as we have been able to in prisons, we would have seen a dramatically higher number of COVID-19 cases in the public and a much lower rate of death from COVID-19.

In the early stages of the pandemic, 81% of deaths from COVID-19 in the public were among those over the age of 65. At the end of 2023, the percentage of all COVID-19 deaths where the individual is over 65 years of age is 74.75%, with an additional 18.46% of deaths being among those aged 50 to 64 years old, for a combined total of 93% of COVID-19 deaths occurring in individuals over the age of 50. While we do not have exact percentages for the entire prison population, the Federal Bureau of Prisons indicates that only 2.7% of federal prisoners are over 65, with only an additional 16.6% being between the ages of 51 and 64. This shows that the group most at risk of death from COVID-19 in the general population, the elderly, is dramatically underrepresented in the prison population. Saloner et al. (2020) indicate that individuals 65 or older make up more than 15% of the public, so they are more than five times as common in the public than in prison populations.

COVID-19 Case Rates and Fatalities for Prison Staff

Prison staff members are also at substantial risk for infection from COVID-19 and may serve as crucial transmission vectors between the community and prison populations (Novisky et al., 2021; Wallace et al., 2021). According to the U.S. Bureau of Labor Statistics, there are almost 440,000 correctional officers in the country, in addition to administrative and support staff, totaling over 500,000 correctional workers (Montoya-Barthelemy et al., 2020). Among all prison staff, there have been almost 247,000 confirmed COVID-19 cases (COVID Prison Project, 2022). Much like with inmates, these rates indicate a higher case rate than the general public's known case rate, regardless of whether the rates are higher because of mandatory testing following an outbreak in a facility. That said, the prison staff case rate is dramatically higher than the case rates in the general population.

A notable issue with those higher case rates is that they are even higher than those for inmates, who should, in theory, be tested roughly as frequently. However, correctional staff are exposed to more than one source of potential COVID-19 transmission: inside the prison and outside in public. Correctional officers may be contributors to an outbreak in a prison facility, by importing the disease from the outside or by contracting it inside and transferring it to other portions of the facility. This supposition is supported by the fact that in roughly half of instances where a first case was identified in a correctional facility, a correctional worker had the first case (Novisky et al., 2021). Additionally, when incarcerated individuals are quarantined, the correctional officers and service providers treating them or providing them with food or other necessities would become the only vector of transmission out. The combination of these factors could explain a higher case rate for staff than for incarcerated individuals, who are directly exposed only to the prison environment.

Additional Health Challenges of COVID-19

Death from COVID-19 is a rare event, and it becomes even rarer when we consider the potential rates of asymptomatic cases that do not get tested and are not included in statistics. While COVID-19 has caused many deaths, many diseases kill a much higher percentage of those who become infected. Death is not, however, the only negative outcome possible from COVID-19, so even if we accept the relative rarity of deaths (as a low percentage of cases), it is important to understand other short- and long-term impacts of COVID-19.

There have been reports of individuals in the general population experiencing what has been termed "Long COVID," where the symptoms of COVID-19 persist long after an individual ceases being able to transmit the disease to others (Callard & Perego, 2021; Sudre et al., 2021). Over 10% of individuals who survive a COVID-19 infection indicate experiencing symptoms for at least a month after the onset of the disease. Those who experience more severe symptoms are more likely to experience Long COVID. Fatigue and frequent headaches are the most common symptoms, with loss of smell and respiratory problems being somewhat less common (Sudre et al., 2021). While more significant symptoms, such as cardiac problems and memory issues, have been relatively uncommon (4%–6%), they have been significantly more common in those who experienced symptoms for a shorter period (0.2%–0.5%). Given the challenges of controlling disease spread in carceral institutions and of providing inmates with quality health care, there is strong potential for Long COVID and accompanying health problems in populations of the correctional system.

Institutional Challenges in Managing COVID-19

The prevalence of COVID-19 among those who work in and those who are housed in correctional institutions is not surprising given the nature and structure of the institutions. Many reasons contribute to the spread, severity, and impact of COVID-19.

Transmissibility

As COVID-19 is an airborne disease, it presents greater challenges for containment compared to diseases transmissible only through the exchange of bodily fluids or even those diseases that can spread from surface contact. Prisons provide an environment ripe for the transmission of many communicable diseases, as evidenced by the increased spread of airborne diseases such as the flu or tuberculosis. Easier transmission extends to COVID-19 as well. Some issues that allow easier transmission are close contact with other individuals, substantial use of communal spaces (such as cafeterias or bathrooms), and shared cells.

Social distancing is one of the best ways to prevent or decrease COVID-19 transmission, but this is the form of prevention that prisons have the most difficulty implementing. While prisons are often strict about their distribution of cleaning supplies or sanitizer (Montoya-Barthelemey et al., 2020), they can provide them to inmates. Still, prisons have limited space and are not designed to allow for social distancing, so the environmental design of prisons can encourage the spread of COVID-19 and other diseases (Henry, 2020).

Import and Export

Standard prison system policies can contribute to the spread of disease beyond just the prison setting itself. The common control measures for COVID-19 of self-isolation and especially social distancing are less available to incarcerated individuals (Parsons & Worden, 2021). Additionally, the standard practice of transferring inmates between prisons is a clear vector for transmission. Again, given the high rates of asymptomatic but transmissible COVID-19 infection, it would be easy for an individual who is infected to be approved for transportation to a new prison and introduce the disease there.

Notable as well, cases in prisons can be exported to nearby communities, whether through inmate releases or daily travel between the community and prison. Counties with state prisons located within them had almost 10% more COVID-19 cases than those without one, even after accounting for population size (Sims et al., 2021). Furthermore, for every 1,000 people a state prison could hold, there was a 5% increase in COVID-19 cases in the surrounding county. This finding also provides evidence of effectiveness in our most robust pandemic management recommendations. Federal prisons instituted much more serious lockdowns than other prisons did, and there was no relationship between the presence of a federal prison and the COVID-19 case rates in the surrounding area (Sims et al., 2021).

Overcrowding

Overcrowding is a substantial problem in prisons and can lead to higher transmission rates of COVID-19 (Parsons & Worden, 2021; Udwadia et al., 2020). In one study, individuals who were incarcerated and living in dorm-style rooms with multiple other residents were more likely to be infected than those in cells with fewer residents (Chin et al., 2021). Increasing the number of individuals sharing a room is a clear mechanism to manage overcrowding and is tied to a heightened risk of infection.

While rare, some states had begun addressing overcrowding before COVID-19 arrived, with California even being ordered by its state court system to lower the prison population (Newman & Scott, 2012). Generally, states were slow to reduce their prison populations or had increased them before the pandemic. While there has been a general reduction in the prison population through the pandemic, this is due less to the intentional release of inmates and more to typical releases combined with a lower intake (Nowonty & Piquero, 2020). This means that the prison reductions we see are less a result of prisons' own policies and have more to do with the policies and practices of the courts and law enforcement.

There is also a substantial difference between the slower trend toward reducing prison populations practiced by some states and the rapid decarceration suggested as a suitable response to COVID-19 (Parsons & Worden, 2021; Udwadia et al., 2020). Even under demands by public health officials, some states have resisted decarceration despite the well-stated need to decarcerate. Efforts to halt decarceration have gone so far as to appeal court decisions on the matter, and these stalling attempts have continued even during repeated outbreaks of COVID-19 in prisons (Parson & Worden, 2021). The first year of the pandemic saw some initial efforts to decarcerate and reduce prison populations, but in 2021, 19 states and the federal government increased the number of people incarcerated (Kang-Brown, 2022). In Alaska, the incarceration levels returned to the levels that existed before COVID-19. Although the rest of the states reduced their prison populations enough to decrease the national population of incarcerated individuals, these other states continued to resist decarceration.

In-Prison Health Care

Due to costs, crowding, and demand, prison health care can quickly become overburdened by a surge or disease outbreak. Even hospitals for the public have experienced substantial strain during the pandemic, in some cases running out of emergency room beds. Since prison cell density was linked to infectious disease rates even before the pandemic, an especially infectious disease could spread easily and substantially tax the prison health care system (Abraham et al., 2020). These systems may lack personnel and necessary equipment for testing, treatment, or protection, generally and especially in response to the new and rapidly spreading COVID-19 infection (Montoya-Barthelemey et al., 2020).

Private Prison Problems

One issue related to (though distinct from) these problems as they occur within government-run prisons is the problems within private prisons. Our ability to analyze the effectiveness of dealing with COVID-19 and other diseases is challenged by there being no mandated reporting of health-related events in the private system. Private industries maintain more latitude than government facilities regarding which policies to implement and how to do so. This lack of data may explain why it is difficult to find any literature on private prisons and *any* disease, let alone COVID-19. While we cannot make inferences about private facilities' efficacy of response to the pandemic, the focus on profit in private prisons is generally thought to exacerbate the problems (understaffing, overcrowding, lack of services) that public prisons experience (Tartaglia, 2014). This would hold true for COVID-19 responses as well.

Other Impacts of Prisons and COVID-19

The long-term adverse effects of COVID-19 are not limited to physical health alone but extend also to mental health. This is particularly important in a correctional setting, as prior research has found that incarcerated individuals experience significant stress, which increases their likelihood of experiencing infectious diseases later in life (Massoglia, 2008). Therefore, the stress introduced to incarcerated individuals because of COVID-19 can increase the odds that they will contract infectious diseases post-release, such as COVID-19. Additionally, the stress of transitioning from prison life to public life can increase the hardships of formerly incarcerated individuals (Western et al., 2015), so even higher levels of stress in prison could, in theory, further increase post-incarceration hardships.

Stress on Incarcerated Persons

Generally, individuals who are incarcerated have a higher prevalence of mental illness than is found in the public (Montoya-Barthelemey et al., 2020), which could lead to compounding stressors with COVID-19. While research has tracked worsened mental health during the pandemic, worsened mental health is not necessarily connected to worries about vulnerability to COVID-19 but is often tied to the measures taken to combat COVID-19 in prison, namely, restricting those privileges that prisoners value: visitation, counseling, educational opportunities, and yard time (Johnson et al., 2021; Pyrooz et al., 2020).

While some researchers have logically argued that individuals who are incarcerated will experience heightened stress directly due to COVID-19 (Johnson et al., 2021; Novisky et al., 2021), the accuracy of this argument is unclear. Persons who are incarcerated generally reported not being worried about COVID-19 but interestingly not because of their having negligible concern over COVID-19 and its impacts. Instead, many recognize that an infectious disease will spread through the system quickly and that there is little use in worrying when contraction is practically unavoidable (Pyrooz et al., 2020). In essence, they perceive that becoming infected is inevitable. Additionally, early responses to COVID-19 were intended to reduce its spread and included measures that prevented engagement in normal day-to-day activities. While these efforts may have reduced the spread, they also would have decreased the quality of life of inmates by curtailing their daily routines (Pyrooz et al., 2020).

Strains on Institutional Staff

There has been strong empirical work on the strains faced by staff in correctional facilities, analyzing their stressors before COVID-19 and the additional anxieties introduced during the pandemic. There has not been substantial work, however, on their perceptions of the efforts made to combat COVID-19; thus it is difficult to make a direct comparison either to the public or to incarcerated individuals. The work done on staff mental health has indicated generally high stressors even before COVID-19 emerged, with high levels of work-related stress and elevated rates of mental health concerns (Johnson et al., 2021; Martin-Howard, 2022; Montoya-Barthelemey et al., 2020). A reduction in the number of correctional staff because of COVID-19 (by voluntary exiting system or from illness) has resulted in increasing burnout among the staff that remains, in addition to their fears of contracting the virus. The combination of enhanced stressors for correctional workers during the pandemic alongside generally weak support for mental health services results in worsened mental health outcomes for correctional workers, similar to individuals who are incarcerated (Martin-Howard, 2022).

Added Strain beyond the Walls

COVID-19 has undoubtedly resulted in increased levels of stress among the public. However, as with those working or living in prisons, it is hard to disentangle the stress rising from the disease from that resulting from measures to address it. While experiences were dramatically different within a prison, the public still experienced efforts to limit the spread, including closing restaurants, clubs, gyms, and other facilities promoting social congregation. Unsurprisingly, mental health outcomes in the public were worsened by the pandemic (Dlugosz, 2021; Flaskerud, 2020; Gallagher et al., 2020). While stress levels for American adults were generally higher in 2020 than in prior years (Flaskerud, 2020), those who lost loved ones or were diagnosed with COVID-19 themselves were particularly likely to experience some form of an emotional disorder (Gallagher et al., 2020). These results are remarkable, as we have not seen any significant shift in the average stress level of American adults since the data were first recorded in 2007, indicating that the added stress was likely due to the uniquely powerful nature of COVID-19. Young adults indicated the worst mental health on account of COVID-19, which follows a general trend of worse mental health in young adults than in others (Dlugosz, 2021). However, it is also possible that this trend was exacerbated by closing pro-social environments and facilities, which young adults are particularly likely to attend.

Individuals with family members in prison also experience significant mental distress, particularly when they are concerned about the well-being of their incarcerated relative (Testa & Fahmy, 2021). Importantly, this heightened level of concern was associated with more use of dysfunctional coping mechanisms but not functional coping strategies. This may be because prison visitation was severely restricted through the early and middle stages of the COVID-19 pandemic, with most prisons stopping in-person visitation to minimize the spread of infection. Moreover, not every prison was equipped with the right tools to implement virtual visitation (either by phone or videoconference) as an alternative, and these are not perfect replacements for in-person visitation even in the best of circumstances (Dallaire et al., 2021).

COVID-19 Compared with Other Diseases

It should not be surprising that the transmission of COVID-19 was intensified in correctional institutions, as this has been a common issue with many other outbreaks, including tuberculosis and swine flu (Nowonty & Piquero, 2020). Prisons were well recognized as environments conducive to disease transmission even before COVID-19 emerged (Adimora & Schoenbach, 2005; Thomas & Sampson, 2005; Thomas et al., 2008; Van't Hoff et al., 2009). In some instances, prisons recorded disease rates 10–100 times as high as the public, which may aid in explaining why we have seen such a high COVID-19 case rate for prison inmates and correctional staff compared to the public. Furthermore, a better understanding of the spread and prevalence of COVID-19 and other diseases can aid in understanding the policies that effectively respond to infectious disease outbreaks and thereby craft even better responses in the future.

Including a review of other major diseases that have impacted the correctional system puts COVID-19 in a larger context of disease in corrections and may suggest how we could use this information to combat future pandemics, epidemics, or even everyday diseases of concern. Even for those who deny a moral requirement to care for those who are incarcerated or who think that we should not provide health care to inmates at taxpayers' expense, it is undeniable that prisons act as incubators for serious diseases and serve to introduce or reintroduce infectious diseases to the public outside their walls (Adimora & Schoenbach, 2005; Thomas & Sampson, 2005; Thomas et al., 2008; Wolfe et al., 2001). Therefore, for any number of diseases, prisons are critical locations for intervention, potentially changing the long-term trajectory of epidemics.

Tuberculosis is likely the most apt comparison to COVID-19 within the correctional system. Both were present outside the prison system but were magnified within it, and both are respiratory diseases transmitted through droplets in the air and have potentially long-lasting consequences. While tuberculosis received strong initial research attention during outbreaks in the 1980s and 1990s, it has generally been ignored in the criminological and correctional literature since then.[1] Drug-resistant tuberculosis is less of a threat today, largely due to the interruption in its spread and to direct observation therapy, where health workers observe patients taking their medication to ensure no missed doses (Frieden et al., 1995).

Tuberculosis can inform much of our understanding of COVID-19 in corrections, given some similarities and differences between the two diseases. Like asymptomatic cases of COVID-19, not everyone carrying the organism that causes tuberculosis will have an active infection. An estimated one-third of people with tuberculosis are not aware of the infection. Numerous additional factors may increase the likelihood of having an active infection (Mueller, 1996; Saunders & Evans, 2020). Unlike COVID-19, in which asymptomatic individuals can spread the disease, it is rare for an asymptomatic tuberculosis-infected individual to transmit the bacterium, as transmission is usually limited to those who are symptomatic (Udwadia, 2020). However, potentially due to a slower buildup, the number of expected cases to result from a single infectious individual in a vulnerable population is substantially higher for tuberculosis than it is for COVID-19. There is another major difference in lethality. While COVID-19's death rate in the early stages of the pandemic, at its highest, was around 2%, untreated tuberculosis kills around half of those it infects. Notably, before COVID-19 emerged, tuberculosis was the world's leading infectious disease that resulted in death, but COVID-19 began killing more per day as early as April 2020 (Saunders & Evans, 2020).

Tuberculosis was nearly eliminated at one point (though this outcome is unlikely for COVID-19) but reemerged in the 1980s and 1990s. This outbreak also included the introduction of a more severe strain of tuberculosis and multiple-drug-resistant tuberculosis, which was highly resistant to the standard pharmaceutical treatments used to manage the infection. The resulting spread of tuberculosis had a lopsided impact, with a substantially higher number of infections in correctional settings. In 1985, inmates were almost four times more likely to have tuberculosis than the public (Snider & Hutton, 1989). Its reemergence in corrections was stronger than may have been expected, partially due to the close nature of incarceration and the higher prevalence of HIV/AIDS (another disease that has more noticeable impacts and spread in correctional settings), which exposed an individual to a greater risk of active tuberculosis infection (Snider & Hutton, 1989). The elevated risk of exposure to tuberculosis in prisons remains, with studies indicating at least an order of magnitude increase in the likelihood of infection for those in prisons compared with the public (Baussano et al., 2010).

Much like COVID-19, tuberculosis was recognized as a threat within prisons and to the communities beyond them. A tuberculosis outbreak in corrections could easily cross over to the community through staff or through recently released inmates (Nowotny et al., 2021). Inmates are often young upon release, so substantial lifetime impacts may exist (Snider & Hutton, 1989). Prisons were noted as being critical sources in maintaining high rates of tuberculosis in non-white and inner-city populations, just as they have been sources of COVID-19 for the public.

By the mid-1990s, new cases of tuberculosis reached over 24,000 a year in the public, though the rate of infection was five times higher for persons who were incarcerated (Mueller, 1996). While this is low in absolute terms compared with COVID-19, it is significant for a disease that was considered practically eliminated, especially given the significant negative impacts it can have, including lasting respiratory problems, compromised lung function, and death (Saunders & Evans, 2020; Udwadia et al., 2020). Management of the disease includes isolation of the infected individual during the contagion period (the duration varies from person to person), placement in an area where air does not return to the rest of the prison, and attempts at drug treatments (Mueller, 1996). These strategies may even be more effective in dealing with COVID-19 infections, as individuals with COVID-19 are infectious for shorter lengths of time than those with tuberculosis. Additionally, COVID-19 has a much more consistent and predictable time of infectiousness than tuberculosis does.

Both tuberculosis and COVID-19 interact substantially with other diseases or conditions to cause the most harm. Notably, there is evidence of a heightened risk of COVID-19 infection among those who have tuberculosis (Visca et al., 2021). Even those who have recovered from tuberculosis may be at greater risk for adverse outcomes from COVID-19 (Saunders & Evans, 2020; Udwadia et al., 2020), including more time on a ventilator, long-term pulmonary fibrosis, and long-term lung damage. While this is not exclusive to correctional facilities, the historical connection between tuberculosis and prisons, combined with the current connection between prisons and COVID-19, creates a prominent overlap of respiratory diseases that can have devastating consequences.

Finally, tuberculosis and COVID-19 can co-occur in an individual at the same time. Both primarily impact the respiratory system, so co-occurrence may be particularly dangerous. While we lack current data for understanding the full interaction between the two, the determinants for COVID-19 mortality are similar to some determinants of tuberculosis mortality, such as HIV infection, diabetes, malnutrition, and being impoverished, many of which may apply to individuals who are incarcerated or recently released.

Sexually transmitted infections (STIs) are (depending on the specific infection) relatively widespread beyond corrections facilities. However, they are of particular concern in prisons, given the generally restricted access to safer sex practices or supplies (such as condoms) and the increased coercive potential for rape (Thomas et al., 2008). This concern around STIs in prisons is not new (Beltrami et al., 1997; Moran & Peterman, 1989); STIs hold a longer-lasting position in prisons than tuberculosis or COVID-19. Despite their name, STIs can spread in ways other than sexual intercourse. Most relevant here is needle-sharing among users of intravenous drugs (Pala et al., 2018).

As with COVID-19, many individuals may enter prisons with STIs (Hammett, 2009; Moran & Peterman, 1989), and prisons are likely to increase their spread. New cases of both STIs and COVID-19 in individuals who have been incarcerated for some time signal one of two things: either the prison failed to detect the disease during intake or the individuals engaged in activity in the prison that transmitted the disease, or both.

Increasing screening and testing for STIs, as with COVID-19, would help to understand their spread within prisons better, improve treatment among the infected, and potentially limit their spread. However, measures to prevent and reduce STIs have been limited in their implementation despite the relative ease of access and use of prevention and reduction strategies and a much longer history of their recommendation. While some institutions are highly effective at implementing recommendations, such as wide-scale STI testing and treatment (Beltrami et al., 1997; Hammett, 2009), others are less so, and it is rare for there to be STI screens once an individual has gone through an intake evaluation.

While the recommendations for preventing STIs in prisons are different in some respects (provision of condoms, needle exchange programs) from preventing other diseases, including COVID-19, there are some commonalities. First, there is a general resistance to implementing these measures, as they may cost more up front, although they may also save money in the long run. Second, screening for more infections could be applied across all of the diseases of interest. Lastly, screening more commonly within a facility would help to minimize the spread of most diseases. The simple fact is that these diseases are being spread within the facilities, so acting as though they are not will result in the continuation of the cyclical pattern of spread and exportation to the general public.

Improving Institutional Responses to Disease in Corrections

COVID-19 has had clear effects within correctional settings, and its recent history provides important lessons about infectious disease prevention, control, and mitigation in prisons. While tuberculosis is now a minor disease in the United States, it remains a serious concern in developing nations, particularly in their correctional systems. STIs remain a vital concern in corrections, including in the United States. New variants of COVID-19 are expected to continue to emerge. However, some concerns about the lethality of the disease have faded with the introduction and acceptance of vaccines.

While STIs will likely always exist in our correctional system, other diseases can be defeated. There is a potential to eradicate tuberculosis now as it nearly was before. Early strains of COVID-19 have been largely replaced by weaker strains that have less impact on those they infect. There is hope to be found in these factors. More than that, there are lessons to be learned and applied from our understanding of public health challenges in carceral settings.

Prisons populations are generally vulnerable to diseases, which can emerge as localized epidemics in society, but we can minimize these impacts. Decarceration is a key mechanism to do so, not just as a near-panic response to an emerging disease but as a policy. As already discussed, quick decarceration does not generally occur; prisons do not voluntarily begin to release more inmates than usual. They did not do so on a large scale through COVID-19 or other epidemics, so there is little reason to expect them to do so in the future. Instead, the trends in changes to court procedures and law enforcement actions offer the potential of leading to a policy of decarceration that will alleviate the problematic overcrowding of prisons in the United States.

Following through on a policy of decarceration would also aid with other problems in prisons, especially where health care is concerned. Fewer inmates would mean less of a demand for essential services, and health care workers in a facility would not be overwhelmed and so could comprehensively address the health needs of the inmates. Given that prisons cause disease transmission beyond the prison itself, decarceration could help to reduce diseases in the public as well, particularly in the most disadvantaged communities with the highest rates of incarceration.

Despite rhetoric in favor of decarceration across the country, sustained efforts to do so are few, and research on their effects is similarly scarce. There is one good example to examine. In 2009, California was subject to a court order in *Brown v. Plata*, wherein the state was required to reduce its prison population by 25% in two years (Petersilia, 2016). The state succeeded in doing so, remaining the primary example of decarceration in the United States. Decarceration as a policy often carries concerns about increases in crime rate, but after California released almost 30,000 incarcerated individuals within approximately a year, there was virtually no rise in violent crime (Henry, 2020; Petersilia, 2016). Additionally, in the first several months of the pandemic, those prisons that had reduced their prison populations the most in the years prior to the pandemic avoided COVID-19 outbreaks in their facilities. Unfortunately, the minimal amount of decarceration that has occurred in the United States does not provide substantial evidence of the results of decarceration other than a few instances.

Overall, the successes and missteps of responses to tuberculosis and STIs provide significant information that can help inform our responses to disease outbreaks in the future, both in correctional settings and in the public. These lessons can be combined with new knowledge from responses to the COVID-19 pandemic, a far more widespread problem than either tuberculosis or STIs. First, proactive screening of individuals being introduced to a prison—whether upon transfer from another facility or upon initial admission—can potentially prevent a disease from gaining a foothold in the prison in the first place. While transfers and admissions are not the sole mechanism by which diseases may enter a correctional setting (correctional officers, vendors, and visitors also can introduce them), they serve as a key way that diseases can enter a facility. We also need better information from correctional institutions, particularly private prisons, to understand when and where to intervene effectively in order to minimize the spread and impact of infectious diseases.

Additionally, improved screening could work in concert with another important way to reduce the spread of diseases in correctional settings: specialized housing separate from the general population. With dedicated housing for individuals sick with an infectious disease, spread can be limited (to an extent, given the potential for their being asymptomatic and infectious). Both individuals entering a facility for the first time and those incarcerated there for a longer period should be screened. The potential for a dormant infection, such as tuberculosis, provides an additional opportunity to reduce spread. When tuberculosis is latent, infected individuals rarely transmit it, but it is still treatable. The period between infection and transmissibility allows for a robust public health intervention in a correctional setting without separating the infected individual. Other diseases with similar latent periods could be managed the same way, but this requires adequate and consistent testing *before* the disease is known to be present in a correctional setting.

Conclusion

COVID-19 will not be the last major disease to impact our correctional institutions. Between drug-resistant tuberculosis, STIs, and now COVID-19, there has been a significant concern over specific communicable diseases in corrections roughly every 15 years for the past 45 years. Their highest infection rates tend to last a while; some diseases may never disappear entirely. By taking the proper steps and applying lessons from these three diseases, we can ensure that we are better prepared for the next serious wave of disease in correctional settings, reducing its impact and potentially delaying it. Additionally, by taking preventive actions, we can reduce the transmission from prisons to society, thus curtailing the introduction or reintroduction of disease, helping to save lives, and minimizing suffering. Lastly, the applicability of these lessons extends far beyond just major disease outbreaks. It can help us ensure proper care for inmates, which also impacts the communities to which most will return.

COVID-19 was unique in that the very existence and spread of the disease became highly controversial. With other diseases, controversy tends to revolve around its treatment or prevention, such as with condom provision in prisons or needle exchange programs in general. These examples show how political arguments have historically derailed efforts to control disease, and this has been the case for COVID-19. It is important to recognize how political barriers can stymie solutions and prolong harm from a disease. There must be a strong agreement moving forward on the value of human life, even for those denied their freedom, and on preventing dangerous and damaging conditions in order to enact public health policies. There is room for debate around how we treat or prevent diseases, but at the base of these debates should at least be an acknowledgment that the disease exists and holds the potential to cause serious harm to individuals and to society.

Note

1. There is a small literature on tuberculosis from the early 2000s to the 2010s, but these studies are primarily focused on developing nations. Their direct applicability to considerations of disease spread in a wealthy nation like the United States is limited.

9. Parole Granted? COVID-19's Impact on Parole Decision-Making and Legislative Change

Angela S. Murolo

Introduction

The COVID-19 pandemic created an unsafe prison environment, where disease is well known to spread quickly. Prisons are overcrowded, making it difficult to provide adequate space for social distancing or quarantine (Hawks et al., 2020; Novisky et al., 2021; Pyrooz et al., 2020). This public health crisis has created an urgent need to reconsider what is the proper size of a prison population and who can safely return to the community. Because older people are a growing proportion of the prison population and have an increased likelihood of multiple morbidities, they are particularly vulnerable to illness and death (Binswanger et al., 2009; Loeb & Steffensmeier, 2006; National Academies, 2021; Williams & Abraldes, 2007; Williams et al., 2012). This has prompted lawmakers to seek efficient and safe ways to reduce the prison population. Compassionate release and medical or geriatric parole have been touted as an appropriate harm reduction mechanism to decrease the infirm incarcerated population, but it is scarcely utilized (The Crime Report Staff, 2022; Murolo, 2020, 2022; Riley, 2021; Tinto & Roberts, 2021). Many states, including Virginia, proposed new legislation during the pandemic to decrease time served and decrease the prison population. New legislative attempts and traditional release mechanisms, including parole, conditional release, or geriatric parole, were used to achieve this end.

The objectives of this chapter are threefold: one, to review legislative attempts by the State of Virginia to reduce the prison population during the first year of the pandemic (2020); two, to compare regular parole and geriatric conditional release (geriatric parole) decisions in 2020 compared to prior years to determine what types of inmates were released in 2020;

three, to establish how COVID-19 impacted the Virginia prison population's size and to determine whether those changes were significant. The overall goal of this study is to understand legislative and parole-based attempts to decarcerate in an effort to improve contingency plans in future public health crises and to decrease prison populations safely.

Background

Incidence and Prevalence

While preliminary research has estimated the prevalence and incidence of COVID-19 in prisons (see Equal Justice Initiative, 2021; Li et al., 2020; Marquez et al., 2021), these estimates should be viewed with caution. Early data provided by the Marshall Project found that one in five prisoners were infected with COVID-19 (The Crime Report Staff, 2021a). However, the Marshall Project also found that 43 states would not provide demographic information, including race or age, on people "tested for, diagnosed with or killed by COVID-19" (Chammah & Meagher, 2020, para. 3). One state (Kansas) released general age information, and nine state agencies did not respond to requests for information from the Marshall Project, making it incredibly difficult to understand who specifically was impacted by COVID-19 in prison and what mediations may have been needed (National Academies, 2021). However, based on what data were available, Black people were disproportionately likely to be infected with COVID-19 in Michigan, Missouri, and Vermont prisons. They were disproportionately likely to die in Michigan prisons (Chammah & Meagher, 2020).

Data collected by the COVID Prison Project indicated that as of January 27, 2021, 370,546 people in prison had contracted COVID-19 and 2,287 had died from the virus (Pettus-Davis et al., 2021). LeMasters et al. (2020) used these data to compare the infection and death rates of the prison population with those of the free-world population. They found great disparities in testing, positivity, and fatality rates in the prison population compared to the free world, with greater levels of testing and infection in the prison population.

The Marshall Project's findings have some corroboration. Researchers at the COVID Behind Bars Data Project of the University of California–Los Angeles found that data reporting for infections and deaths has waned over time and has ended in some states altogether (LeMasters et al., 2020; Ollove, 2021). Reasons for this are varied, but some states acknowledged that sharing this information with the public does not "look good" and will be "used against them"; another reason for the failure to report COVID-19 data was that doing so was deemed "not necessary" (Ollove, 2021). Interestingly, the COVID Behind Bars Data Project and the Prison Policy Initiative scored states on their level of transparency. No state scored above a C, and most states were graded D or F (Herscowitz, 2021; Ollove, 2021), signaling unknowns about the incidence and prevalence of COVID-19 infections and deaths in prison.

COVID-19 and the Aging Prison Population

Over time, the prison population has grown older and will continue to do so in the foreseeable future. In 2013, inmates over the age of 55 represented 10% of the total prison population (Carson & Sabol, 2016). By 2017, 20.3% of the state and federal prison populations were over 50, and approximately 12% were over 55 (Bronson & Carson, 2019). By 2019, 22% of the incarcerated populations in state and federal prisons were over 50, with projections indicating that, by 2030, one-third of people in prison will be over the age of 50, indicating growing health care challenges for correctional officials (Carson, 2020; Chettiar et al., 2012; West et al., 2010). As the prison population grays, the COVID-19 pandemic has shed light on the challenges of maintaining a safe and healthy environment for older and infirm prisoners.

Elderly and sick people are more likely to fall ill and die from COVID-19, especially those 65 years old and above (Li et al., 2020; Mayo Clinic Staff, 2022). This is especially true among the elderly and ill incarcerated population (Baumgartner et al., 2021; Equal Justice Initiative, 2021). Older incarcerated people have disproportionately high rates of chronic health conditions compared to younger incarcerated people and older people in the free world, making them especially vulnerable to COVID-19 (Akiyama et al., 2020; Alexander et al., 2020; Li et al., 2020; National Academies, 2021; Prost et al., 2021). While data are limited, there is some research available on rates of illness and death. Incarcerated people of all ages were infected at five times the national rate and had 2.7 times the mortality rate of nonincarcerated people during COVID-19's peak (Equal Justice Initiative, 2021; Marquez et al., 2021). By April 2021, people in prison were 3.3 times more likely to contract and 2.5 times more likely to die from COVID-19 (Marquez et al., 2021). This created a pressing need to release older people who are most at risk of illness or death (Tinto & Roberts, 2021). It is known that older people in prison are especially likely to be affected. However, information on illness and death from COVID-19 among prisoners according to age is hard to come by (Equal Justice Initiative, 2021; LeMasters et al., 2020).

Preventive Measures

According to the Centers for Disease Control and Prevention (2022c), there are many ways to protect oneself from COVID-19. Early in the pandemic, wearing a face mask, washing hands, social distancing, cleaning and disinfecting, avoiding poorly ventilated spaces, testing for COVID-19, and quarantining when the virus was contracted were the best ways to prevent the spread of infection. Later, vaccines were added to the regimen to improve protection from COVID-19. However, the very nature of prison presents problems for protecting oneself from disease (Dutheil et al., 2020). Access to personal protection equipment is restricted. The use of face masks creates security risks, and hand sanitizer has a high alcohol content, creating additional safety and security challenges in institutional settings (Liu et al., 2022; Novisky et al., 2021). At the onset of the pandemic, the resources for self-protection were in limited supply, making their distribution challenging for all populations. Unsurprisingly, social distancing is difficult, if not impossible, in overcrowded prisons (National Academies, 2021; Simpson et al., 2019).

Attempts in prisons to quell the spread of COVID-19 largely mimicked attempts to contain the illness in the free world, with great variation across states and institutions. Pettus-Davis et al. (2021) conducted interviews with 327 people incarcerated in three states to determine what strategies prisons and people in prison used to protect themselves from COVID-19. Results indicated that most people wore face masks (85%), washed their hands (84%), and socially distanced when possible (66%). In their research on 788 incarcerated people in California's jails, Liu et al. (2022) found that questionnaire respondents thought they were not getting new masks frequently enough (39%), and 33% reported receiving only one mask from March 2020 until the period under study (July 8, 2020–April 30, 2021).

Novisky et al. (2021) reviewed state and federal responses to containment strategies to prevent the spread of COVID-19. They found a range of responses to maintaining clean environments, with some states providing specific protocols and others providing vague references to cleaning. Novisky and colleagues also found that mask use across institutions was inconsistent. Some states did not allow masks for security reasons (Nevada), some states did not provide masks to the entire incarcerated population (Delaware), and some did not require the use of face masks by incarcerated populations (Oregon, Pennsylvania, South Carolina), demonstrating an inconsistent response across correctional jurisdictions. Lastly, hand sanitizer was not always available to incarcerated people because of the high alcohol content; its availability was limited to prevent its possible misuse. In many states, inmates were not allowed to use hand sanitizer that they produced (Novisky et al., 2021).

Prisons took additional steps to prevent the spread of COVID-19 by eliminating visits to incarcerated people (Akiyama et al., 2020). All correctional districts (state and federal) suspended prisoner visitation beginning in March 2020 (Novisky et al., 2021; Pettus-Davis et al., 2021). The elimination of visits was aimed at reducing contact between people inside and outside prisons, in effect socially distancing incarcerated and free people (Pettus-Davis et al., 2021). However, people in prison were also concerned about contact with correctional officers who could potentially bring COVID-19 into the prison (National Academies, 2021; Novisky et al., 2021; Pyrooz et al., 2020). To mitigate isolation and to promote the social connectedness needed to maintain prisoners' well-being, many states provided free phone calls, video visits, teleconferences, and postage stamps to help prisoners maintain connections with the outside world (Akiyama, 2020; Novisky et al., 2021).

Social distancing is necessary to prevent the transmission of communicable diseases, including COVID-19 (Esposito et al., 2022). In a systematic review, Simpson et al. (2019) found evidence supporting the association between prison cell spatial density and the transmission of communicable diseases. Although their research design has limitations, their findings are congruent with public health recommendations for social distancing as an effective measure to prevent the spread of COVID-19 (Centers for Disease Control and Prevention, 2022c). Excessive crowding in jails and prisons makes social distancing challenging, despite it being an optimal public health strategy (Akiyama et al., 2020; Cloud et al., 2020). According to the Prison Policy Initiative, during the initial phase of the pandemic, 41 states were operating at or above 75% of their capacity, and nine states and the Federal Bureau of Prisons were operating above capacity. These circumstances provided little room for social distancing in most states (Widra, 2020). However, Pyrooz et al. (2020) found that 75% of respondents housed in isolation units had reduced their risk of infection.

Testing for COVID-19 is a necessary prevention strategy inconsistently utilized during the pandemic and with wide-ranging results (Esposito et al., 2022). According to research by LeMasters et al. (2020), there was great variation in states' testing information, with some states reporting as few as 6 tests per 1,000 people (Hawaii). Ten states' prison systems reported no testing. Novisky et al. (2021) found that 35% of jurisdictions had no public information on how many people in prison were tested for COVID-19. Minnesota administered more than one test per person, and several states had tested at least half of the prison population at the time of research (LeMasters et al., 2020). Because of the wide variation in testing, positivity percentages ranged from 0% to 42%, and the smaller the proportion of those tested, the larger the positivity rate (LeMasters et al., 2020). In Ohio's Marion Correctional Institute, mass testing efforts revealed 79% of the inmate population and 35% of the prison staff were infected with COVID-19 (KhudaBukhsh et al., 2023; Simpson et al., 2021). According to Pettus-Davis et al. (2021), between 15.5% and 28.2% of participants requested testing as a preventive measure to reduce the risk of COVID-19 infection, and between 23% and 26.5% of respondents reported that correctional facilities provided information on how inmates could get tested for COVID-19. Additionally, between 30.8% and 51.5% of respondents said that correctional facilities offered testing for COVID-19.

Vaccines to protect against COVID-19 were approved for emergency use authorization on December 11, 2020, and were made available to the public beginning December 15, 2020. While availability was prioritized based on age and health risk in the free community, incarcerated people were frequently not prioritized based on their "environmental risk" (Strodel et al., 2021, p. 1). This is despite the World Health Organization's recommendation that people in prison be prioritized for vaccination (Simpson et al., 2021). Strodel et al. (2021) analyzed vaccine distribution and prioritization documents across the 50 states and the District of Columbia and found that 47% of states did not include incarcerated people in prioritized categories. Among the states that did prioritize people for vaccination based on incarceration status, 22% of them prioritized incarcerated people in phase one, 29% in phase two, and 2% in phase three. During the same period under study, 63% of states prioritized law enforcement officers, and 49% of states prioritized jail and prison workers during phase one of vaccine distribution (Strodel et al., 2021).

It is unclear how many incarcerated people have been vaccinated across the country in federal and state prisons, as states vary in the degree to which they are forthcoming with vaccination data beyond the level of the general population. According to the COVID-19 Behind Bars Data Project, many states are delaying or failing to update their public-facing COVID-19 data information, including vaccination progress, and data about correctional staff are even scarcer (Widra, 2021). However, some states, such as Virginia, Pennsylvania, and Massachusetts, provided incentives to persuade people in prisons to get vaccinated (Bozelko, 2021).

Containment Measures

Once COVID-19 has entered a community or institution, there are options for containing the disease. According to the Centers for Disease Control and Prevention (2022c), infected people should quarantine or socially isolate themselves from others. This is complicated in prison and raises ethical issues discussed below. Additionally, contact tracing was used by the Centers for Disease Control and Prevention (2002a) early in the pandemic to slow the spread of COVID-19 and contain the illness among those in close contact with the infected person. Once someone comes into contact with someone who has COVID-19, contact tracing can guide the best steps to prevent the spread of infection. Clarke et al. (2020) investigated in-prison contact tracing in Ireland. Contact tracing teams were set up in prisons with collaboration from various community-based public health agencies. Contact tracing was effectively implemented in 12 prisons, and contact tracing teams were able to identify and isolate people with COVID-19 and monitor people who had come in contact with them. This promising finding indicates COVID-19 can be contained in a prison environment.

The Centers for Disease Control and Prevention (2022d) recommends quarantining if one is exposed to or has been in close contact with someone infected with COVID-19. It further recommends self-isolating if one tests positive for the illness. However, isolation in prisons is equated with punishment (solitary confinement) and may have ethical issues associated with its use for medical purposes. Solitary confinement is known to exacerbate mental and physical health issues; the elimination of prison visits might amplify feelings of social isolation (Alexander et al., 2020; Cloud et al., 2020). Consequently, prisoner rights advocates voiced the need to avoid solitary confinement as a tool to prevent the spread of COVID-19 in prison (Cloud et al., 2020). Conversely, prisoners may fail to or choose not to report symptoms of COVID-19 to prevent isolation, thereby contributing to the spread of illness (Cloud et al., 2020).

Beyond traditional prevention and containment methods outlined by the Centers for Disease Control and Prevention (2022a, 2022c), prisons have other levers to pull for lowering the likelihood of spreading illness, including reductions in prison populations. This can take many forms, including compassionate release, parole, medical parole, or geriatric release. Before the COVID-19 pandemic, release mechanisms like compassionate release, medical parole, and geriatric parole were seldom used and failed to reduce prison populations effectively and efficiently (Murolo, 2020, 2022; Wylie et al., 2018).

Prison Population Reduction Measures

Aside from preventive and containment measures in prison, a way to decrease the spread of illness is to decarcerate (National Academies, 2021; Vella et al., 2022). Vest et al. (2021) found that prisons with less than 85% occupancy were less likely to have outbreaks and deaths from COVID-19. At the height of the pandemic, both activists and incarcerated individuals called for the increased use of compassionate release to reduce prison populations. Compassionate release is "the release of chronically ill and aging inmates prior to completing their sentence" (Wylie et al., 2018, p. 216). Compassionate release encompasses several mechanisms that address various issues related to age and illness. It typically provides the opportunity for people who have a terminal illness and are near death to return to the community for their final days (Pro & Marzell, 2017). Medical parole is also associated with "end of life and hospice care and targets persons who are incarcerated and have a terminal illness with less than six months to live" (Murolo, 2022, p. 45). Geriatric parole is a release mechanism predicated on age and time served, not on a physical illness (Maschi et al., 2015; Murolo, 2022).

Before the pandemic, compassionate release mechanisms were rarely utilized and were riddled with bureaucratic entanglements. Ethridge and White (2015) studied Texas's Medically Recommended Intensive Supervision program from 2007 to 2012. During the period under study, there was an initial increase in the number of people reviewed and approved for release under this program in 2007. However, over time, political winds shifted, and the percentage of people being approved for release had declined by approximately 58% in 2012. In 2013, Texas legislators wanted to remove an age component from the provision altogether (Ethridge & White, 2015) and preferred to focus on infirm individuals. Families Against Mandatory Minimums (2021a, 2021b) reported on the various compassionate release mechanisms and often found that less than 10% of people considered for such release had it approved (Price, 2018).

Compassionate release took on a new urgency with the rise of COVID-19 cases in prison. According to the Federal Bureau of Prisons, 30% of federal inmates tested positive for COVID-19 in 2020, indicating a need to consider compassionate release for people at the highest risk of infection (The Crime Report Staff, 2021b). The pandemic led to the approval of nearly 21% of federal-level petitions for early release, higher than the 6% of releases approved from 2013 to 2017 (The Crime Report Staff, 2021b). However, there were great disparities in the results of motions to release relative to the location of federal courts, facts of the case, and when motions were filed. Tolan (2021) indicated that most approvals for compassionate release occurred early in the pandemic (early to mid-2020) but waned over time. This is consistent with the findings of Miller, Martin, and Topaz (2022) on jail releases in New York City during the pandemic. Many advocates for compassionate release argued that this does not go far enough to address the sick and elderly in prison (Alexander et al., 2020; Brobst, 2021; Tinto & Roberts, 2020). Furthermore, Brobst (2021) argued that decisions on compassionate release focused on public safety risk instead of other variables like community impact, victim impact, or prisoner health, which effectively puts prisoners at risk of illness or death (Riley, 2021).

Virginia's Release Mechanisms

Virginia abolished parole in 1995 as part of the "truth in sentencing" movement, making anyone convicted of a crime after January 1, 1995, ineligible for parole (Murolo, 2022; Virginia Department of Corrections, 2011). However, geriatric conditional release was an exception to this rule, which provided a release mechanism for the aging prison population (Dujardin, 2017; Murolo, 2022). According to Virginia statute § 53.1–40.1, any elderly person who was not convicted of a Class 1 felony could apply for conditional release if the person was at least 60 years old and had served a minimum of 10 years or was 65 years old and had served a minimum of 5 years. Due to low release numbers under this statute and the rapid growth of the aging correctional population, in 2013 the Virginia Finance Subcommittee examined the impact of releasing older offenders (Chiu, 2010; Virginia Parole Board, 2013). Based on estimated savings from releasing older people, the State Budget Bill of 2014 required all "truth in sentencing" geriatric inmates to have an automatic parole board review starting on July 14, 2014 (Murolo, 2022). Prior to this, people wishing to be considered for geriatric conditional release had to apply for consideration and would not be considered if they were applying for discretionary parole at the same time (Virginia Parole Board, 2014).

Research by Murolo (2022) investigated the impact of this policy change. With publicly available data from the Virginia Parole Board's website, geriatric parole decisions before and after the statute change were analyzed to understand how this policy change impacted parole releases and the elderly prison population in Virginia. Results indicated that geriatric parole reviews and releases increased after the statute change but were not statistically significant. Importantly, the elderly prison population increased during the period under study (2013–2018). Those increases *were* significant, indicating that the requirement that all elderly people eligible for geriatric conditional release should have a hearing was hardly effective at reducing the aging prison population. Because of this, it is important to investigate how COVID-19 further impacted attempts to reduce the elderly prison population in Virginia.

Theoretical Frameworks

One of the principles of punishment is incapacitation, or removing people from society so they can no longer commit crimes (Blumstein, 1983). Based on what is understood about crime and recidivism, it is expected that most people will reoffend and return to prison, so incarceration is also preventive in nature (Seiter, 2008). As Brobst (2021) points out, this notion of selective incapacitation to ensure public safety indicates how courts and parole boards have reacted to compassionate release during the COVID-19 era. Both may fear an uptick in violence and crime, and therefore they may see no upside to releasing people from prison regardless of inmate health concerns (Murolo, 2022).

Conversely, the initial push to release people from prison during the pandemic can be viewed from a harm reduction perspective. Harm reduction principles were initially applied to users of injected drugs to prevent the spread of HIV/AIDS (Roe, 2005). Community-based organizations provided drug paraphernalia to users of injected drugs, which was used as a work-around to prevent the spread of illness while violating what many considered unfair laws. Those viewing harm reduction from a critical perspective argue that harm reduction as a preventive practice should be a "platform for broader structural social change" (Roe, 2005, p. 244). Specifically, Miller (2001) argues that harm reduction allows "society to continue causing harm to individuals without accepting responsibility for or acknowledging the social, legal and economic source of those harms" (quoted in Roe, 2005, p. 245).

The Current Study

Some may argue that compassionate release is the harm reduction band-aid of mass incarceration that fails to address the need for broader structural reform of criminal justice and is a tool to exert further control over the correctional population (Mugford, 1993). In this view, "true harm reduction" would come from changing sentencing policies that will make compassionate release less necessary. It is from the perspective of selective incapacitation and compassionate release that this study investigates the following questions:

Research Question 1: What were the legislative attempts made in Virginia to reduce the prison population during COVID-19, and what was the outcome of those attempts?

Research Question 2: Did the use of regular and geriatric parole during the first year of the pandemic increase compared with previous years?

Research Question 3: Were prison population changes during 2020 significant?

Data

This study used publicly available data from multiple sources. To answer RQ1, transcripts were obtained from Virginia's Legislative Information System (LIS), a searchable database that provides access to legislative bills and codified laws (https://lis.virginia.gov). To answer RQ2, regular parole and geriatric conditional release data were obtained from the Virginia Parole Board website.[1] Each record in this dataset represents one individual hearing. The sample for these analyses consists of 23,391 regular parole and geriatric conditional release hearings.

To answer RQ3, prison population data were obtained from multiple publicly available sources on the Virginia Department of Corrections website. Prison population data from 2013 to 2019 were obtained from the Virginia Department of Corrections "Offender Population Trends" reports (2011–2015, 2015–2019).[2] Prison population data for 2020–2021 were obtained from the Virginia Department of Corrections website.[3] The institutional average prison populations were used to calculate prison populations from year to year.

Methods

A multi-methods approach was taken to understand this issue holistically. To answer RQ1, a content analysis of legislation considered during the COVID-19 period (2020) was conducted to determine the parameters of legislation and its potential impact. A search using LIS was conducted for 2020 to find legislation that would decarcerate the prison population in Virginia. A manual search of related bills and resolutions was conducted by subject, focusing on prisons and other correction methods. This led to 14 proposed bills in 2020 Special Session 1 and to 37 proposed bills in the 2020 Session. To determine whether the legislation was appropriate for this analysis, documents were uploaded into a Word document, and the key-in-word context method was used based on the following search terms: medical, geriatric, parole, public health, COVID-19, release, credits, and conditional release. The search terms were selected based on prior literature on this topic. Key-in-word context provides the opportunity to review words in the context of sentences to understand the variation of meaning of the word(s), as well as whether the meaning of words is dependent on their use in phrases or idioms (Weber, 1990, p. 44).[4] After data gathering, the sources were searched for key terms to make meaning of themes across the legislation. Ultimately, there were 13 relevant bills up for review during the 2020 Session and the 2020 Special Session. Four legislative bills and documents that were passed and relevant to this research were analyzed, namely, HB33, SB5018, SB5034, and HB5148.

To answer RQ2, parole decision data were gathered for the same period under study to understand whether COVID-19 impacted parole decisions. Using both regular parole and geriatric conditional release decisions provided a greater understanding of who was granted release under both mechanisms during the first year of the COVID-19 pandemic. Finally, to answer RQ3, prison population data from 2013 to 2021 were analyzed to determine if the change in the prison population was significant for 2020. Descriptive statistics were used to understand who among the incarcerated were released during the pandemic. A two-sample proportions z-test determined whether the changes from 2013–2019 (before the pandemic) and 2020 (year one of the pandemic) were significant by testing whether the proportions of the two groups were the same or significantly different (Ritchey, 2000).

Results

Legislation

The appendix summarizes all the legislative bills considered during the study period. With the use of key-in-word context, 13 bills were related to the research terms. Four bills were passed in 2020. The first bill (HB33) expanded access to parole by addressing the Supreme Court of Virginia's decision in *Fishback v. Commonwealth*, which held that because juries were not instructed that parole was abolished in Virginia, people still incarcerated on July 1, 2020, who had committed a felony on or after 1995 would be eligible for parole consideration. However, there are eligibility exceptions based on the nature of their offenses, including Class 1 felonies (first-degree and capital murder), a victim who was a minor, offenses sexual in nature, or with "carnal knowledge."

The second bill (SB5018) was passed during the 2020 Special Session as an amendment for the conditional release of terminally ill prisoners. The bill defines terminally ill as "having a chronic or progressive medical condition caused by injury, disease, or illness where the medical prognosis is the person's death within 12 months." There are exceptions to eligibility based on the nature of offenses, including Class 1 felonies, sexual offenses, kidnapping, felonious assault, lynching, stalking, and several other felony offenses.

The third bill to pass during the pandemic was SB5034, which also considered terminally ill prisoners. SB5034 and the fourth bill to pass (HB5148) created a "four-level classification system for the awarding and calculation of earned sentence credits" in addition to the consideration of conditional release for a terminal illness. Both SB5034 and HB5148 allow research through a "work group" to study the impact of earned sentence credits, with a report to be submitted to the governor.

The passage of the four bills described above indicates an increased willingness to provide the possibility of parole. However, there are limitations, based on the offense, on who can be considered for release. These changes can be viewed from both a harm reduction and selective incapacitation standpoint. The state chose to continue to selectively incapacitate those convicted of the most serious felonies. The state also employed a harm reduction strategy to expand consideration of parole and compassionate release. By employing a work group strategy, the state is considering how this legislation will impact public safety and how the use of compassionate release mechanisms can reduce harm.

Prison Population Changes over Time

Table 9.1 displays changes in the prison population over time. To answer RQ2, yearly average prison populations were reviewed from 2013 to 2021. Results indicate that the prison population remained relatively stable from 2013 to 2019, with the biggest increase in the prison population occurring from 2013 to 2014 and the biggest decrease occurring from 2015–2016. The prison population increased by 112 people from years 2013–2019. The prison population decreased by 2,701 people from 2019 to 2020 and 3,065 from 2020 to 2021. The two-sample z-test of proportions indicates that the differences between 2013–2019 and 2020–2021 institutional average prison populations are statistically significant ($z = 109.32, p = 0.000$), whereby the prison population decreased significantly during COVID-19.

Table 9.1 Virginia Prison Population Changes

Year	Institutional average prison population	Year-to-year change in population	Change in population during study periods
2013	29,883		
2014	30,342	+495	
2015	30,326	−16	
2016	30,101	−225	
2017	30,049	−52	
2018	29,959	−90	
2019	29,995	+36	+112*
2020	27,294	−2,701	
2021	24,229	−3,065	−3,065**

* Difference from 2013 to 2019
** Difference from 2020 to 2021
Differences between 2013–2019 and 2020–2021: $z = 109.31768, p = 0.000$

Unfortunately, broader demographic data on the prison population during 2020 and 2021 are not currently available. The Virginia Department of Corrections publishes Offender Population Reports, but data are provided only up to 2019 (https://vadoc.virginia.gov). Greater transparency for current data would provide an understanding of specifically who was released during the pandemic beyond parole release data.

Parole Decisions

Descriptive statistics were generated to determine if the COVID-19 era impacted parole decisions, and the percentage and rate of release were calculated and compared before and after COVID-19 (Table 9.2). The percentage of people paroled for 2013–2019 was 7.11% and increased to 10.34% during COVID-19 (2020). The release rate for 2013–2019 was 232 people released per year, which increased to 249 people released on parole in 2020. The two-sample z-test of proportions indicates that the differences between 2013–2019 and 2019–2021 parole release approvals were statistically significant ($z = -5.684$, $p = 0.000$), whereby the percentage of people paroled increased significantly during COVID-19.

Table 9.2 Virginia Parole Decisions

Years	Total parole decisions	Parole granted (n)	Parole granted (%)
2013–2019	19,357	1,376	7.11%
2020	2,409	249	10.34%

Differences between 2013–2019 and 2019–2021: $z = -5.684$, $p = 0.000$

If we consider parole decisions by type separately (regular and geriatric), more people were granted parole through both release mechanisms during the COVID-19 period, and four people were released through dual eligibility consideration (Table 9.3). Releases through regular parole increased from 6.63% approved before the pandemic to 9.86% during the first year of the pandemic. The two-sample z-test of proportions indicates that the differences between 2013–2019 and 2019–2021 parole release approvals are statistically significant ($z = -4.9$, $p < 0.00001$), whereby the percentage of people released through regular parole increased significantly during the COVID-19 period. Releases for geriatric conditional release (geriatric parole) also increased during the first year of the pandemic. Geriatric parole approvals increased from 5.82% approved before the pandemic to

Table 9.3 Virginia Parole Decisions by Type

Panel A

Years	Type of review	Total parole decisions	Parole granted (n)	Parole granted (%)
2013–2019	Regular	17,635	1,170	6.63%
2020	Regular	1,845	178*	9.86%

Differences between 2013–2019 and 2019–2021: $z = -4.9$, $p < 0.00001$
*Four people were dual eligible

Panel B

Years	Type of review	Total parole decisions	Parole granted (n)	Parole granted (%)
2013–2019	Geriatric	3,060	178	5.82%
2020	Geriatric	924	67	7.25%

Differences between 2013–2019 and 2019–2021: $z = 43.4$, $p = 0.000$

7.25% during the first year of the pandemic. The two-sample z-test of proportions indicates that the differences between 2013–2019 and 2019–2021 parole release approvals were statistically significant ($z = 43.4$, $p = 0.000$), whereby the percentage of people released through geriatric parole increased significantly during COVID-19.

Table 9.4 displays the demographic variables of those released in 2020 under regular parole and geriatric conditional release. Males accounted for most regular ($n = 177$, 99.4%) and geriatric ($n = 61$, 91%) releases. Among those who were released under regular parole, 78% of released incarcerated individuals were Black, with an average age of 53 years old (standard deviation = 12.57, range = 18–79). People who were released through the geriatric conditional release provision had an average age of 65 (standard deviation = 4.85, range = 60–83). Therefore, demographic data indicate that a predominantly male African American population over age 50 returned to the community in 2020.

Discussion

Initial legislative efforts in Virginia to reduce the prison population during the pandemic were ambitious, but only a handful of bills were passed. The bills passed allowed for greater consideration of whom could be reviewed

Table 9.4 Virginia Parole Approvals in 2020—Demographics

Parolees	n / %	Mean age	SD	Age range
Regular releases	178*	53	12.56833	18–79
Male	177 / 99.4%			
Female	1 / 0.06%			
Race				
Black	139 / 78%			
White	39 / 22%			
Geriatric releases	67	65	4.84719	60–83
Male	61 / 91%			
Female	6 / 9%			
Race				
Black	44 / 65.7%			
White	22 / 32.8%			
Asian / Pacific Islander	1 / 1.5%			

* Four persons were dual eligible
SD = standard deviation

for parole, compassionate release, or earned sentence credits. However, all the bills had exceptions based on the crime committed, notably limiting who would have a chance to be released. This is consistent with selective incapacitation and legislators' concern that people who commit felonies are an ongoing risk to society, regardless of age or assessed likelihood of reoffending. Additionally, the bills passed are open to the critique leveled at harm reduction. That is, the bills passed reduce harm to older people in prison but fail to address broader structural issues. Because the bills were written so narrowly, they cannot adequately address mass incarceration in Virginia and continue to inflict harm or false hope of early release.

The results of analyzing the parole data indicate that there was a statistically significant increase in both regular and geriatric parole during the first year of the pandemic. This may be comforting to some. However, less than 10% of people were released through parole, which is consistent with prior research on geriatric release and medical parole

(Families Against Mandatory Minimums, 2021a, 2021b; Price, 2018). The results of parole releases also support selective incapacitation and critical harm reduction perspectives. According to Roe (2005), harm reduction principles were initially accepted even though they circumvented the law because they "reduced the medical and political burden on the state and divert certain segments of the drug-using population out of the legal system" (p. 247). Considering the high cost of incarcerating an elderly prison population, it is not likely a coincidence that most parole approvals diverted this segment of the population out of prison. However, with the vast number of crime-type exceptions that limit eligibility for release, this measure does not effect real change. Admittedly, though, reducing the elderly prison population will reduce the number of a prison's most vulnerable demographic during a public health crisis. Having complete prison population data would provide a clearer sense of whether parole adequately reduced the aging population or if it continued to grow as it had in the past (Murolo, 2022). Lastly, there was a significant reduction in the prison population beyond parole releases, signaling that the earned sentence credit bill may have had a bigger influence on prison populations than parole release mechanisms.

Limitations

The data and research presented in this chapter include several limitations that should be acknowledged. Publicly available data provide a sense of transparency and an opportunity for "secondary analysis that is replicable, efficient and affordable" (Murolo, 2022, p. 45). However, data for this study were obtained from multiple sources, providing an opportunity for inconsistencies or missing information. For example, prison population data were obtained from two sources. For 2013–2018, data were obtained from "State Responsible Offender Population Trends" for fiscal years 2011–2019, which provides age, sex, and race data (Virginia Department of Corrections, 2017, 2020a). However, prison population data for the years 2020 and 2021 were obtained from "Monthly Population Summaries," which provide no demographic information (Virginia Department of Corrections, 2020b, 2021), making it difficult to ascertain how parole releases impacted the overall prison population during COVID-19. Murolo's (2022) research on geriatric release determined that the elderly population continued to grow while efforts were made to review more people for geriatric conditional release, which was not possible to determine in this study based on currently available data. Parole decision data should also be reviewed with caution. The Virginia Parole Board releases monthly parole decisions; however, a supplemental file was added to the board's website that included missing parole decisions from 2012 to 2017 that were not initially contained in posted monthly parole decisions. Additionally, there are minimal reasons provided for parole denials or information on crimes committed.

Policy Implications

Several policy implications should be considered to improve responses to public health emergencies and to address the failings of criminal justice policy. First, states should have an emergency plan for public health crises and pandemics. According to research by Henry and Wachtendorf (2020), parole policies in Texas, Louisiana, and Florida failed to provide guidance on how parolees should respond to parole-based concerns during emergencies, leaving many parolees in violation of parole. Planning for public health emergencies should begin in prison and continue when one is released on parole. That is where community support and wrap-around services are necessary for the continuance of care, especially among the over-50 incarcerated and paroled population (Bedard et al., 2022; Murolo, 2022). State departments of corrections should build collaborative relationships with public service providers to ensure a seamless transition from prison to community.

Legislatively, the "abolition of parole" should be abolished. Virginia is trying to pursue a harm reduction model of parole where the state continues to increase the number of incarcerated individuals eligible for release through geriatric conditional release due to the ruling in *Fishback v. Commonwealth*, but this is a tepid response to the larger issue. Parole should be a consideration regardless of the crime; the fact that this is not possible reflects a limited understanding of the age-crime curve and recidivism rates among people convicted of homicide. The relationship between age and cessation of criminal activity is well established (Farrington, 1986). While Virginia's effort to decrease the elderly population was statistically significant, parole approvals were still less than 10% of the reviewed population. Additionally, data indicate that people convicted of homicide are the least likely to reoffend (La Vigne, 2021). Providing no option for parole among this population fails to provide the opportunity for rehabilitation and motivation to participate in prison programs that provide an avenue to parole.

Many advocates and scholars called for increased use of compassionate release during the pandemic (Nowotny et al., 2020; Simpson & Butler, 2020; Tinto & Roberts, 2020). Clearly, compassionate release was designed to be a harm reduction tool to mitigate the harm of prisons on older people, and that is the problem. A true harm reduction model would put limits on incarceration terms as suggested by The Sentencing Project (Mauer, 2016) and put into practice in prisons in places like Norway and Sweden, where incarceration is used as a tool to separate and reform, not to take revenge (Montross, 2021). Having release mechanisms like compassionate release "reduces the incentive to fundamentally change damaging policies" (Roe, 2005, p. 247).

Conclusion

Because of the scope of the pandemic, prison population reduction was the primary prevention goal among Virginia's legislators, corrections officials, and the parole board. Virginia successfully reduced prison populations during this period, with many limitations on who could be considered for sentence reduction measures. However, many people were sent to prison for technical violations, and there is no clear indicator that the elderly population was significantly reduced (Ollove, 2021). Furthermore, the prison population has since grown between 2021 and 2023, indicating that any changes were temporary. As pandemic fatigue sets in and crime rates rise, prison officials are less willing to release people solely based on pandemic status, and many are being returned to prison for minor parole violations (The Crime Report Staff, 2021b, 2022; Johnson, 2022). However, research on the federal level indicates that of 11,000 people released during COVID-19, only 17 individuals reoffended (Gill, 2022). This indicates that more can be done to reduce prison populations while protecting public safety. Releasing people during the pandemic was a harm reduction measure, but these necessary strategies for protecting health create an opportunity to implement broader structural change (Roe, 2005).

Appendix

Table 9.5 Virginia Proposed Legislation (2020 Session, 2020 Special Session)

Legislative code	Description of bill*	Status	Key terms
HB33/SB793/SB821	Parole; exception to limitation on the application of parole statutes. Provides that a person is eligible to be considered for parole if (i) such person was sentenced by a jury prior to the date of the Supreme Court of Virginia decision in *Fishback v. Commonwealth*, 260 Va. 104 (June 9, 2000), in which the Court held that a jury should be instructed on the fact that parole has been abolished, for a felony committed on or after the abolition of parole going into effect (on January 1, 1995); (ii) the person remained incarcerated for the offense on July 1, 2020; and (iii) the offense was not one of the following: (a) a Class 1 felony; (b) if the victim was a minor, rape, forcible sodomy, object sexual penetration, or aggravated sexual battery or an attempt to commit such act; or (c) carnal knowledge. The bill also requires the Parole Board to establish procedures for consideration of parole of persons entitled to it and also provides that any person who is eligible for parole as of July 1, 2020, shall be scheduled for a parole interview no later than July 1, 2021, allowing for extension of time for reasonable cause.	Passed April 22, 2020, identical to SB793/SB821	parole
HB281	Prisoners; medical care. Eliminates the Department of Corrections prisoner co-payment program for nonemergency health care services.	2/7/20 Passed House	medical
HB431	Provides that any person serving a sentence imposed upon a conviction for a felony offense, other than a Class 1 felony, (i) who has reached the age of 65 and older and who has served at least 15 years of the sentence imposed or (ii) is 50 years of age or older and has	02/11/20 House: Left in Public Safety	conditional release, geriatric, prisoners, parole

Table 9.5 (continued)

Legislative code	Description of bill*	Status	Key terms
	served at least 20 years of the sentence imposed may petition the parole board for conditional release.		
HB915	Allows any person serving a sentence imposed upon a conviction for a felony offense, other than a Class 1 felon, who (i) is 55 years of age or older and has served at least 15 years of the sentence imposed or (ii) is 50 years of age or older and has served at least 20 years of the sentence imposed to petition the parole board for conditional release.	01/31/20 House: Continued to 2021 in Courts of Justice by voice vote	conditional release, geriatric, prisoners, parole
HB1224	Prohibits persons serving a sentence imposed upon a conviction of murder in the first degree or a sexually violent offense, if the offense resulting in such conviction occurred on or after July 1, 2020, from petitioning the Parole Board for conditional release. Under current law, such persons may petition the Parole Board when such persons reach age 65 and have served at least five years of their sentence or reach age 60 and have served at least 10 years of their sentence. The prohibition does not apply to any person who is serving a life sentence for any crime other than homicide and who was under the age of 18 at the time of the commission of the offense.	01/31/20 House: Continued to 2021 in Courts of Justice by voice vote	conditional release, geriatric, prisoners, parole
HB1370/HB1532	Rate at which sentence credits may be earned. Increases the maximum number of sentence credits that may be earned by a person convicted of any felony that is not a violent felony, committed on or after January 1, 1995, from four and one-half credits for each 30 days served to 10.5 credits for each 30 days served.	02/05/20 House: Incorporated by Courts of Justice (HB1523-credits Scott) by voice vote	credits
SB91	Application of parole statutes. Repeals the abolition of parole. The bill also provides that the Virginia Parole Board shall establish procedures for consideration of parole for persons who were previously	02/03/20 Senate: Continued to 2021 in Judiciary (15-Y O-N)	parole

Table 9.5 (continued)

Legislative code	Description of bill*	Status	Key terms
	ineligible for parole, because parole was abolished, to allow for an extension of time for reasonable cause.		
HB5016†	Application of parole statutes for juveniles and persons committed upon felony offenses committed on or after January 1, 1995. Repeals the abolition of parole. The bill also provides that the Virginia Parole Board shall establish procedures for consideration of parole for persons who were previously ineligible for parole, because parole was abolished, to allow for an extension of time for reasonable cause.	08/26/20 Senate: *Passed by indefinitely* in Judiciary with letter (14-Y 0-N)	parole
SB5018†	Provides that any person serving a sentence imposed upon a conviction for a felony offense, other than those enumerated in the bill as exceptions to eligibility and who is terminally ill as defined in the bill is eligible for consideration by the Parole Board for conditional release.	Passed October 28, 2020	terminally ill, conditional release, parole
HB5035†	Any person serving a sentence imposed upon a conviction for a felony offense, other than (1) a Class 1 felony: (i) if the offense was committed on or after January 1, 2021, murder in the first degree in violation of §18.2–32; or (11) if the offense was committed on or after January 1, 2021, a sexually violent offense as defined in §37.2–900, (i) (a) who has reached the age of 65 or older and who has served at least five years of the sentence imposed or (II) (b) who has reached the age of 60 or older and who has served at least ten 10 years of the sentence imposed may petition the Parole Board for conditional release. The exclusion set forth in clause (II) shall not apply to any person who is serving a life sentence for any crime other than homicide and who was under the age of	11/9/2020 Left in Court of Justice	conditional release, geriatric prisoners

Table 9.5 (continued)

Legislative code	Description of bill*	Status	Key terms
	18 at the time of the commission of the offense. The Parole Board shall promulgate regulations to implement the provisions of this section. 2. That the provisions of this act may result in a net increase in periods of imprisonment or commitment. (The prohibition does not apply to any person who is serving a life sentence for any crime other than homicide and who was under the age of 18 at the time of the commission of the offense.)		
SB5034†	Release of prisoners. Provides that any person serving a sentence imposed upon a conviction for a felony offense other than those enumerated in the bill as exceptions to eligibility and who is terminally ill as defined in the bill is eligible for consideration by the Parole Board for conditional release.	Passed 11/9/2020	terminally ill, prisoners, conditional release, credits
SB5103	Eligibility for parole; murder. Provides that any person convicted of murder where the location of the body of the victim is unknown and the Parole Board has probable cause to believe that such person convicted has information concerning the location of the body is not eligible for parole. The bill contains technical amendments.	08/24/20 Senate: *Passed by indefinitely* in Rehabilitation and Social Services (8-Y 6-N)	parole
HB5148†	Establishes a four-level classification system for the awarding and calculation of earned sentence credits. The bill also specifies certain crimes that are subject to the maximum 30 days served that is permitted under current law. The bill provides that the Department of Corrections shall convene a work group to study the impact of the sentence credit amendments in the act.	Passed. The remainder of the bill is delayed, effective date of July 1, 2022, and requires the calculation of earned sentence credits to apply retroactively to the entire sentence of any	earned sentence credits

Table 9.5 (continued)

Legislative code	Description of bill*	Status	Key terms
		inmate who is confined in a state correctional facility and participating in the earned sentence credit system on July 1, 2022.	

* Text excerpts from bills on Virginia's Legislative Information System
† Bill up for review in Special Session 1

Notes

1. "The [Virginia Parole Board] provides monthly parole board decisions for regular and geriatric conditional release reviews, as well as decisions related to revocation hearings and violation hearings" (Murolo, 2022, pp. 44–45). Five years of downloadable files are available by month, including data for the current year. Data provided by the VPB includes demographic variables, "case type (regular parole and geriatric conditional release, etc.), decision date, decision (grant / not grant), and reasons for parole not granted" (Murolo, 2022, p. 45). Administrative data for January 1, 2013–December 31, 2020 (including a supplemental file that provided prior missing parole review decisions) from the website of the Virginia Parole Board were included in this study. Data before January 1, 2013, do not include type of parole decision and therefore were not included in the study. For this study, both regular parole and geriatric conditional release reviews were examined.

2. The "State Responsible Offender Population Trends" reports provide Department of Corrections' daily average populations of offenders for the fiscal year (July 1– June 30).

3. "Monthly Population Summary" reports were downloaded for the months of June 2020 and 2021, which is the end of the fiscal year.

4. By using key-in-word context, one can determine whether the words used agree with the operationalization of the terms used to decipher relevant legislation.

10. Stress and Well-Being: Assessing the Impact of COVID-19 on Community Supervision Officers

Lucas Alward, Ashley Lockwood, Holly Macleod,
Sarah Ackerman, and Jill Viglione

Introduction

Community supervision is the largest arm of the United States correctional system, with approximately 3.74 million adults in the United States under some form of community supervision at year-end of 2021 (Kaeble, 2023). The genesis of community supervision stems from a "helping" role rooted in a belief that not all individuals convicted of a crime should be incarcerated (Petersilia, 1997). Today, individuals under supervision must adhere to a set of guidelines and requirements (i.e., conditions) typically imposed by the court or a parole board (Petersilia, 1997). Traditional conditions of supervision include reporting to the supervisor's office, drug and alcohol monitoring, location and behavioral monitoring, appearing in court, and avoiding new criminal behavior. Supervised clients may also be required to adhere to special conditions such as attending work and treatment programs, paying restitution, undergoing electronic monitoring, and obeying curfews (Klingele, 2013).

To manage clients in the community, probation and parole officers (PPOs) are tasked with job demands that include monitoring behavior and providing assistance and support to those on their caseload (Gayman & Bradley, 2013). Over time, expectations and associated roles of PPOs have evolved, often attributed to the job's complexity and shifting ideologies (Hsieh et al., 2015). Historically, there has been tension in defining the responsibilities and goals of supervision officers and over whether the focus should be on public safety or the treatment of clients (Skeem & Manchak, 2008). Over the last decade, efforts to reimagine community supervision through adopting evidence-based practices have resulted in revised roles of PPOs that integrate law enforcement, rehabilitation, and behavioral change goals (Taxman, 2008).

With the push for community correction agencies to implement principles of effective intervention, PPOs must fulfill an increased number of job roles and demands (White et al., 2015), such as monitoring clients' adherence to supervision requirements, conducting validated risk/needs assessments, and providing effective interventions (i.e., cognitive behavioral therapies) (Andrews & Dowden, 2006; Gendreau et al., 2010). While job demands have changed over time, PPOs have always been responsible for ensuring that individuals on their caseload do not present a threat to public safety. The strategies for achieving that goal have waxed and waned over time between focusing on functions that punish and monitor and those that rehabilitate and assist. The work has involved in-person interactions between the PPO and the client in the office and in the community (e.g., home visits). The onset of the COVID-19 pandemic introduced immediate challenges to this traditional structure of community supervision, limiting the ability of agencies to conduct business as usual.

Impact of COVID-19 on
Community Supervision Work

The COVID-19 pandemic quickly resulted in changes to the way PPOs approached their job. The pandemic and associated mitigation strategies (e.g., social distancing requirements) that began in March of 2020 forced some probation and parole departments to close their doors completely, decreasing their face-to-face contact with clients (Marcum, 2020; Schwalbe & Koetzle, 2021; Viglione et al., 2021). Officers across the country had to discontinue physical check-ins with their clients to practice social distancing, and new agency-enforced protocols shifted check-ins to a virtual platform (e.g., videoconferencing or telephone visits) (Marcum, 2020; Schwalbe & Koetzle, 2021; Viglione & Nguyen, 2022). The shift to virtual supervision contact was a major change in how community supervision is traditionally conducted. Both within the United States and internationally, supervision agencies reported that the ability to leverage technology to continue supervising clients allowed them to maintain contact and relationships with clients during the pandemic (Galleguillos et al., 2022; Schwalbe & Koetzle, 2021; Viglione et al., 2021), while one study found PPOs believed they lost personal connections with their clients (Phillips et al., 2021). Additionally, PPOs reported that the use of virtual contact was less disruptive to their clients and their prosocial networks (e.g., work and family) (Schwalbe & Koetzle, 2021).

One major challenge that agency directors reported was the inability to hold clients accountable when they were not in compliance with their supervision conditions (Lockwood et al., 2023; Viglione et al., 2021). As one example, Ainslie and colleagues (2023) examined the impact of COVID-19 on community sanctions in England and Wales and revealed that proceedings for formal breaches or supervision violations were halted altogether during the initial lockdown in March 2020. This resulted from multiple factors: court backlogs, courts not prioritizing violation hearings, limited space in jails, inability to utilize warrants, and lack of drug testing (Nunphong et al., 2023; Rapisarda & Byrne, 2021; Viglione et al., 2021). As a result, agency directors reported that they and their staff were unable to do a key part of their jobs. They noted concerns over public safety and client well-being (e.g., concerns for drug overdose). In a study of Texas PPOs for adults and juveniles, the officers reported that agency policies changed quickly throughout the pandemic, making it challenging for them to adjust to any one strategy (Martin & Zettler, 2022).

Research on the effects of the pandemic on PPOs is still accumulating, but existing research suggests that officers were subject to drastic and frequent changes to their job expectations. As the pandemic brought about unforeseen, paradigmatic changes to how supervision officers fulfilled their responsibilities, several studies noted how PPOs adapted to such changing circumstances. A qualitative study by Phillips and colleagues (2021) revealed how probation staff felt alone and unable to support their colleagues while working from home. Additionally, they found PPOs struggled to balance family and home life with work as they had to take care of their children while engaging in remote learning and completing their job duties. These findings were largely echoed by Norman and colleagues (2021) in their qualitative analysis of community parole officers in Canada. For instance, thematic results indicated that alterations to work routines, such as work-from-home policies, introduced new stressors, including balancing supervision duties and childcare responsibilities, especially as most schools and day cares were closed. Similarly, Martin and Zettler (2022) found that 30% of PPOs reported feeling overwhelmed with their current workload and frequent changes in supervision practices, and they reported decreases in their productivity.

Given the pandemic's notable impacts to date (e.g., changes in contact standards, use of technology, changes in responses to noncompliance) in conjunction with the fact that PPOs' traditional work expectations have not changed (e.g., public safety), more research is needed to understand the experiences of PPOs throughout the pandemic and its impacts on their well-being and job stress. Job stress refers to "the response people may have when presented with work demands and pressures that are not matched to their knowledge and abilities and which challenge their ability to cope" (Leka et al., 2003, p. 3). Job stress among correctional workers occurs because of job-related anxiety and frustration, often in response to negative stimuli or role stressors (Griffin et al., 2010; Lambert et al., 2015). Research on stress among PPOs has highlighted several organizational job-related factors, including high caseloads, large amounts of paperwork, and the challenge of meeting unexpected and often unreasonable deadlines, as being major antecedents to PPO job stress (Finn & Kuck, 2005; Simmons et al. 1997). Additionally, when PPOs felt limited in assisting their clients, they often experienced greater job stress (Studt, 1972). Heightened job stress can result in negative health outcomes: for example, higher blood pressure and increased rates of depression (Gayman & Bradley, 2013; Gould et al., 2013; Ricciardelli et al., 2020), greater family conflict and marital problems (Obidoa et al., 2011), increased turnover (Lee et al., 2009; Simmons et al., 1997), and burnout (Gayman & Bradley, 2013; Lambert et al., 2015). Research on PPOs found higher job stress was linked to post-traumatic stress disorder, turnover intent, and reduced life satisfaction (Gayman & Bradley, 2012; Lewis et al., 2013; White et al., 2015). In addition, burnout can negatively impact an employee's willingness to engage in their work or to make an effort, potentially compromising organizational effectiveness (Salyers et al., 2015).

This chapter explores how PPOs experienced well-being and job stress during the COVID-19 pandemic.

Methods

Data Collection

Data for this study are part of a larger, longitudinal project designed to examine how community correction agencies responded to the COVID-19 pandemic. A key component of this study focused on examining PPOs' experiences working during the pandemic. (For a full description of project methodology, see Viglione et al. [2021].) Three waves of data were collected, including self-reported survey responses of community supervision agency administrators and qualitative interviews with PPOs from across the United States. The current analysis draws from interview data collected during wave one of the study, which occurred from July through November 2020. The interviews focused on PPOs' experiences at work during the pandemic, including assisting clients, monitoring and responding to noncompliance, and the impact of COVID-19 on their personal and professional well-being. The interview protocol primarily consisted of open-ended questions developed specifically for this study and several closed-ended validated measures to assess PPO well-being and mental health. Participants were asked to reflect on the strategies and techniques they used to help manage feelings of stress and burnout and whether their respective agencies had implemented policies to improve officer well-being.

Recruitment of PPOs for participation in the qualitative interviews occurred in several stages. Community correction administrators who completed the electronic survey component of this project were asked to share a flyer for interview recruitment with officers in their agency. In total, 57 agency directors agreed to share the flyer with their staff along with an electronic link to schedule an interview. In response, 49 PPOs signed up to participate in interviews. Seven PPOs were excluded from the study because they had no active supervision caseload, resulting in a final sample of 42 PPOs. Interviews were conducted over the telephone and were not recorded. Instead, interviewers used the "jotting" method to compile field notes directly onto the interval protocol while focusing on building rapport with respondents (Emerson et al., 2001). The interviewers tried to record exact quotations during the interviews. Immediately following each interview, the interviewers reviewed and expanded on the field notes. On average, the interviews lasted 76 minutes, ranging from 50 to 131 minutes.

Sample

Of the 42 PPOs who participated, the majority supervised adults (90%) and had an average caseload of 71 individuals. Approximately 55% of the PPOs indicated they supervised at least one special population (e.g., mental health). Most of the sample identified as female (67%) and white (88%) and were, on average, 43 years old. Over half of the sample held a bachelor's degree (60%), while 33% had completed a master's degree. See Table 10.1 for descriptive statistics on the participants.

Table 10.1 Characteristics of the Sample (N = 42)

Variable	% (n)	M (SD)	Minimum	Maximum
Age	100% (42)	42.6 (10.5)	22	59
Gender				
Male	33% (14)	—	—	—
Female	67% (28)	—	—	—
Supervision type				
Adult PPO	90% (38)	—	—	—
Juvenile PPO	10% (4)	—	—	—
Race/ethnicity				
White	88% (37)	—	—	—
Black	2% (1)	—	—	—
Hispanic/Latino	10% (4)	—	—	—
Education level				
High school / GED	2% (1)	—	—	—
Associates	5% (2)	—	—	—
Bachelors	60% (25)	—	—	—
Masters	33% (14)	—	—	—
Caseload		71	1	280
Special population				
Yes	55% (23)	—	—	—
No	38% (16)	—	—	—

M = mean; SD = standard deviation

Measures

The analysis to follow drew on a combination of data collected via open-ended questions as well as three closed-ended validated measures: the General Well-Being Schedule, the Patient Health Questionnaire, and the General Anxiety Disorder assessment.

General Well-Being Schedule. The General Well-Being (GWB) Schedule (Fazio, 1977) was used to assess the psychological well-being and distress, generalized anxiety and depression, and physical health of the participants during the COVID-19 pandemic. The GWB Schedule consists of 18 items spanning six dimensions: positive well-being, self-control, vitality, depression, anxiety, and general health. Participants were asked to indicate the frequency with which they experienced each feeling during the past month. The first 14 questions on the GWB are rated on a six-point response scale with three different sets of response options (1 = not at all, 6 = yes, definitely so; 1 = not at all, 6 = extremely so; 1 = in very low spirits, 6 = in excellent spirits), with the remaining four items rated from 0 to 10 (0 = very relaxed, 10 = very tense). A total GWB score was calculated by summing each of the items after reverse-scoring negatively worded items (a = 0.83). Following the cut points outlined in the GWB scoring protocol, scores ranging from 0 to 60 reflect severe distress, 61 to 72 moderate distress, and 73 to 110 positive well-being (Fazio, 1977).

Depression and Anxiety. Participants (*n* = 14) who indicated they felt distressed either "a good bit of time," "most of the time," or "all of the time" on at least three items on the GWB schedule were given an additional set of questions to explore their psychological distress further. First, the Patient Health Questionnaire (PHQ-9) was administered to measure possible depression-related symptoms in the last two weeks (Kroenke et al., 2001). Participants were asked to report the frequency with which they experienced a range of symptoms (e.g., feelings of hopelessness, poor appetite) (0 = not at all, 3 = nearly every day). Items included in the PHQ-9 are based on the criteria for depressive disorders from the *Diagnostic and Statistical Manual of Mental Disorders*, fourth edition. A variable measuring the presence of depressive symptoms was calculated by summing the scores on each of the PHQ-9 items (a = 0.61).

Second, the General Anxiety Disorder (GAD-7) assessment was administered to examine the presence of anxiety symptoms within the last two weeks (Spitzer et al., 2006). The GAD-7 consists of seven items based on the criteria for anxiety disorders from the *Diagnostic and Statistical Manual of Mental Disorders*, fourth edition. Participants were asked to report the frequency with which they experienced a range of symptoms (e.g., persistent worrying, restlessness) (0 = not at all, 3 = nearly every day). A variable measuring the presence of anxiety symptoms was calculated by summing the scores of each of the GAD-7 items (a = 0.90).

Job Stress and Burnout. The analyses also drew from qualitative data collected during semi-structured interviews to supplement the quantitative measures described above. These interviews aimed to understand the experience of working during a pandemic from the perspective of PPOs supervising active caseloads. Because the interviews were semi-structured, the researchers were trained to utilize probing to gain in-depth knowledge and understanding of work conditions during the pandemic. While no questions were designed to measure job stress and burnout directly, these were common themes that arose across the interviews.

Analytic Strategy

Quantitative measures (GWB, GAD-7, PHQ-9) were entered into SPSS statistical software. A series of descriptive analyses were conducted to assess participants' scores on each measure. Due to the small sample size, inferential statistics were not conducted. All open-ended data were transcribed in Microsoft Word and linked to ATLAS.ti, a software commonly used for data management (Muhr, 1991). Two researchers completed independent inductive, iterative, line-by-line coding to identify emergent themes and patterns present in the data (Glaser & Straus, 1967). Throughout this process, the research team utilized a memo strategy in which the researchers drafted analytical memos detailing their reflections throughout coding. This strategy is useful for recording and clarifying ideas and aids in documenting ideas that may become prevalent throughout the entire dataset (Glaser, 1978). Once this coding was complete, the full research team reviewed the transcripts for intercoder reliability. This review revealed an agreement rate of 96%, with all disagreements resolved through an analysis by the full research team. Once this process was complete, the research team reflected on the analytical memos guiding the querying process. As a result, the team queried the data for themes and patterns relating to job stress, well-being, and burnout. The following section details the findings.

Results

Quantitative Results

Descriptive analyses revealed that the overall mean score on the GWB Schedule was 72.02 (standard deviation [SD] = 8.72), suggesting moderate distress. Of those who met the criteria for further assessment using the PHQ-9 and GAD-7, their scores indicated mild symptoms of depression (mean [M] = 6.29; SD = 3.27) and anxiety (M = 9.13; SD = 4.76). While the quantitative measures collectively revealed that the PPOs were moderately distressed, data from interviews provided a more in-depth understanding of their experiences during the pandemic.

Community Supervision, COVID-19, and Stress

Analysis of qualitative data revealed similar findings. Many of the PPOs who participated in interviews reported that the onset of the COVID-19 pandemic did not increase their stress. However, they explained how their experience of working in community corrections had helped to prepare them for the pandemic. Their jobs typically carry a high level of stress that they were used to facing. These stressors include concern over noncompliance and public safety and adapting to policy and procedural changes. Being used to operating under stress, the onset of the COVID-19 pandemic did not dramatically increase stress for participants in our sample. The following quote from PPO Baker provides a representative example of this finding:

> I have been around a long time and have got accustomed to feelings of stress. This is not a job with peaks and valleys like law enforcement where you might have an incredibly single stressful event. Rather with probation you almost always have a certain moderate level of stress that is on you all the time.

As this statement from PPO Baker suggests, PPOs are accustomed to operating under a consistent level of stress on the job. Another PPO in our sample, PPO Berger, discussed how she and the majority of her colleagues had been working in probation for at least 20 years, and the onset of the COVID-19 pandemic actually decreased their workloads. That is, they became less busy during the pandemic as normal operations halted. They were not meeting face-to-face with clients or conducting in-person field visits, and they were either not attending court or doing so much less frequently. This could help explain PPOs' moderate levels of distress as reported in the quantitative results. It seems that officers in our study had become used to operating under steady stress before the pandemic. And for some, the transition to remote supervision reduced some stressful aspects of their job.

The ability for PPOs to work from home seemed to reduce preexisting stress levels for some officers. As one PPO explained, "there aren't people on top of you watching what you're doing and not doing." Other PPOs described how working from home in conjunction with reductions to their other work-related duties (e.g., travel, home visits) allowed them to work at a slower pace than they did pre-pandemic. Additionally, no longer having to commute to work was a stress reducer for many PPOs. As PPO Welch put it, "the commute into the office is deplorable at best, so for many of us, getting to work from home has actually served to improve our quality of life." Officers expressed an overall reduction in stress during the pandemic due to having more flexibility and to working at a slower pace. The pandemic removed some typically frustrating parts of the work (e.g., commutes, micromanaging by supervisors) and allowed officers to work flexibly. Thus, COVID-19 changed the sources and intensity of stress for many officers in the study rather than adding to their stress.

COVID-19 and Increased Stress

While they represented a smaller portion of study participants, some PPOs in our study reported experiencing increased job stress from work during the pandemic. All of these officers attributed their feelings of added stress to changes in agency operations that impacted how they performed their job. The main stressor was the inability to meet in person with individuals on their caseload and the need to learn a new way of supervising (i.e., virtually). Officer Urban noted, "It has been exhausting at times especially when we were adapting in real time and changing daily."

Officer Miller also described stress in this experience:

> My experience as a community supervision officer is 100 times more stressful. We're not seeing people in office right now, which makes it difficult to do what I was doing, which was to personally interact with people with substance abuse issues. Everything is being done remotely. We aren't drug testing unless there is a specific issue or a judge has said they want them tested right now. It is very difficult for some of them to get their conditions done because places aren't open, parks aren't open for community service. Even if I am able to find them a site, a lot of them are unwilling to go to the site because of COVID-19.

In this excerpt, PPO Miller highlights the challenges associated with the shifts to remote supervision. The shift to remote supervision resulted in a lack of drug testing, which made it challenging for him to monitor his substance use caseload. Additionally, he notes a challenge other PPOs described facing, namely, greater difficulty for probationers to complete their supervision conditions. While sometimes this was due to things in the individual's control (e.g., unwilling to go to a site), often it was due to shutdowns of community resources. This was a significant challenge because a PPO's job is to monitor and encourage individuals to complete their supervision conditions.

Likewise, many PPOs value interaction in the community as a key component of their job. Social distancing made this challenging during the pandemic. Officer Styles discussed how she views her job as a "community member"; before the pandemic, she was always out of the office and communicating with clients, so "when everything was shut down to a halt, and there were no face-to-face contacts, it was very difficult." In this regard, PPOs felt they were not able to perform their job fully without the ability to interact with their clients in-person. For these PPOs, the reduction in face-to-face interactions increased their stress as they felt they were no longer performing their job to the best of their ability.

Officers also noted that efforts across the country to decrease jail and prison populations to prevent the spread of COVID-19 had affected community supervision. In consequence, their supervision caseloads had increased, both pretrial and post-conviction. Officers noted that these increases in caseloads, or even changes in the composition of their caseloads (more pretrial, for example), were exhausting. A representative example from PPO Kaiser illustrates this finding:

> We have more people on supervision than we have officers or budget, but now we can't even hire people because we have a hiring freeze. . . . We have two pretrial folks who can't breathe. It's like constant "I can't keep up.".. . . There are so many more people. It feels like, maybe it's my perception. But now the people are being released from jail or being kept on pretrial. The courts are just putting everyone on pretrial.

Thus, PPOs described a noticeable divergence between changes in sentencing practices and funding for community corrections agencies. Despite courts sending more individuals to community corrections, the agencies responsible for their supervision did not receive adequate resources to support those increases. In these situations, the burden was passed down to the PPOs, who had to supervise a larger caseload without additional support.

Beyond job-related factors, PPOs also reported increased stress outside work. For example, PPO Muncy described how she was more stressed because she was always worrying that her vulnerable mother would contract COVID-19 in the nursing home where she lived. Another officer, PPO Styles, described a similar challenge:

I would say what is most challenging is supervising clients and making sure you are still healthy and not bringing the virus home to family members. My husband is high risk and my daughter just left for graduate school, and I cannot ruin that for her.

PPOs identified the fear of contracting COVID-19 on the job and bringing it home to their family members. PPO Styles noted that because she could not prevent interactions with individuals while on the job, she implemented social distancing at home to keep her family safe.

Additionally, those PPOs who reported feeling stressed and burned out also reported that their agency did nothing to support staff or mitigate stress during the pandemic. For example, PPO Black described how his agency verbally encouraged staff to support one another but did not implement a formal policy or adjust pay to provide professional support. He noted, "It is like, oh yeah, this is a great idea and we support it, but you all go figure it out yourselves." Another officer echoed this finding, stating they felt their agency was "not concerned with the employees at all."

Beyond lack of support, PPOs noted that poor agency communication was a precursor to increased stress. There was a lack of communication about policy changes and/or frequent changes to policies and procedures. As PPO Marsh put it, "It seemed like the agency was changing things every hour," while PPO Jackson described how he felt the information he received was always "premature":

> They would send out an email and then 40 minutes later recall what they had just disseminated to staff. For example, they sent out an email about providing time off if we were waiting on a COVID test, that we had the COVID relief package where you could take days off while you wait for results. But then another email was sent basically saying anything after five days is actually not going to be covered, and if you take more than five days off, you will only get two-thirds of your pay.

As a result of frequently changing policies, PPOs reported feeling like communication was often confusing, contradictory, and sporadic.

While frustrated, PPOs often still believed their agency was doing the best it could under the circumstances. Officer Kaiser expressed this belief:

> I think the department is doing the best they can, but it seems like they are changing things on the fly. Not necessarily for the worst, but just on the fly. For example, for a while we were not conducting any

drug tests. Then, it was suddenly like we could do oral swabs, but no urine drug tests.

The frequency of changes made PPOs unsure about how they could fulfill their job responsibilities. They were often concerned that they would have to shift gears soon after they had adjusted to a new work method. While many expected changes to occur, they largely wished their agencies communicated more clearly about the changes as they occurred. Most of the PPOs who reported feeling more stressed and exhausted also reported experiencing a lack of agency support and poor communication.

Given that a larger proportion of PPOs in our study said they did not experience increased stress during COVID-19, with some even reporting reductions in stress, the next step of our analyses was to identify potential explanations for PPOs' experiences. The following subsections identify strategies reported by PPOs for coping with stress. These strategies include coping mechanisms employed by individuals as well as agency strategies to support staff during the pandemic.

Individual-Level Coping Mechanisms

Interestingly, most PPOs in our sample associated their limited stress and burnout during the pandemic with the fact that they had already developed coping mechanisms. They described how they had developed strategies to manage stress in their jobs long before the pandemic. These preexisting coping strategies provided a foundation for helping them balance the changes and adaptations required during COVID-19. Officers described a series of helpful coping strategies, including personal coping techniques, reliance on peer support networks, and agency-related support.

At the individual level, PPOs highlighted the importance of having coworkers they could rely on to talk to, commiserate with, and rely on for feedback and of having a strong support system outside work. For example, PPO Hunt described the importance of both a positive working environment and a support structure outside work:

> This is one of the least stressful jobs I've had. I have a good support system at home, and I have good coworkers, and we all talk it out. We all work together really well, and I think that helps reduce our stress significantly.

Other PPOs echoed the importance of the work environment for mitigating officer stress levels. Officers described how key components of agency culture (e.g., supportive, positive leadership) helped to establish a positive working environment. In a representative example from the field notes, PPO Powers discussed how officers in his agency were able to manage work during the pandemic:

> My coworkers would help and step up as best they can, would be really willing to help. We really try to foster a family atmosphere here; we know we can talk to our supervisor if needed to lift that burden.

In agencies where PPOs felt they could lean on their colleagues and supervisors for support, whether physical or emotional assistance, they managed the stress associated with their job and the additional stress posed by COVID-19. In some agencies, PPOs described how they would take breaks during the day or hold employee get-togethers to increase morale. For example, PPO Prince said, "On more than one occasion, as an office, we have been watching movies together—we all watched *The Social Dilemma* on Zoom and then discussed our thoughts afterward." Officers highlighted how activities like this helped to take their minds off work-related stressors.

In addition to support at work, most PPOs emphasized the importance of having a social support network to counter job-related stress. For coping with stress, officers described the importance of spending time with family and friends and telling them about work issues. For many officers, it was crucial to have time to decompress. For example, PPO Gordon noted, "Every now and then, a couple of my close friends sit outside on the deck and chit chat and eat some food and try to breathe after the week." PPO Lowry explained that "being with your circle of people and supporting each other both inside and outside of work" helps manage their stress levels. Having support networks to lean on outside work proved immensely valuable for PPOs' ability to find balance and manage work-related stressors.

Officers also discussed the importance of self-care during the pandemic. In particular, PPOs described how they developed personal strategies focused on their mental and physical well-being. For example, PPO Munson stated, "For me, I really try to practice taking intentional breaks and do stretching and physical therapy for my shoulder." Other PPOs incorporated meditation into their day or alone time to decompress. Officer Stevens described how she took personal time to "do a lot of reading; you know, the self-help books to keep my mind right." Officers also described the helpfulness of engaging in physical activity (e.g., hiking, walking their dog, exercising) to decrease stress levels. Physical activity was noted as an effective strategy to boost overall well-being and take their mind off work. The following representative example from the field notes highlights this finding:

> For myself personally, I do meditation. I listen to music. I have gone to the beach carefully a few times when I know it won't be busy. I have carefully ventured out to walk the dogs in one of our favorite towns that is nearby. Stuff like that. I turn off the news.

PPOs also commonly had picked up a new hobby during the pandemic. For example, PPO Gordon noted she "started working on house projects, which has been helping distract from challenges of work." Several officers noted the importance of focusing on a project or new hobby to serve as an outlet for stress reduction. While not always feasible, PPOs noted that vacations or even "stay-cations" were critical for resetting and alleviating stress.

Overall, results indicate several individual-level coping strategies that helped PPOs manage challenges presented at work after the onset of the COVID-19 pandemic. Relying on social networks for emotional support played a crucial role for PPOs in managing operational changes and mitigating feelings of stress and burnout. Officers also engaged in self-care activities such as physical exercise and meditation techniques to reduce stress.

Agency-Level Strategies to Mitigate Stress

PPOs also described strategies their agencies implemented during the COVID-19 pandemic to provide support and manage stress. For example, some agencies implemented weekly Zoom check-ins where PPOs could receive or provide emotional support, vent, and problem-solve new challenges they were facing. In some instances, agencies created emotional support teams to help staff. Similarly, some agencies implemented formal peer-support group sessions led by trained therapists. PPO Prince described how this worked in her agency: "We have therapists who are running these support groups. Anyone can sign into a session. It might be focused on dealing with COVID-19, how to work at home with kids, or how to support a kid's Zoom learning." Agencies sought to provide support not just for job-related stress but for other sources of stress for staff.

Our analysis suggests that when agencies recognized that the pandemic had impacts beyond the job alone, they could better support their staff. Recognition of the new challenges made PPOs feel heard and supported by their agency. Officers whose agencies committed to supporting a work-life balance during the pandemic reported beneficial effects. The ability to work from home was critical in this regard. Officer Smith described how new policies for remote work were helpful: "working from home at least a day or two a week made me less anxious. It was great for my mental health." This quotation encapsulates the sentiment of many PPOs who believed that working from home improved their well-being, made them feel valued by their agency, and reduced their fears of contracting the virus.

Discussion

This study aimed to understand the experience of PPOs working during the COVID-19 pandemic and its impact on PPOs' well-being and stress. Prior research has identified sources of job stress and occupational exhaustion among criminal justice employees, yet we know relatively little about how a global pandemic impacts the work of PPOs and their well-being on the job.

Interestingly, results revealed that increased stress and burnout related to the pandemic were not universally experienced by those in our sample. Most of the PPOs interviewed reported that the pandemic did not dramatically increase their stress level. Instead, these officers discussed having experienced a generally high level of stress pre-pandemic. That is, the COVID-19 pandemic did not necessarily increase stress across the board for PPOs in our study; rather, it altered the sources and intensity of stress. Being used to working in a high-stress field, many PPOs said they were prepared for dealing with challenges and already had coping strategies in place. This finding points to the importance of understanding job stress and mitigation techniques among community corrections professionals, especially since previous research found that PPOs experience higher levels of job stress than do police and correctional officers (Patterson, 1992). Given the negative consequences associated with job stress (e.g., health problems, turnover), the findings from this study suggest promising avenues for mitigating some of that stress, even during a generally stressful global health emergency.

PPOs relied on several individual and agency-level strategies to alleviate feelings of stress and burnout, which is consistent with prior research (Finn & Kuck, 2005; Salyers et al., 2015; White et al., 2015). Officers identified the importance of personal "mental health" days, physical exercise, and social support from peers and family as strategies that helped to mitigate the challenges of the pandemic and to reduce feelings of stress. Officers also described their organization's role in helping protect against stress and burnout. In particular, PPOs who worked for agencies that provided formal support mechanisms experienced a more positive working environment and felt more supported by their colleagues. This finding is supported by previous research that found agency supervisory support and peer network connections represented critical organizational attributes associated with reduced job stress for correctional and probation officers (Lambert & Hogan, 2010; Rhineberger-Dunn & Mack, 2020; Whitehead & Lindquist, 1985). Officers who felt supported by their supervisors and colleagues were less likely to feel alone or isolated at work, which can mitigate work-related stressors (Iliffe & Steed, 2000).

Of the PPOs who reported experiencing increased stress because of the pandemic, the majority attributed their increased emotional exhaustion and stress to frequent policy changes, poor communication about those changes, and the elimination of face-to-face contact with individuals under their supervision. That these experiences led to increased stress is not surprising as research consistently finds that greater role ambiguity and role conflict influence officer attitudes and can lead to increased job stress and burnout (Lambert et al., 2015; Rhineberger-Dunn & Mack, 2020). These results largely affirm Norman and colleagues' (2021) analysis of Canadian community parole officers. Inconsistent messaging and limited agency communication generated ambiguity about what PPOs were expected to accomplish during the pandemic. When employees experience unclear agency directives or new policies that conflict with established agency goals, employees are significantly more likely to report negative outcomes, including increased feelings of stress and burnout (Alward & Viglione, 2023; Lambert et al., 2015; Matz et al., 2014; Salyers et al., 2015).

Some PPOs said their agencies provided little to no support in mitigating job stress during the pandemic. This finding accords with previous evidence showing that inadequate administrative support was among the strongest predictors of probation officer job stress (Slate & Johnson, 2013). This finding also supports the work of Phillips and colleagues (2021), which indicated that probation staff were experiencing greater emotional exhaustion and decreased support with the removal of in-person work. These findings suggest the importance of developing a positive, supportive work environment, which may be more challenging with remote work. For agencies that continue to incorporate remote work into their operations, they should seek to develop strong, clear communication strategies and techniques to promote employee interaction and collaboration.

Several policy implications can be drawn from the experiences of both PPOs who experienced increased stress and those who did not. First, findings suggest the important role of agency leadership and culture in combating staff stress. The existing literature corroborates these as key agency attributes for improving staff health and well-being (Gayman & Bradley, 2013; Matz et al., 2014; Lambert et al., 2015). In the current study, PPOs were less stressed when their agencies provided formal support mechanisms, clear communication about policy changes, and a positive working environment characterized by collegiality and staff helping one another. Second, PPOs who were meaningfully engaged in activities outside work reported they were better able to cope with job stress. Third, PPOs argued that being able to work remotely improved their quality of life and reduced their job stress. This is perhaps the most important takeaway from the study, as participating officers noted that even working remotely one to two days a week reduced their stress. While remote work was not a common agency practice before the pandemic, nearly all PPOs in every agency across the country worked remotely in some capacity during the pandemic. This has provided an opportunity to test out a new strategy for community supervision that may ultimately make the job more attractive, increase the pool of applicants, and reduce turnover. This area deserves further evaluation to understand whether and how remote work can be sustained for community supervision.

The current study has several limitations. First, the results presented here are cross-sectional and were collected early in the pandemic. Thus, the findings do not represent trends, nor can they speak to whether and how PPOs' experiences and stress may have changed over the course of the pandemic. As part of our larger study, we are collecting such data and will examine officer well-being and stress longitudinally. Second, this study relied on the experiences of 42 PPOs who were primarily white and female and supervised adult caseloads. Additionally, there is also a possibility for selection bias. PPOs who were inherently less stressed may have been more likely to participate in interviews. Despite this possibility, our sample did include individuals with a mixture of experiences and reported levels of stress.

Future research should incorporate more diverse samples to gain a holistic understanding of the impact of the pandemic on PPO well-being and stress.

Conclusion

The current study contributes to a growing body of research that examines the impact of the COVID-19 pandemic on community corrections. This study affirms the stressful nature of community corrections work and the need for PPOs to have access to strategies (whether individual or agency-level) to mitigate those stressors. Officers in this study reported a moderate stress level, with qualitative findings indicating that PPOs operate under consistent stress on the job. Given this high-stress environment, the pandemic did not necessarily increase stress for all PPOs. Rather, the pandemic reduced some sources of pre-COVID-19 stress (e.g., by decreasing time spent traveling) while also introducing new sources of stress (e.g., an inability to see clients in-person and reduced support from the agency). While these findings provide a preliminary understanding of potential avenues for reducing PPO stress (e.g., remote work, improved agency communication), more research is needed to examine sources of stress and mitigation techniques. Given the large size of the community supervision workforce in the United States and the important role that PPOs play in assisting individuals to succeed in the community, a better understanding of how to reduce their job stress could improve supervision effectiveness and boost recruitment and retention of quality staff.

11. Cybercrime: Offending and Victimization during the COVID-19 Pandemic

Jin R. Lee, Jennifer M. Ayerza, Wei-Gin Lee,
Vahid Jadidi, and Thomas J. Holt

Introduction

The growth and pervasiveness of computers and the internet have altered how society functions, including how individuals communicate, exchange information, and engage in commerce (Holt, Bossler, & Seigfried-Spellar, 2022; Yar, 2013). The ubiquity of digital technology is evident in the fact that approximately two-thirds (65.7%) of the global population is connected to the internet, of which 57% gains access through mobile devices (Statista, 2023). In the United States, almost 92% of the population uses the internet and regularly connects with others in online spaces (Statista, 2023).

Despite the benefits of technology, including more efficient communications and the globalization of commerce, its use has simplified some aspects of criminality, such as easing access to vulnerable populations for the purpose of committing fraud (Holt, Bossler, & Seigfried-Spellar, 2022; Wall, 2007). At the same time, technology has created new forms of misuse, such as compromising computer systems and accessing sensitive electronic data without authorization. All of these behaviors fall under the umbrella term of *cybercrime*, which covers the wide range of offenses that occur in online environments or that use computer technology to do harm (Furnell, 2002; Holt, Bossler, & Seigfried-Spellar, 2022; Lee, 2022; Wall, 2007). One of the most common cybercrime classification frameworks used by scholars recognizes four categories of offending: (1) cyber-trespass involving computer hacking and unauthorized network access; (2) cyber-deception/theft offenses encompassing fraud and the acquisition of data or intellectual property; (3) cyber-porn/obscenity, which includes all manner of sexual offenses; and (4) cyber-violence including online acts of bullying, harassment, stalking, and related behaviors targeting individuals in virtual and real settings.

Using this framework, research has found that cybercrimes involving human subjects or nonhuman targets (e.g., computer systems, sensitive data) have risen exponentially over the past two decades (Holt & Bossler, 2015). The spread of COVID-19 and the resulting government lockdowns and stay-at-home orders transformed individuals' daily routines, leading them to spend more time on the internet while decreasing their physical mobility (Gartner, 2020; Interpol, 2020). The increased reliance on both the internet and digital technology to accomplish common tasks and mundane activities (e.g., leisure, education, finances, and work) increased people's exposure to online environments, which appears to have facilitated a rise in cybercrime behaviors during the COVID-19 pandemic (see Buil-Gil, Miró-Llinares, et al., 2021; Hawdon et al., 2020; Interpol, 2020).

Given the COVID-19 pandemic's impacts on society and technological dependency, we must understand how cybercriminality may have changed. This chapter provides an overview of cybercrime behaviors during the COVID-19 pandemic. Specifically, this chapter identifies several prominent cybercrime behaviors (e.g., computer hacking, online fraud, online interpersonal violence) and examines any noteworthy shifts in patterns of offending and victimization during the pandemic. These changes' short- and long-term implications for our understanding of cybercrime offending and victimization are also discussed.

Computer Hacking

Hacking is classified under the general notion of cyber-trespass in Wall's (2001) typology of cybercrime and is generally defined as the act of modifying a system's software and/or hardware in ways that were neither proposed by the creator nor in line with the creator's intentions (Holt, 2020; Jordan & Taylor, 1998; Lee & Holt, 2020; Wall, 2001). Hacking is often associated with malicious, criminal activity because individuals gain access to sensitive networks and attempt to steal valuable data they may store as a form of cyber-theft (Furnell, 2002; Grabosky, 2016; Holt, 2007; Wall, 2001). Despite its application for legitimate purposes (i.e., identifying software vulnerabilities, penetration testing), hacking behaviors are commonly perceived as a serious threat to both the public and private sectors due to the costs associated with victimization, including damages to the target's reputation and the loss of time, data, and money involved in the resolution of hacking incidents (Chan & Yao, 2005; Grabosky, 2016; Lallie et al., 2021; Lewis & Baker, 2013).

It is important to note that the definition of hacking does not imply nor focus on the criminal intent of the actor but on the act itself. Extant literature suggests hackers are driven by various motivations, with criminal hackers representing only a minority subset of the hacker community (Holt, 2007, 2020; Steinmetz, 2015, 2017). Hackers are primarily interested in advancing hardware and software technology and may use their skills to solve technical security problems (Coleman, 2012, 2013; Levy, 1984; Steinmetz, 2015; Taylor, 1999). This does not negate the fact that various hackers may engage in malicious or criminal hacks driven by politics (McKenzie, 1999; Meikle, 2002; Taylor, 2005), online thrill-seeking (Holt, Lee, et al., 2022; Lee & Holt, 2023), and the development of different types of malicious software (Jordan & Taylor, 1998; Steinmetz et al., 2017; Turgeman-Goldschmidt, 2008; Wall, 2007). In these malicious acts, individuals may be inspired by creativity, ambition, or the desire for technological development (Levy, 1984; Steinmetz, 2015). A substantive proportion of hackers also monetize their skills by selling stolen data and hacking tools to less skilled actors for a fee (Holt, 2013; Lee, 2023).

Hacking also captures a wide range of behaviors that vary in technological sophistication and expertise (Holt, Bossler, & Seigfried-Spellar, 2022; Robalo & Abdul Rahim, 2023). For instance, offenders can acquire individuals' personal information through shoulder-surfing, or watching an individual's device, screen, or keypad as they input personal data and sensitive information. Others use more technical methods, such as procuring sensitive data by writing malware code to infiltrate and compromise computer systems (Holt, Bossler, & Seigfried-Spellar, 2022). Various hacking tools and prepackaged services can even be purchased through the online illicit marketplace in the event that offenders do not possess the skills or have the time to develop their own tools (Décary-Hétu & Dupont, 2013; Décary-Hétu & Leppänen, 2016; Ianelli & Hackworth, 2005).

Since most societies worldwide shifted from physical activities to virtual meetings and cloud applications during the COVID-19 pandemic, the opportunities to target individuals, businesses, and governments alike increased dramatically. One of the most common offenses during this period was distributed denial of service (DDoS) attacks. A DDoS attack involves using software-based tools or other methods of hacking to send malicious traffic to servers and other online infrastructure. Most attacks can send a high volume of traffic that overwhelms the server's ability to handle legitimate requests and renders the associated website, gaming platform, or other online resources unusable (Holt, Lee, & Smirnova, 2023; Hyslip & Holt, 2019).

While DDoS attacks were widespread even before the COVID-19 pandemic, they grew in both frequency and severity during the pandemic, targeting critical organizations such as government servers, educational platforms (e.g., universities/colleges, research institutions), and health care networks (e.g., hospitals, pharmaceutical labs) and causing significant disruptions to organizations fighting the pandemic (Osborne, 2020; Palmer, 2020; World Health Organization, 2020). One such incident targeted Jisc, a nonprofit company based in the United Kingdom that specializes in providing digital network resources and information technology services for both higher education institutions and other public sector organizations. The attacks caused restrictions and delays in student and staff access to the internet and information technology resources through school servers (Hale, 2020). Relatedly, several French hospitals were targeted by DDoS attacks, followed by further attacks that led to the loss of restricted access to patient data (Hale, 2020). Similar cyberattacks on the U.S. Department of Health and Human Services resulted in significant server damage (Stein & Jacobs, 2020).

Numerous health care institutions reported hacking attacks during the early months of the pandemic. These attacks were thought to come from nation-state-sponsored hackers seeking access to sensitive data on pandemic responses. For instance, an American pharmaceutical company developing a therapeutic drug for COVID-19 was targeted. Similar attacks targeted universities engaged in COVID-19 drug and vaccine research in order to access proprietary information that could be used to gain an advantage and slow the pandemic's spread (Grierson & Devlin, 2020; Osborne, 2020).

Another common hacking technique during the pandemic involved attacks against videoconferencing platforms like Zoom, Cisco WebEx, and Google Meet. The shift to online meeting tools during the pandemic was critical for enabling remote work and virtual education, all dependent on access to personal computers and online networks (Borkovich & Skovira, 2020). Attackers targeted this infrastructure for so-called Zoombombing, where offenders gained unauthorized access to private online meetings covertly or overtly (Robalo & Abdul Rahim, 2023). Though some instances of

Zoombombing focused on annoying and harassing legitimate participants, others used the opportunity to steal individuals' private credentials and gain access to open workstations during the sharing of screens in virtual meetings (Mandal & Khan, 2020).

Online Fraud

The pandemic also saw a rise in various forms of cyber-theft, generally defined as acquiring and misusing an individual's private information for personal and/or financial gain (Holt, Bossler, & Seigfried-Spellar, 2022). Online fraud offenses have been a persistent problem since the development of the internet. This is evident in estimates from the Federal Trade Commission (2020) of 2.46 million cases of fraud reported in the United States, with $3.5 million in total losses, in 2020 alone. These figures increased in 2021 during the peak of the COVID-19 pandemic, with over 3 million reported fraud cases causing approximately $6.1 million in losses.

Online fraud offenses can be categorized into several subgroups based on their outcomes, including (1) unauthorized transactions using financial information, (2) unauthorized transactions using identity information, (3) authorized transactions without fraudulent intent, and (4) authorized transactions with fraudulent intent (Ma & McKinnon, 2022). The first category of fraud includes only compromised financial data, such as stealing credit and debit card information to make unauthorized purchases, whereas the second category involves using personally identifiable information to accomplish various objectives, including impersonation behaviors and creating new accounts or compromising existing accounts. Identifying information comprises various types of sensitive data, such as an individual's legal name, date of birth, billing address, email address, and account usernames and passcodes.

The third category contains offenses where individuals authorize transactions without having any fraudulent intent or awareness that they are committing fraud. An example of this is when individuals deposit counterfeit money or fraudulent bank checks that they received without knowing they were derived from stolen or illegal funds. The fourth category includes intentional online fraud committed for financial gain, especially in a context of organized crime.

Research has found that many online fraud offenses adopt social engineering tactics to acquire sensitive data or compromise network systems

(Holt & Bossler, 2015). Social engineering is a strategy of manipulating individuals into violating security protocols and thereby gaining unauthorized access to protected computer networks (Mitnick & Simon, 2002). These techniques aim to deceive unsuspecting individuals into divulging confidential and personally identifying information through emails, text messages, or fraudulent websites (Borkovich & Skovira, 2020).

Social engineering is commonly employed by scammers in an attempt to obtain useful information from potential victims. To that end, research found that bank loan fraud proliferated at the peak of the COVID-19 crisis, focusing on deceiving individuals into giving over money and personal information (Alawida et al., 2022). Noteworthy instances include bank clients receiving text messages instructing them to reschedule a package delivery online, leading some to disclose their banking information unwittingly and subsequently falling victim to account breaches (Alawida et al., 2022). In another development, two Indonesian hackers were apprehended in 2021 for orchestrating a $60 million fraud operation that targeted around 30,000 Americans. This fraudulent scheme involved deceiving individuals into providing both personal and financial data on a deceptive website under the pretense of receiving $2,000 as part of an unemployment relief program (CBS News, 2021). These dishonest strategies were effective during the pandemic given increased unemployment and financial stress.

Another type of fraud that increased during the COVID-19 pandemic was romance fraud (Buil-Gil & Zeng, 2022), where offenders manipulated and exploited victims into sending them money and sensitive data after establishing a trusting relationship with them. Many romance fraud schemes begin on social media or by email, typically through innocuous requests for friendship or discussions of perceived common interests. Once offenders have gained the trust of their victims, they use emotive language to develop a deeper emotional or romantic relationship (Button & Cross, 2017). After some time, scammers then request funds from their targets, usually to resolve a fabricated urgent situation like a health crisis or travel problem (Action Fraud, 2020). Requests for funds continue until victims are either unable to make additional payments or realize they have been defrauded (Button & Cross, 2017). Research suggests romance fraud behaviors were prevalent during the pandemic, partly due to increased physical and social isolation from lockdown restrictions, particularly among younger adults (Buil-Gil & Zeng, 2022; Ma & McKinnon, 2022). This behavior demonstrates another instance where offenders exploited the unique conditions of the pandemic to target people vulnerable to these abrupt changes (BBC News, 2020).

Another common form of online fraud that flourished during the pandemic was online shopping scams, which generally involve perpetrators pretending to be legitimate vendors with quality products on fake websites or fraudulent ads within a genuine retailer site (e.g., Amazon). Buil-Gil, Miró-Llinares, et al. (2021) conducted a time-series analysis to examine the short-term effects of COVID-19 and lockdown restrictions on online fraud behaviors, finding that the number of frauds linked with online shopping and auctions had the most substantial increase. Additionally, Kemp and colleagues (2021) examined whether any increases in online fraud during the first months of the COVID-19 lockdown in the United Kingdom were beyond expected crime variability. They found that several online fraud behaviors (e.g., online shopping, auction, and dating fraud) significantly increased during this period, while many offline fraud behaviors (e.g., door-to-door fraud) decreased.

In addition to online shopping fraud, a spike was also observed in online fraud related to fake vaccines, proof of vaccination (i.e., vaccination cards or records), and virus testing kits. Many of these cases involved offenders generating fraudulent information about a COVID-19 cure or selling fake vaccination cards that could be used by the unvaccinated to enter restricted physical spaces. Listings and advertisements for fake vaccination cards surfaced on numerous online platforms, including Twitter, Instagram, and eBay (Frias, 2021). Several initiatives were carried out to prevent sales of fake vaccination cards, including the National Association of Attorneys General urging the CEOs of Twitter, eBay, and Shopify to better monitor their sites for fraudulent COVID-19-related products. The Federal Bureau of Investigation disseminated information advising the general public against uploading images of their vaccination cards on social media platforms, arguing that doing so could provide scammers with the personal information needed to generate fake vaccination cards and records (Frias, 2021).

Cyber-porn and Online Interpersonal Violence

Criminology literature has tracked the impact of COVID-19 on offline interpersonal violence behaviors, and several studies have found evidence of similar behavioral patterns in online spaces. There is substantive evidence to suggest that forms of cyber-enabled abuse increased during the pandemic. Wall's (2001) classification of cyber-porn and obscenity includes the production of child sexual exploitation materials, including images and videos of children engaging in sexual situations or acts. Such content is heavily criminalized around the world and is used by offenders for personal gratification or for grooming children to engage in sexual contact in offline environments (Holt, Bossler, & Seigfried-Spellar, 2022).

Given that children were isolated at home during pandemic lockdowns or placed in situations outside the home due to changes in routine, there were increased opportunities for their victimization by adults (Harris et al., 2021). Children had more unsupervised time online during the pandemic, creating opportunities for exposure to offenders who might victimize them. Official data sources in the United States and United Kingdom noted an increase in child sex offenses reported during the pandemic, particularly involving sexual exploitation images (Harris et al., 2021; Junewicz et al., 2022).

The behaviors that fall in the category of cyber-violence share some commonalities with online child sexual exploitation in that victims may be affected by images and videos that they produce voluntarily or against their will. Other behaviors are essential analogs to offline interpersonal violence, including intentional harm or aggression facilitated by the internet or the use of digital technology against another person, such as online harassment, cyberbullying, cyberstalking, and online sexual violence (Henry & Powell, 2018; Henson et al., 2013). While online interpersonal violence shares many characteristics with its offline counterpart, it is distinctive in that the internet serves as the primary conduit for facilitating violence, which may alter other dimensions of the offense.

Specifically, online interpersonal violence allows perpetrators to access a wider pool of potential targets in that anyone who uses the internet could potentially be a target of online interpersonal violence. In addition, technology increases the ease with which perpetrators commit these harms because of online artifacts' permanence. For instance, damaging pictures and harmful texts may never be fully removed from the internet, even if the initial post is taken down. Relatedly, the relative anonymity provided by the internet allows offenders to conceal their offline identity, making it harder for both victims and law enforcement to identify and apprehend offenders.

Though online interpersonal violence existed before the COVID-19 pandemic, research revealed increases in both its frequency and severity during the pandemic. For example, a survey by Pew Research Center found that 28% of Americans in 2021 reported experiencing multiple forms of online abuse (Vogels, 2021), which is nearly double the amount reported in 2014 (Duggan, 2017). Results also revealed that 41% of Americans experienced some form of online harassment during the pandemic, with purposeful embarrassment and name-calling being the two most common forms of online harassment (Vogels, 2021). Similarly, Huiskes and colleagues (2022) found that 69.9% of participants reported experiencing at least one form of online interpersonal violence behavior (i.e., online sexual harassment, image-based sexual abuse, sexual aggression or coercion, or sexuality-based harassment) during the COVID-19 pandemic. In addition, 86.1% of respondents reported experiencing multiple victimization experiences during this time period. The most common form of victimization was receiving unwanted sexually explicit images and comments (53.3%), followed by receiving repeated and/or unwanted sexual requests online (42.9%; Huiskes et al., 2022).

Surveys conducted by Pew Research Center further revealed a significant increase in the number of women who had reported being sexually harassed online during the pandemic (Duggan, 2017; Vogels, 2021). Research suggests women were significantly more likely than men to report experiencing online sexual harassment, receiving unwanted sexually explicit images and content, and receiving repeated and/or unwanted sexual requests online (Huiskes et al., 2022). Further, people identifying as LGBTQ+ reported experiencing higher rates of online harassment during the COVID-19 pandemic, with 7 out of 10 respondents experiencing a form of online harassment and 50% describing the harassment as having to do with their sexual identity (Huiskes et al., 2022; Vogels, 2021).

Cyberbullying and cyberstalking also became increasingly pervasive during this time period (Bussu et al., 2023; Martellozzo et al., 2022). Cyberbullying increased especially for individuals identified as Asian American (Patchin & Hinduja, 2023; Schilling & Wang, 2023). This increase in cyberbullying incidents toward Asian Americans was attributed to the hostile language and sentiments expressed during the COVID-19 pandemic (Lee et al., 2023).

An increase in sextortion, involving the threat of disseminating explicit sexual images to procure additional images, sexual acts, or money, was also observed during the COVID-19 pandemic, especially for minority populations (Eaton et al., 2023). The term *sextortion* is a combination of *sexual* and *extortion* and involves the offender pressuring a victim into sexual cooperation (Barak, 2005). Offenders often employ bribery, blackmail, or threats to release a person's explicit content to the public (Clevenger & Navarro, 2021; Powell & Henry, 2019; Wolak et al., 2018). Making the threat gives the offender power and control over the victim (O'Malley & Holt, 2022). In this way, perpetrators do not have to release these private images to constitute an act of sextortion. While some cases of sextortion are motivated by financial gain, many are conducted to solicit more sexual images and favors and could be perpetrated by individuals who wish to reestablish a relationship or to force a partner's continual compliance in a relationship (Clevenger & Navarro, 2021; O'Malley & Holt, 2022; Wolak & Finklehor, 2016).

Though sextortion offenses were common before the COVID-19 pandemic, the financial demands behind some sextortion were harsher during this time period as victims who were unemployed or struggling financially due to the pandemic had fewer options to resist their victimization. Specifically, victims were faced with the difficult choice of either paying the perpetrator to stop the abuse, thereby exacerbating their financial vulnerability, or refusing to pay the ransom and risking the release of their private images. Some individuals were limited to only one option as they did not have the financial means to pay their offenders. Regardless of whether individuals had the financial means to stop their abuse, sextortion incidents worsened the financial straits brought on by COVID-19.

Conclusion

The growth and ubiquity of technology have presented challenges for various stakeholders in addressing the threat of cybercrime (Nhan & Huey, 2013). Consumers' lack of cybercrime awareness, perceptions of cybercrime's low seriousness, and law enforcement's inability to effectively respond to calls for service for all forms of cybercrime have contributed to the difficulties in apprehending offenders and mitigating victimization (Chan & Yao, 2005; Fissel & Lee, 2023; Holt & Bossler, 2015; Lee, 2022). These challenges were exacerbated by the social changes compelled by the pandemic, putting additional strain on various stakeholders to respond to cybercrime inquiries effectively.

The global shift toward remote work and online dependencies accelerated by the pandemic is expected to persist beyond the pandemic (Gafni & Tal,

2022). This necessitates an increased awareness among organizations and employees of the inherent risks of remote work and the need for heightened cybersecurity measures, such as using cyber-hygiene protocols within both home and work settings (Gafni & Tal, 2022). To that end, governments must play a central role in ensuring transparent communication with the public and delivering accurate information through streamlined channels (Nugroho & Chandrawulan, 2023). Specifically, governments must recognize the influence of social media and foster partnerships with popular social media platforms to mitigate the spread of misinformation that leads to online fraud incidents.

Overall, the pandemic and its numerous consequences underscore the multifaceted approach needed to avert and mitigate cybercrime risks in a post-pandemic society (Nugroho & Chandrawulan, 2023). Since many of these cybercrimes were opportunistic offenses by individuals taking advantage of rapid societal transformations, more effort is required to develop proactive solutions to cybersecurity problems and to improve victim resources. Given these alarming trends, future research is urgently needed to develop effective strategies to counter online offenders and lower victimization, particularly during crises (Alawida et al., 2022).

Contributors
References
Index

Contributors

Sarah Ackerman is a doctoral student in the Clinical Psychology PsyD Program at Nova Southeastern University. She received her bachelor of science degree in psychology from the University of Central Florida.

Lucas Alward is an assistant professor in the Department of Criminal Justice at Boise State University. His primary research interests include the perceptions and experiences of people under correctional supervision and the design, implementation, and effectiveness of correctional interventions. Some of his research has appeared in the *Journal of Criminal Justice and Behavior* and *Crime & Delinquency*.

Jennifer M. Ayerza is a PhD student in the Department of Criminology, Law and Society at George Mason University. Her research interests are in cyber-violence, sexual offending, technology-facilitated sexual violence, computer-mediated communications, deviancy, and online victimization.

McKenna Bennett received her master's degree in criminology and criminal justice from Southern Illinois University Carbondale. Her research interests include corrections and reentry in the midst of a technological society, with a particular focus on barriers to employment in an increasingly digital world.

Shannon Christensen is a doctoral student at Southern Illinois University Carbondale. Her interests include security threat groups, health care in correctional facilities, and systematic responses to emergencies.

Rachele J. DiFava is a clinical psychology PsyD candidate at Nova Southeastern University, pursuing a concentration in forensic psychology. She is also a current affiliate of the P.L.E.A. Lab led by Dr. Miko M. Wilford. Her research focuses on factors that affect individuals' legal decision-making, such as the impacts of false confessions and defense attorney recommendations.

Jacob W. Forston graduated from Arizona State University with a master's degree in criminology and criminal justice. His research interests include plea bargaining, specifically in the context of legal decision-making.

Janne E. Gaub is an associate professor in the Department of Criminal Justice and Criminology at the University of North Carolina at Charlotte. Her research centers on policing, specifically technology (particularly body-worn cameras), misconduct, specialty units, and gender.

Taylor Gerry received her master of arts degree from Southern Illinois University Carbondale, studying criminology and criminal justice. Her research interests are within the realm of juveniles.

Andrew Hartung earned his master's degree in criminal justice administration in 2022. His thesis, "The Impact of Covid-19 on Campus Police," focused largely on campus police, job commitment, and newly conceptualized measures for containing COVID-19. He is currently employed with the City of Big Rapids, Michigan, as its code official.

Erin C. Heil received her PhD in criminal justice from the University of Illinois–Chicago in 2008. She has focused her research and teaching on the exploitation of vulnerable populations and relevant intersections with the law, in the context of labor trafficking, illegal international adoption, trafficking through religion, and sex trafficking of Native people. She has published extensively on the topic of human trafficking, authoring the book *Sex Slaves and Serfs*, coauthoring *Human Trafficking in the Midwest*, coediting *Broadening the Scope of Human Trafficking Research: A Reader*, and coediting *Social Work Practice with Survivors of Sex Trafficking and Commercial Sexual Exploitation*.

Thomas J. Holt is a professor in the School of Criminal Justice at Michigan State University. His research focuses on cybercrime, cyberterrorism, and the policy response to these issues. His recent work has been published in various journals including *Crime & Delinquency*, the *Journal of Criminal Justice*, and *Terrorism & Political Violence*.

Rasheed Babatunde Ibrahim is a doctoral candidate in criminology and criminal justice at Southern Illinois University Carbondale. His research focuses on the police, police-community relations, police-citizen encounters, and public perceptions of the police.

Vahid Jadidi is a PhD student in the Department of Criminology, Law and Society at George Mason University. His research interests are in gender-based violence, social inequality, political sociology and social movements, and social network analysis.

Marthinus C. Koen is an associate professor of criminal justice in the Criminal Justice Department at the State University of New York at Oswego, where he teaches classes on research methods, criminological theory, policing, and criminal profiling. His research interests lie in organizational change, pandemic policing, police technology, and criminal justice education. Dr. Koen's most recent published works have focused on the impacts of body-worn cameras, discovery reforms, and COVID-19 on prosecutorial organizational structures, practices, and perceptions.

Jin R. Lee is an assistant professor in the Department of Criminology, Law and Society at George Mason University. His research interests are in cybercrime, online interpersonal violence, cybersecurity, cyberpsychology, computer-mediated communications, and big data. His recent work has appeared in numerous peer-reviewed journals, including *Criminology & Public Policy, the American Journal of Criminal Justice, Computers in Human Behavior, and Crime & Delinquency.*

Wei-Gin Lee is a PhD student in the Department of Criminology, Law and Society at George Mason University. His research interests are in policing, cybercrime, crime investigation and prevention, gender and crime, quantitative methods, and criminal victimization.

Ashley Lockwood is a doctoral student in the Department of Criminal Justice at the University of Central Florida. Her primary research interests are the intersections of the criminal justice system with mental health and trauma and with disadvantaged groups. Her recent research has appeared in the *Journal of Police and Criminal Psychology, Victims & Offenders*, and *Perspectives.*

Holly Macleod is a victim witness specialist at the State Attorney's Office in Florida. She graduated with a bachelor's of science in criminal justice from the University of Central Florida.

Angela S. Murolo is an assistant professor at St. Francis College in Brooklyn, New York. Her dissertation investigated older people's experiences on parole and parole officers' views on working with them. Dr. Murolo has written several articles on correctional responses to geriatric inmates, the increasingly older prison population, and geriatric parole.

Ismail Ayatullah Nasirudeen is currently a master's student in the Department of Sociology, Bayero University, Kano, Nigeria. His research interests include gender-based violence, juvenile delinquency and youth crimes, law enforcement, and child abuse.

Andrea J. Nichols is a lecturer at Washington University in St. Louis, Missouri. Dr. Nichols's teaching and research interests broadly include sex trafficking, commercial sexual exploitation, sex work, and intimate partner violence.

James A. Plank is an assistant professor of practice at Texas A&M University–Kingsville and teaches undergraduate criminal justice courses.

Dr. Plank's research interests are in policing and community relations. He is a former police officer for the City of Killeen, where he worked for 12 years. He was a parole officer for the State of Texas and a probation officer in Bell County for six years.

Breanne Pleggenkuhle is an associate professor at Southern Illinois University Carbondale. Her research primarily focuses on corrections, particularly the experiences of formerly incarcerated persons, the collateral consequences of a felony conviction, and how community impacts post-conviction experiences. Her recent projects have focused on the evaluation of the implementation, process, and outcome of the R3 (Restore. Reinvest. Renew) Illinois programs in southern Illinois.

Joseph A. Schafer is a professor at Arizona State University. His research focuses on policing, organizational change, leadership, police officer perceptions and behavior, and future issues in crime and justice. He has served as a visiting scholar in the Behavioral Science Unit of the FBI Academy, a fellow with the Australian Institute of Police Management, and a commissioner with the Commission on Accreditation for Law Enforcement Agencies.

Ben Stickle is a professor of criminal justice administration at Middle Tennessee State University. His research focuses on property crime and policing; he is widely recognized through his research contributions on metal theft, package theft, and emerging crime trends, including crime during the COVID-19 pandemic.

Matthew Vanden Bosch is a doctoral candidate in the College of Criminology & Criminal Justice at Florida State University. His research focuses on bias offenses, sexual violence, and public opinion on crime and criminal justice. His research has been published in *Crime & Delinquency* and *The Mid-Southern Journal of Criminal Justice.*

Jill Viglione is an associate professor in the Department of Criminal Justice at the University of Central Florida. Her research focuses on examining the processes associated with the implementation of evidence-based practices in criminal justice settings. Her recent research has appeared in *Criminal Justice and Behavior, Psychology, Crime & Law,* and the *International Journal of Offender Therapy and Comparative Criminology.*

David R. White is a retired assistant chief of police with nearly 20 years of experience in law enforcement. He is an associate professor of criminal justice at Ferris State University. Dr. White's research interests include issues of police culture, organizations, and legitimacy as well as individual motivations and job fit in criminal justice organizations.

Miko M. Wilford is an associate professor in the Department of Psychology at Iowa State University. Her research interests lie under the umbrellas of human memory and decision-making. She is particularly interested in the impact of social-cognitive psychological phenomena on plea decision-making and eyewitness memory. She has served as an expert consultant on several cases involving potentially false guilty pleas or strangers' eyewitness identifications.

Shi Yan is an assistant professor in the School of Criminology and Criminal Justice, Arizona State University. He studies guilty pleas and the decision-making of courtroom actors. He is also interested in studying community-based sanctions and programs.

References

Abraham, L. A., Brown, T. C., & Thomas, S. A. (2020). How COVID-19's disruption of the US correctional system provides an opportunity for decarceration. *American Journal of Criminal Justice, 45*, 780–792.

Abramis, D. J. (1994). Work role ambiguity, job satisfaction, and job performance: Meta-analyses and review. *Psychological Reports, 75*(3), 1411–1433.

Abrams, D. S. (2021). COVID and crime: An early empirical look. *Journal of Public Economics, 194*, 104344.

Action Fraud. (2020). *Romance fraud.* www.actionfraud.police.uk/a-z-of fraud/dating-fraud

Adanu, E. K., Brown, D., Jones, S., & Parrish, A. (2021). How did the COVID-19 pandemic affect road crashes and crash outcomes in Alabama? *Accident Analysis & Prevention, 163*, 106428.

Adimora, A. A., & Schoenbach, V. J. (2005). Social context, sexual networks, and racial disparities in rates of sexually transmitted infections. *Journal of Infectious Diseases, 191*(Suppl. 1), S115–S122.

African American Policy Forum. (2022). *#SayHerName.* https://www.aapf .org/sayhername

Agnew, R. (1992). Foundation for a general strain theory of crime and delinquency. *Criminology, 30*(1), 47–88.

Agnew, R. (1999). A general strain theory of community differences in crime rates. *Journal of Research in Crime and Delinquency, 36*(2), 123–155.

Agnew, R. (2006). *Pressured into crime: An overview of general strain theory.* Roxbury.

Agrawa, S., Kirchmaier, T., & Villa-Llera, C. (2022). *Covid-19 and local crime rates in England and Wales—two years into the pandemic.* Centre for Economic Performance. https://cep.lse.ac.uk/pubs/download/cepcovid-19 -027.pdf

Ahmed, I., Nawaz, M. M., Ali, G., & Islam, T. (2015). Perceived organizational support and its outcomes: A meta-analysis of latest available literature. *Management Research Review, 38*(6), 627–639.

Ainslie, S., Fowler, A., Phillips, J., & Westaby, C. (2023). COVID-19 and community sanctions. In C. Kay & S. Case (Eds.), *Crime, justice and COVID-19* (pp. 50–75). Bristol University Press.

Akiyama, M. J., Spaulding, A. C., & Rich, J. D. (2020). Flattening the curve for incarcerated populations—Covid-19 in jails and prisons. *New England Journal of Medicine, 382*(22), 2075–2077.

Alawida, M., Omolara, A. E., Abiodun, O. I., & Al-Rajab, M. (2022). A deeper look into cybersecurity issues in the wake of Covid-19: A survey. *Journal of King Saud University–Computer and Information Sciences, 34*(10, Part A), 8176–8206.

Alexander, A. A., Allo, H., & Klukoff, H. (2020). Sick and shut in: Incarceration during a public health crisis. *Journal of Humanistic Psychology, 60*(5), 647–656.

Allen, A. (2020). *Restaurant coronavirus timeline.* Aaron Allen & Associates. https://aaronallen.com/blog/restaurant-industry-coronavirus

Altheimer, I., Duda-Banwar, J., & Schreck, C. J. (2020). The impact of COVID-19 on community-based violence interventions. *American Journal of Criminal Justice, 45*, 810–819.

Alward, L. M., & Viglione, J. (2023). Individual characteristics and organizational attributes: An assessment of probation officer burnout and turnover intent. *International Journal of Offender Therapy and Comparative Criminology.* https://doi.org/10.1177/0306624X23115988

Andresen, M. A., & Hodgkinson, T. (2020). Somehow, I always end up alone: COVID-19, social isolation and crime in Queensland, Australia. *Crime Science, 9*, 1–20.

Andrews, D. A., & Dowden, C. (2006). Risk principle of case classification in correctional treatment: A meta-analytic investigation. *International Journal of Offender Therapy and Comparative Criminology, 50*(1), 88–100.

Anti-Slavery International. (2020, July 15). *Covid-19 and slavery: The five big impacts.* www.antislavery.org/covid-19-and-slavery-the-five-big-impacts/

Armed Conflict and Location Data Project. (2021). *US Crisis Monitor releases full data for 2020.* https://acleddata.com/2021/02/05/us-crisis-monitor-releases-full-data-for-2020/

Ashby, M. (2020). Initial evidence on the relationship between the coronavirus pandemic and crime in the United States. *Crime Science, 9*(1), 1–16.

Associated Press. (2020, May 25). *A "perfect storm" for car break-ins: Vehicle theft spikes across the US amid COVID-19 pandemic.* NBC News. https://www.nbcnews.com/news/us-news/perfect-storm-car-break-ins-vehicle-theft-spikes-across-u-n1214236

August Homes. (2016, October 24). *Research: Package theft report.* https://august.com/blogs/home/research-package-theft-report

Baidoo, L., Zakrison, T. L., Feldmeth, G., Lindau, S. T., & Tung, E. L. (2021). Domestic violence police reporting and resources during the 2020 COVID-19 stay-at-home order in Chicago, Illinois. *JAMA Network Open, 4*(9), e2122260.

Baker, K. (2022, April 21). Police chief: Crime rise a return to normal from pandemic. *News-Times.* https://www.newstimes.com/news/article/Danbury-police-chief-Rise-in-crime-reflects-17084449.php

Bakst, B. (2021, June 30). *Owners of burned and looted businesses plead for state help.* Minneapolis Public Radio. https://www.mprnews.org/story/2021/02/16/owners-of-burned-looted-businesses-plead-for-state-help

Baldwin, J. M., Eassey, J. M., & Brooke, E. J. (2020). Court operations during the COVID-19 pandemic. *American Journal of Criminal Justice, 45,* 743–758.

Balmori de la Miyar, J. R., Hoehn-Velasco, L., & Silverio-Murillo, A. (2021a). The U-shaped crime recovery during COVID-19: Evidence from national crime rates in Mexico. *Crime Science, 10*(14), 1–23.

Balmori de la Miyar, J. R., Hoehn-Velasco, L., & Silverio-Murillo, A. (2021b). Drug lords don't stay at home: COVID-19 pandemic and crime patterns in Mexico City. *Journal of Criminal Justice, 72,* 101745.

Barak, A. (2005). Sexual harassment on the internet. *Social Science Computer Review, 23*(1), 77–92.

Barnes, S. R., Beland, L. P., Huh, J., & Kim, D. (2020). *The effect of COVID-19 lockdown on mobility and traffic accidents: Evidence from Louisiana.* Global Labor Organization Discussion Paper Series 616. https://ideas.repec.org/p/zbw/glodps/616.html

Barnes, S. R., Beland, L. P., Huh, J., & Kim, D. (2022). COVID-19 lockdown and traffic accidents: Lessons from the pandemic. *Contemporary Economic Policy, 40*(2), 349–368.

Barrett, C. D., & Yaffe, M. B. (2020). COVID-19: All the wrong moves in all the wrong places. *Science Signaling, 13*(649). https://doi.org/10.1126/scisignal.abe424

Baumgartner, F. R., Daniely, T., Huang, K., McGloin, P., Vattikonda, N., Washington, K., Johnson, S., Swagert, A., Love, A., & May, L. (2021, August 26). Thousands of prisoners have died of Covid-19. Because of the "tough on crime" era, there's worse to come. *The Washington Post.* https://www.washingtonpost.com/politics/2021/08/26/thousands-prisoners-have-died-covid-because-tough-crime-era-theres-still-worse-come/

Baussano, I., Williams, B. G., Nunn, P., Beggiato, M., Fedeli, U., & Scano, F. (2010). Tuberculosis incidence in prisons: A systematic review. *PLOS Medicine, 7*(12), e1000381.

Baxter, H. (2021, August 12). Rand Paul and the COVID drug stocks that everyone should know about. *Independent.* https://www.independent.co.uk/voices/rand-paul-wife-covid-stocks-b1901580.html

BBC News (2020). *Coronavirus: Loneliness and lockdown exploited in romance scams.* British Broadcasting Corporation. www.bbc.com/news/business-52664539

Becker, G. S. (1968). Crime and punishment: An economic approach. *Journal of Political Economics, 76*(2), 169–217.

Bedard, R., Vaughn, J., & Murolo, A. S. (2022). Elderly, detained, and justice-involved: The most incarcerated generation. *CUNY Law Review, 25*(1), 161–197.

Been Verified. (2021). *Catalytic converter thefts more than quadrupled last year.* https://www.beenverified.com/data-analysis/catalytic-converter-theft-state-rankings/.

Beer, T. (2021, January 6). Trump called BLM protesters "thugs" but Capitol-storming supporters "very special." *Forbes.* https://www.forbes.com/sites/tommybeer/2021/01/06/trump-called-blm-protesters-thugs-but-capitol-storming-supporters-very-special/?sh=7256bd303465

Behne, F. (2021, July 21). *States halt COVID data publication.* COVID Prison Project. https://covidprisonproject.com/blog/

Belson, K., & Draper, K. (2020, July 13). Washington NFL team to drop name. *The New York Times.* https://www.nytimes.com/2020/07/13/sports/football/washington-redskins-new-name.html

Beltrami, J. F., Cohen, D. A., Hamrick, J. T., & Farley, T. A. (1997). Rapid screening and treatment for sexually transmitted diseases in arrestees: A feasible control measure. *American Journal of Public Health, 87*(9), 1423–1426.

Bernauer, W., & Slowey, G. (2020). COVID-19, extractive industries, and indigenous communities in Canada: Notes towards a political economy research agenda. *Extractive Industries and Society, 7*(3), 844–846.

Bhatia, S., Sikka, U., Trivedi, I., Uppal, S., Brockley, J., & Navaneeth, N. (2021). *A world of no lockdowns.* Ideas for India. https://www.ideasforindia.in/topics/macroeconomics/a-world-of-no-lockdowns-the-case-of-south-korea-and-sweden.html

Bhuptani, P. H., Hunter, J., Goodwin, C., Millman, C., & Orchowski, L. M. (2022). Characterizing intimate partner violence in the United States during the COVID-19 pandemic: A systematic review. *Trauma, Violence, & Abuse, 24*(5), 3220–3235.

Bibas, S. (2004). Plea bargaining outside the shadow of trial. *Harvard Law Review, 117*(8), 2464–2547.

Binswanger, A., Krueger, P. M., & Steiner, J. F. (2009). Prevalence of chronic medical conditions among jail and prison inmates in the USA compared with the general population. *Journal of Epidemiology and Community Health, 63*(11), 912–919.

Blankenberger, B., & Williams, A. M. (2020). COVID and the impact on higher education: The essential role of integrity and accountability. *Administrative Theory & Praxis, 42*(3), 404–423.

Blumstein, A. (1983). Selective incapacitation as a means of crime control. *American Behavioral Scientist, 27*(1), 87–108.

Boman, J. H., & Gallupe, O. (2020). Has COVID-19 changed crime? Crime rates in the United States during the pandemic. *American Journal of Criminal Justice, 45*, 537–545.

Boman, J. H., & Mowen, T. J. (2021). Global crime trends during COVID-19. *Nature Human Behaviour, 5*(7), 821–822.

Borkovich, D. J., & Skovira, R. J. (2020). Working from home: Cybersecurity in the age of COVID-19. *Issues in Information Systems, 21*(4), 234–246.

Borrion, H., Kurland, J., Tilley, N., & Chen, P. (2020). Measuring the resilience of criminogenic ecosystems to global disruption: A case study of COVID-19 in China. *PLOS One, 15*(10), e0240077.

Bottoms, A., & Tankebe, J. (2012). Beyond procedural justice: A dialogic approach to legitimacy in criminal justice. *Journal of Criminal Law & Criminology, 102*(1), 119–170.

Boyatzis, R. E. (1998). *Transforming qualitative information: Thematic analysis and coding development.* Sage.

Bozelko, C. (2021, November 18). Vaccine mandates should cover the incarcerated, too, not just prison guards and workers. *STAT.* https://www
.statnews.com/2021/11/18/vaccine-mandates-should-cover-inmates-too
-not-just-prison-guards-and-workers/

Bradbury-Jones, C., & Isham, L. (2020). The pandemic paradox: The consequences of COVID-19 on domestic violence. *Journal of Clinical Nursing, 29*(13–14), 2047–2049.

Bradford, B., & Quinton, P. (2014). Self-legitimacy, police culture and support for democratic policing in an English constabulary. *British Journal of Criminology, 54*(6), 1023–1046.

Brantingham, P. J., & Brantingham, P. L. (1984). *Patterns in crime.* Macmillan.

Brantingham, P. J., Tita, G. E., & Mohler, G. (2021). Gang-related crime in Los Angeles remained stable following COVID-19 social distancing orders. *Criminology & Public Policy, 20*(3), 423–436.

Braun, V., & Clarke, V. (2006). Applied qualitative research in psychology. *Applied Qualitative Research in Psychology, 3*(2), 77–101.

Bright, C. F., Burton, C., & Kosky, M. (2020). Considerations of the impacts of COVID-19 on domestic violence in the United States. *Social Sciences & Humanities Open, 2*(1), 1–5.

Brobst, J. A. (2021). The revelatory nature of COVID-19 compassionate release in an age of mass incarceration, crime victim rights, and mental health reform. *University of St. Thomas Journal of Law and Public Policy, 15*(1), 200–258.

Bronskill, J., Perkel, C., & Casey, L. (2020, June 5). *Prime Minister Justin Trudeau takes a knee at anti-racism demonstration.* CTV News. https://www.ctvnews.ca/canada/trudeau-takes-a-knee-at-anti-racism-demonstration-1.4970650?cache=%3FclipId%3D104070

Bronson, J., & Carson, A. (2019). *Prisoners in 2017.* Bureau of Justice Statistics. https://bjs.ojp.gov/content/pub/pdf/p17.pdf

Brooks, S. K., Webster, R. K., Smith, L. E., Woodland, L., Wessely, S., Greenberg, N., & Rubin, G. J. (2020). The psychological impact of quarantine and how to reduce it: Rapid review of the evidence. *The Lancet, 395*(10227), 912–920.

Brown, J., & Fleming, J. (2022). Exploration of individual and work-related impacts on police officers and police staff working in support or frontline roles during the UK's first COVID lockdown. *The Police Journal, 95*(1), 50–72.

Buchanan, M., Castro, E. D., Kushner, M., & Krohn, M. D. (2020). It's f**ing chaos: COVID-19's impact on juvenile delinquency and juvenile justice. *American Journal of Criminal Justice, 45*, 578–600.

Buil-Gil, D., Miró-Llinares, F., Moneva, A., Kemp, S., & Díaz-Castaño, N. (2021). Cybercrime and shifts in opportunities during COVID-19: A preliminary analysis in the UK. *European Societies, 23*(Suppl. 1), S47–S59.

Buil-Gil, D., & Zeng, Y. (2022). Meeting you was a fake: Investigating the increase in romance fraud during COVID-19. *Journal of Financial Crime, 29*(2), 460–475.

Buil-Gil, D., Zeng, Y., & Kemp, S. (2021). Offline crime bounces back to pre-COVID levels, cyber stays high: Interrupted time-series analysis in Northern Ireland. *Crime Science, 10*(1), 1–16.

Bullinger, L. R., Carr, J. B., & Packham, A. (2021). COVID-19 and crime: Effects of stay-at-home orders on domestic violence. *American Journal of Health Economics, 7*(3), 249–280.

Bureau of Transportation Statistics. (2020). *Daily vehicle travel during the COVID-19 public health emergency.* https://www.bts.gov/covid-19/daily-vehicle-travel

Burke, L. (2020, October 14). Alternatives to austerity? *Inside Higher Ed.* https://www.insidehighered.com/news/2020/10/14/college-staff-face-layoffs-some-argue-against-budget-cuts

Bushway, S. D., Redlich, A. D., & Norris, R. J. (2014). An explicit test of plea bargaining in the "shadow of the trial." *Criminology, 52*(4), 723–754.

Bussu, A., Ashton, S. A., Pulina, M., & Mangiarulo, M. (2023). An explorative qualitative study of cyberbullying and cyberstalking in a higher education community. *Crime Prevention and Community Safety, 25*(4), 359–385.

Button, M., & Cross, C. (2017). *Cyber frauds, scams and their victims.* Taylor & Francis.

Byrne, J., Rapisarda, S. S., Hummer, D., & Kras, K. R. (2020). An imperfect storm: Identifying the root causes of COVID-19 outbreaks in the world's largest corrections systems. *Victims & Offenders, 15*(7–8), 862–909.

Callard, F., & Perego, E. (2021). How and why patients made Long Covid. *Social Science & Medicine, 268*, 113426.

Campedelli, G. M., Aziani, A., & Favarin, S. (2021). Exploring the immediate effects of COVID-19 containment policies on crime: An empirical analysis of the short-term aftermath in Los Angeles. *American Journal of Criminal Justice, 46*(5), 704–727.

Campedelli, G. M., Favarin, S., Aziani, A., & Piquero, A. R. (2020). Disentangling community-level changes in crime trends during the COVID-19 pandemic in Chicago. *Crime Science, 9*(1), 1–18.

Cannon, R. T. (2020). Sick deal: Injustice and plea bargaining during COVID-19. *Journal of Criminal Law and Criminology Online, 110*, 91–115.

Cantarelli, P., Belardinelli, P., & Belle, N. (2016). A meta-analysis of job satisfaction correlates in the public administration literature. *Review of Public Personnel Administration, 36*(2), 115–144.

Caridade, S. M. M., Vidal, D. G., & Dinis, M. A. P. (2022). Climate change and gender-based violence: Outcomes, challenges and future perspectives. In W. L. Filho, D. G. Vidal, M. A. Pimenta Dines, & R. C. Dias (Eds.), *Sustainable policies and practices in energy, environment and health research: Addressing cross-cutting issues* (pp. 167–176). Springer.

Carlsen, J. (2022, November 5). *Worst metro cities for package theft for 2021.* https://www.safewise.com/blog/metro-areas-porch-theft/

Carson, E. A. (2020). *Prisoners in 2019.* U.S. Department of Justice. https://bjs.ojp.gov/library/publications/prisoners-2019

Carson, E. A., & Sabol, W. J. (2016). *Aging of the state prison population, 1993–2013.* U.S. Bureau of Justice Statistics. https://bjs.ojp.gov/content/pub/pdf/aspp9313.pdf

Carter, D. P., & May, P. J. (2020). Making sense of the U.S. COVID-19 pandemic response: A policy regime perspective. *Administrative Theory and Praxis, 42*(2), 265–277.

238 *References*

Cass, M. H., Siu, O. L., Faragher, E. B., & Cooper, C. L. (2003). A meta
-analysis of the relationship between job satisfaction and employee health
in Hong Kong. *Stress and Health: Journal of the International Society for
the Investigation of Stress, 19*(2), 79–95.

Castle Rock v. Gonzales, 545 U. S. 748 (2005). https://www.supremecourt.gov
/opinions/boundvolumes/545bv.pdf

CBS News. (2021, April 16). *U.S. COVID relief hacking: Hackers arrested in
Indonesia for aid program scam.* https://www.cbsnews.com/news/us
-covid-relief-hacking-hackers-arrested-indonesia-aid-program-scam/

Ceccato, V., Kahn, T., Herrmann, C., & Östlund, A. (2022). Pandemic restrictions and spatiotemporal crime patterns in New York, São Paulo, and
Stockholm. *Journal of Contemporary Criminal Justice, 38*(1), 120–149.

Censky, A. (2020, May 14). *Heavily armed protesters gather again at Michigan
Capitol to decry stay-at-home order.* National Public Radio. https://www
.npr.org/2020/05/14/855918852/heavily-armed-protesters-gather-again
-at-michigans-capitol-denouncing-home-order

Centers for Disease Control and Prevention (2020, April 19). *Coronavirus
disease 2019 (COVID-19) situation summary.* https://stacks.cdc.gov/view
/cdc/87026.

Centers for Disease Control and Prevention. (2022a, January 11). *Contact
tracing.* https://www.cdc.gov/museum/pdf/cdcm-pha-stem-lesson
-contact-tracing-lesson.pdf

Centers for Disease Control and Prevention. (2022b). *COVID data tracker.*
https://covid.cdc.gov/covid-data-tracker/#global-counts-rates

Centers for Disease Control and Prevention. (2022c, February 25). *How to
protect yourself & others.* https://stacks.cdc.gov/view/cdc/114898

Centers for Disease Control and Prevention. (2022d, March 30). *Quarantine
and isolation.* https://stacks.cdc.gov/view/cdc/115903

Chammah, M., & Meagher, T. (2020, May 28). *Is COVID-19 falling harder on
Black prisoners? Officials won't tell us.* The Marshall Project. https://www
.themarshallproject.org/2020/05/28/is-covid-19-falling-harder-on-black
-prisoners-officials-won-t-tell-us

Chan, J., Burke, K., Bedard, R., Grigg, J., Winters, J., Vessell, C., Rosner, Z.,
Cheng, J., Katyal, M., Yang, P., & MacDonald, R. (2021). COVID-19 in
the New York City jail system: Epidemiology and health care response,
March–April 2020. *Public Health Reports (1974), 136*(3), 375–383.

Chan, S. H., & Yao, L. J. (2005). An empirical investigation of hacking behavior. *Review of Business Information Systems, 9*(4), 41–58.

Charles, P., Muentner, L., Jensen, S., Packard, C., Haimson, C., Eason,
J., & Poehlmann-Tynan, J. (2022). Incarcerated during a pandemic:

Implications of COVID-19 for jailed individuals and their families. *Corrections, 7*(5), 357–368.

Chattopadhyay, R., Knüpling, F., Chebenova, D., Whittington, L., & Gonzalez, P. (2022). *Federalism and the response to COVID-19: A comparative analysis.* Routledge.

Cheng, A., Shammas, B., & Beachum, L. (2022, February 16). U.S. is approaching phase where "Covid isn't a crisis," White House official says. *The Washington Post.* https://www.washingtonpost.com/nation/2022/02/16/covid-omicron-variant-live-updates/

Cheng, C., & Long, W. (2022). The effect of highly publicized police killings on policing: Evidence from large U.S. cities. *Journal of Public Economics, 206,* 1–18.

Chettiar, I., Bunting, W., & Schotter, G. (2012). *At America's expense: The mass incarceration of the elderly.* American Civil Liberties Union. https://assets.aclu.org/live/uploads/publications/elderlyprisonreport_20120613_1.pdf

Chetty, R., Friedman, J. N., Hendren, N., & Stepner, M. (2020). *The economic impacts of COVID-19: Evidence from a new public database built from private sector data* [Unpublished paper]. Opportunity Insights Team. https://opportunityinsights.org/wp-content/uploads/2022/10/2020_version.pdf

Cheung, L., & Gunby, P. (2022) Crime and mobility during the COVID-19 lockdown: A preliminary empirical exploration. *New Zealand Economic Papers, 56*(1), 106–113.

Chin, E. T., Ryckman, T., Prince, L., Leidner, D., Alarid-Escudero, F., Andrews, J. R., Salomon, J. A., Studdert, D. M., & Goldhabger-Fiebert, J. D. (2021). COVID-19 in the California state prison system: An observational study of decarceration, ongoing risks, and risk factors. *Journal of General Internal Medicine, 36*(10), 3096–3102.

Chiu, T. (2010). *It's about time: Aging prisoners, increasing costs and geriatric release.* Vera Institute of Justice Center on Sentencing and Corrections. https://www.vera.org/publications/its-about-time-aging-prisoners-increasing-costs-and-geriatric-release

Clarke, M., Devlin, J., Conroy, E., Kelly, E., & Sturup-Toft, S. (2020). Establishing prison-led contact tracing to prevent outbreaks of COVID-19 in prisons in Ireland. *Journal of Public Health, 42*(3), 519–524.

Clevenger, S., & Navarro, J. (2021). The "third-victimization": The cyber-victimization of sexual assault survivors and their families. *Journal of Contemporary Criminal Justice, 37*(3), 356–378.

Cloud, D. H., Ahalt, C., Augustine, D., Sears, D., & Williams, B. (2020). Medical isolation and solitary confinement: Balancing health and

240 References

humanity in US jails and prisons during COVID-19. *Journal of General Internal Medicine, 35*(9), 2738–2742.

Cloward, R. A., & Ohlin, L. E. (1960). *Delinquency and opportunity: A theory of delinquent gangs.* Free Press.

Cohen, L. E., & Felson, M. (1979). Social change and crime rate trends: A routine activity approach. *American Sociological Review, 44,* 588–608.

Coleman, G. E. (2012). Phreakers, hackers, and trolls: The politics of transgression and spectacle. In M. Mandiberg (Ed.), *The social media reader* (pp. 99–119). New York University Press.

Coleman, G. E. (2013). *Coding freedom: The ethics and aesthetics of hacking.* Princeton University Press.

Collica-Cox, K., & Molina, L. (2020). A case study of the Westchester County New York's jail response to COVID-19: Controlling COVID while balancing service needs for the incarcerated—a national model for jails. *Victims & Offenders, 15*(7–8), 1305–1316.

Cook, J. A., & Taylor, T. W. (2023). The effect of COVID-19 on local government policy implementation: Declines in police reports of domestic violence during lockdowns. *Journal of Government and Economics, 11,* 1–9.

Coppins, M. (2020, June 8). Why Mitt Romney joined Black Lives Matter protesters. *The Atlantic.*

Corkery, M., & Maheshwari, S. (2021, December 3). Thefts, always an issue for retailers, become more brazen. *The New York Times.* https://www.nytimes.com/2021/12/03/business/retailers-robberies-theft.html

Council on Foreign Relations. (2020). *The evolution of human trafficking during the COVID-19 pandemic.* https://www.cfr.org/blog/evolution-human-trafficking-during-covid-19-pandemic

COVID Prison Project (2022). Accessed September 14, 2022. https://covidprisonproject.com/

Cox, S. (2021, June 18). *With car prices surging, yours is a prime target for thieves.* CNBC. https://www.cnbc.com/2021/06/18/with-car-prices-surging-yours-is-a-prime-target-for-thieves-.html

The Crime Report Staff. (2021a, January 14). *Beating COVID-19 in prison seen as crucial to ending pandemic.* The Crime Report. https://thecrimereport.org/2021/01/14/beating-covid-19-in-prison-seen-as-crucial-to-ending-pandemic/

The Crime Report Staff. (2021b, June 11). *Feds denied 80% of appeals for compassionate release from inmates during COVID.* The Crime Report. https://thecrimereport.org/2021/06/11/feds-denied-80-of-appeals-for-compassionate-release-from-inmates-during-covid/

The Crime Report Staff. (2022, February 16). *Inmate rights to compassionate release under threat across the U.S.* The Crime Report. https://thecrimereport.org/2022/02/16/defendants-rights-to-compassionate-release-under-threat-across-u-s/

Currie, J. M., Schnell, M. K., Schwandt, H., & Zhang, J. (2021). Trends in drug overdose mortality in Ohio during the first 7 months of the COVID-19 pandemic. *JAMA Network Open, 4*(4), e217112.

Curtis, T., Miller, B. C., & Berry, E. H. (2000). Changes in reports and incidence of child abuse following natural disasters. *Child Abuse Negligence, 24*(9), 1151–1162.

Cyrus, R. (2022, April 18). Police have no duty to protect the public. *The American Prospect.* https://prospect.org/justice/police-have-no-duty-to-protect-the-public/

Daftary-Kapur, T., Henderson, K. S., & Zottoli, T. M. (2021). COVID-19 exacerbates existing system factors that disadvantage defendants: Findings from a national survey of defense attorneys. *Law and Human Behavior, 45*(2), 81–96.

Dallaire, D. H., Shlafer, R. J., Goshin, L. S., Hollihan, A., Poehlmann-Tynan, J., Eddy, J. M., & Adalist-Estrin, A. (2021). COVID-19 and prison policies related to communication with family members. *Psychology, Public Policy, and Law, 27*(2), 231–241.

Daniels, R. A., Miller, L. A., Mian, M. Z., & Black, S. (2022). One size does NOT fit all: Understanding differences in perceived organizational support during the COVID-19 pandemic. *Business and Society Review, 127*(S1), 193–222

Davila, M., Marquart, J., & Mullings, J. (2005). Beyond mother nature: Contractor fraud in the wake of natural disasters. *Deviant Behavior, 26*(3), 271–293.

Dawley, D., Houghton, J. D., & Bucklew, N. S. (2010). Perceived organizational support and turnover intention: The mediating effects of personal sacrifice and job fit. *Journal of Social Psychology, 150*(3), 238–257.

De Camargo, C. (2022). "It's tough shit, basically, that you're all gonna get it": UK virus testing and police officer anxieties of contracting COVID-19. *Policing and Society, 32*(1), 35–51.

Décary-Hétu, D., & Dupont, B. (2013). Reputation in a dark network of online criminals. *Global Crime, 14*(2–3), 175–196.

Décary-Hétu, D., & Leppänen, A. (2016). Criminals and signals: An assessment of criminal performance in the carding underworld. *Security Journal, 29*, 442–460.

Del Pozo, B., & Beletsky, L. (2020). No "back to normal" after COVID-19 for our failed drug policies. *International Journal of Drug Policy, 83.* https://doi.org/10.1016/j.drugpo.2020.102901

Delussu, F., Tizzoni, M., & Gauvin, L. (2022). Evidence of pandemic fatigue associated with stricter tiered COVID-19 restrictions. *PLOS Digital Health, 1*(5).

Demir, M., & Cassino, P. P. (2024). The effect of COVID-19 on police activities: Traffic stops, arrests, and use of force. *Criminal Justice Review, 49*(1), 64–82.

Demir, M., & Park, S. (2022). The effect of COVID-19 on domestic violence and assaults. *Criminal Justice Review, 47*(4), 445–463.

Desai, N., & Tepfer, S. (2017, November). Proactive case identification strategies and the challenges of initiating labor trafficking cases. *United States Attorneys' Bulletin.* https://cclou.org/wp-content/uploads/2018/12/Labor-trafficking-article.pdf

Detsky, A. S., & Bogoch, I. I. (2020). COVID-19 in Canada: Experience and response. *JAMA, 324*(8), 743–744.

de Vries, I., Nickerson, C., Farrell, A., Wittmer-Wolfe, D. E., & Bouché, V. (2019). Anti-immigration sentiment and public opinion on human trafficking. *Crime, Law and Social Change, 72,* 1–19.

Dewinter, M., Vandeviver, C., Dau, P. M., Vander Beken, T., & Witlox, F. (2021). The impact of strict measures as a result of the COVID-19 pandemic on the spatial pattern of the demand for police: Case study Antwerp (Belgium). *Crime Science, 10*(1), 1–12.

Dickerson, C., & Jordan, M. (2020, May 4). South Dakota meat plant is now country's biggest coronavirus hot spot. *The New York Times.* https://www.nytimes.com/2020/04/15/us/coronavirus-south-dakota-meat-plant-refugees.html

Dixon, A., & Farrell, G. (2021). A year of COVID-19 and crime in England and Wales. *Statistical Bulletin on Crime and COVID-19, 14.* http://doi.org/10.5518/100/38

Dixon, A., Farrell, G., & Johnson, S. (2022). Nearly two years in: Pandemic crime in England and Wales to end of 2021. *Statistical Bulletin on Crime and COVID-19, 16.* http://doi.org/10.5518/100/40

Dlugosz, P. (2021). Factors influencing mental health among American youth in the time of the Covid-19 pandemic. *Personality and Individual Differences, 175,* 110711.

Dolovich, S. (2020). Mass incarceration, meet COVID-19: Opportunity to release prisoners with little public safety risk is clear. *Prison Legal News, 31*(5), 4–34.

Draca M., Koutmeridis T., & Machin S. (2015) *The changing returns to crime: Do criminals respond to prices?* Discussion paper no. 1355. Centre for Economic Performance, London School of Economics.

Dragon, S., & Monk-Turner, E. (2023). Police perceptions of defunding and redirecting calls for service: A qualitative analysis. *International Journal of Police Science & Management, 27*(1), 107–117.

Drew, J. M., & Martin, S. (2020). Mental health and well-being of police in a health pandemic: Critical issues for police leaders in a post-COVID-19 environment. *Journal of Community Safety and Well-Being, 5*(2), 31–36.

Drew, J. M., & Martin, S. (2021). A national study of police mental health in the USA: Stigma, mental health and help-seeking behaviors. *Journal of Police and Criminal Psychology, 36*(2), 295–306.

Duggan, M. (2017, July 11). *Online harassment 2017.* Pew Research Center. https://www.pewresearch.org/internet/2017/07/11/online-harassment -2017/

Dujardin, P. (2017). Should Virginia release more older prisoners to make room for younger ones? *Daily Press.* https://www.dailypress.com/news /crime/dp-nws-parole-geriatric-inmates-20170423-story.html

Dutheil, F., Bouillon-Minois, J. B., & Clinchamps, M. (2020). COVID-19: A prison-breaker? *Canadian Journal of Public Health, 111*(4), 480–481.

Easterbrook, F. H. (1992). Plea bargaining as compromise symposium: Punishment. *Yale Law Journal, 101*(8), 1969–1978.

Eaton, A. A., Ramjee, D., & Saunders, J. F. (2023). The relationship between sextortion during COVID-19 and pre-pandemic intimate partner violence: A large study of victimization among diverse U.S men and women. *Victims & Offenders, 18*(2), 338–355.

Edkins, V. A., & Dervan, L. E. (2018). Freedom now or a future later: Pitting the lasting implications of collateral consequences against pretrial detention in decisions to plead guilty. *Psychology, Public Policy, and Law, 24*(2), 204–215.

Edwards, S. B. (2020). *Coronavirus: The COVID-19 pandemic.* Essential Library.

Education Week (2020). *Map: Coronavirus and school closures.* https://www .edweek.org/leadership/map-coronavirus-and-school-closures-in-2019 -2020/2020/03

Egyes, L. (2017). Borders and intersections: The unique vulnerabilities of LGBTQ immigrants to trafficking. In E. Heil & A. Nichols (Eds.), *Broadening the scope of human trafficking* (pp. 107–123). Carolina Academic Press.

Eisenberger, R., Huntington, R., Hutchison, S., & Sowa, D. (1986). Perceived organizational support. *Journal of Applied Psychology, 71*(3), 500–507.

Eisner, M., & Nivette, A. (2020). *Violence and the pandemic: Urgent questions for research*. Harry Frank Guggenheim Foundation.

Elinson, Z., & Chapman, B. (2020, March 27). Coronavirus pandemic changes policing, including fewer arrests. *The Wall Street Journal*. https://www.wsj.com/articles/coronavirus-pandemic-changes-policing-including -fewer-arrests-11585301402

Emerson, R. M., Fretz, R. I., & Shaw, L. L. (2001). Participant observation and fieldnotes. In P. Atkinson, A. Coffey, S. Delamont, J. Lofland, & L. Lofland (Eds.), *Handbook of ethnography* (pp. 160–174). Sage.

Emezue, C. (2020). Digital or digitally delivered responses to domestic and intimate partner violence during COVID-19. *JMIR Public Health and Surveillance, 6*(3), e19831.

Equal Justice Initiative. (2021, April 16). *COVID-19's impact on people in prison*. https://eji.org/news/covid-19s-impact-on-people-in-prison/

Ertan, D., El-Hage, W., Thierrée, S., Javelot, H., & Hingray, C. (2020). COVID-19: Urgency for distancing from domestic violence. *European Journal of Psychotraumatology, 11*(1), 1800245.

Esposito, M. M., & King, A. (2021). New York City: COVID-19 quarantine and crime. *Journal of Criminal Psychology, 11*(3), 203–221.

Esposito, M., Salerno, M., Di Nunno, N., Ministeri, F., Liberto, A., & Sessa, F. (2022). The risk of COVID-19 infection in prisons and prevention strategies: A systematic review and a new strategic protocol of prevention. *Healthcare, 10*(2), 270.

Estévez-Soto, P. R. (2021). Crime and COVID-19: Effect of changes in routine activities in Mexico City. *Crime Science, 10*(1), 1–17.

Ethridge P. A., White T. G. (2015). The use of medically recommended intensive supervision (medical parole) in Texas *Journal of Correctional Health Care, 21*(4), 375–389.

Families Against Mandatory Minimums (FAMM). (2021a). *Medical parole New York*. https://famm.org/wp-content/uploads/New-York_Final .pdf

Families Against Mandatory Minimums (FAMM). (2021b). *Compassionate release Virginia*. https://famm.org/wp-content/uploads/Virginia_Final .pdf

Farmer, A. K., & Copenhaver, A. (2022). Policing in a pandemic: How law enforcement communicates with the public. *Policing: An International Journal, 45*(1), 124–138.

Farrell, A., Dank, M., Kafafian, M., Lockwood, S., Pfeffer, R., Hughes, R., & Vincent, K. (2019). *Capturing human trafficking victimization through crime reporting*. National Institute of Justice.

Farrell, A., McDevitt, J., Pfeffer, R., Fahy, S., Owens, C., Dank, M., & Adams, W. (2012). *Identifying challenges to improve the investigation and prosecution of state and local human trafficking cases.* National Institute of Justice.

Farrell, A., & Pfeffer, R. (2014). Policing human trafficking: Cultural blinders and organizational barriers. *The Annals of the American Academy of Political and Social Science, 653*(1), 46–64.

Farrington, D. P. (1986). Age and crime. *Crime and Justice, 7,* 189–250.

Fattah, E. A. (2020). *A social scientist's look at a global crisis: Reflections on the likely positive impact of the coronavirus.* School of Criminology, Simon Fraser University.

Fazio, A. F. (1977). *A concurrent validational study of the NCHS General Well-Being Schedule.* National Center for Health Statistics.

Federal Bureau of Prisons. (2022). *COVID-19 modified operations matrix.* https://www.bop.gov/foia/docs/attachment2_covid19_modified_ops _matrix_2021_08_16.pdf

Federal Trade Commission. (2020). *Fraud and ID theft maps.* https:// public.tableau.com/app/profile/federal.trade.commission/viz /FraudandIDTheftMaps/AllReportsbyState

Felson, M. (1986). Linking criminal choices, routine activities, informal control and criminal outcomes. In D. B. Cornish & R. V. Clarke (Eds.), *The reasoning criminal: Rational choice perspectives on offending* (pp. 119–128). Springer-Verlag.

Felson, M., & Clarke, R. V. (1998). *Opportunity makes the thief: Practical theory for crime prevention.* Police Research Series, Paper 98. Policing and Reducing Crime Unit. https://popcenter.asu.edu/sites/default/files /opportunity_makes_the_thief.pdf

Felson, M., Jiang, S., & Xu, Y. (2020). Routine activity effects of the Covid-19 pandemic on burglary in Detroit, March, 2020. *Crime Science, 9*(1), 1–7.

Finn, P., & Kuck, S. (2005). *Stress among probation and parole officers and what can be done about it.* National Institute of Justice.

Fisher, B. S. (1995). Crime and fear on campus. *The Annals of the American Academy of Political and Social Science, 539*(1), 88–101.

Fissel, E. R., & Lee, J. R. (2023). The cybercrime illusion: Examining the impact of cybercrime misbeliefs on perceptions of cybercrime seriousness. *Journal of Criminology, 56*(2–3), 150–169.

Flaherty, C. (2020). Shutdown, repeat. *Inside Higher Ed.* https://www .insidehighered.com/news/2020/08/18/unc-chapel-hill-sends-students -home-and-turns-remote-instruction

Flaskerud, J. H. (2020). Stress in the age of COVID-19. *Issues in Mental Health Nursing, 42*(1), 99–102.

Foran, H. K., & O'Leary, D. (2008). Alcohol and intimate partner violence: A meta-analytic review. *Clinical Psychological Review, 28*(7), 1222–1234.

Forrester, A., Maclennand, F., Slade, K., Brown, P., & Exworthy, T. (2014). Improving access to psychological therapies in prison. *Criminal Behavior and Mental Health, 24*(1), 163–168.

Forston, J. (2022). *Pandemic plea bargaining: COVID-19 mitigation strategies and plea decision making* [Doctoral dissertation, Arizona State University]. https://keep.lib.asu.edu/items/168789

Franco-Paredes, C., Jankousky, K., Schultz, J., Bernfeld, J., Cullen, K., Quan, N. G., Kon, S., Hotez, P., Henao-Martínez, A. F., & Krsak, M. (2020). Covid-19 in jails and prisons: A neglected infection in a marginalized population. *PLOS Neglected Tropical Diseases, 14*(6), 1–4.

Frenkel, M. O., Giessing, L., Egger-Lampl, S., Hutter, V., Oudejans, R. R., Kleygrewe, L., & Plessner, H. (2021). The impact of the COVID-19 pandemic on European police officers: Stress, demands, and coping resources. *Journal of Criminal Justice, 72*(2021), 1–14.

Freudenberg, N. (2001). Jails, prisons, and the health of urban populations: A review of the impact of the correctional system on community health. *Journal of Urban Health, 78*(2), 214–235.

Frias, A. (2021, April 6). *FBI warns against fake coronavirus vaccination cards being sold online.* NBC 7 San Diego. https://www.nbcsandiego.com/news/local/fbi-warns-against-fake-coronavirus-vaccination-cards-being-sold-online/2567947/

Frieden, T. R., Fujiwara, P. I., Washko, R. M., & Hamburg, M. A. (1995). Tuberculosis in New York City—turning the tide. *New England Journal of Medicine, 333*(4), 229–233.

Friedman, J., & Akre, S. (2021). COVID-19 and the drug overdose crisis: Uncovering the deadliest months in the United States, January–July 2020. *American Journal of Public Health, 111*(7), 1284–1291.

Friedman, J. R., & Hansen, H. (2022). Evaluation of increases in drug overdose mortality rates in the US by race and ethnicity before and during the COVID-19 pandemic. *JAMA Psychiatry, 79*(4), 379–381.

Fritz, C. E. (1996). *Disasters and mental health: Therapeutic principles drawn from disaster studies.* Disaster Research Center.

Furnell S. (2002). *Cybercrime: Vandalizing the information society.* Addison-Wesley.

Gafni, R., & Tal, P. (2022). Cyberattacks against the health-care sectors during the COVID-19 pandemic. *Information and Computer Security, 30*(1), 137–150.

Gagnon, A., & Alpern, S. (2021). Reimagining youth justice: How the dual crises of COVID-19 and racial injustice inform judicial policymaking and reform. *Juvenile and Family Court Journal, 72*(2), 5–22.

Galea, S., & Abdalla, S. M. (2020). COVID-19 pandemic, unemployment, and civil unrest: Underlying deep racial and socioeconomic divides. *JAMA, 324*(3), 227–228.

Gallagher, M. W., Zvolensky, M. J., Long, L. J., Rogers, A. H., & Garey, L. (2020). The impact of Covid-19 experiences and associated stress on anxiety, depression, and functional impairment in American adults. *Cognitive Therapy and Research, 44*(6), 1043–1051.

Galleguillos, S., Sánchez Cea, M., Koetzle, D., Mellow, J., Piñol Arriagada, D., & Schwalbe, C. (2022). The COVID-19 pandemic and probation in Chile: Remote supervision and regional differences. *International Criminology, 2*(1), 70–83.

Gartner. (2020, March 19). *Gartner HR survey reveals 88% of organizations have encouraged or required employees to work from home due to coronavirus.* Press release. Gartner Newsroom. https://www.gartner.com/en /newsroom/press-releases/2020-03-19-gartner-hr-survey-reveals-88--of -organizations-have-e

Gaub, J. E., Koen, M. C., & Davis, S. (2022). Transitioning from pandemic to normalcy: What police departments can learn from the rank-and-file. *Policing: An International Journal, 45*(1), 91–105.

Gayman, M. D., & Bradley, M. S. (2013). Organizational climate, work stress, and depressive symptoms among probation and parole officers. *Criminal Justice Studies, 26*(3), 326–346.

Gendreau, P., Andrews, D. A., & Theriault, Y. (2010). *Correctional Program Assessment Inventory–2010 (CPAI-2010).* University of New Brunswick.

Germano, R., Lau, T. T., & Garri, K. A. (2022). *COVID-19 and the U.S. district courts: An empirical investigation.* Federal Judicial Center.

Ghaemmaghami, A., Inkpen, R., Charman, S., Ilett, C., Bennett, S., Smith, P., & Newiss, G. (2021). Responding to the public during a pandemic: Perceptions of "satisfactory" and "unsatisfactory" policing. *Policing: A Journal of Policy and Practice, 15*(1), 2310–2328.

Gill, M. (2022, September 29). Thousands were released from prison during COVID. The results are shocking. *The Washington Post.* https://www .washingtonpost.com/opinions/2022/09/29/prison-release-covid -pandemic-incarceration/

Glaser, B. G. (1978). *Theoretical sensitivity: Advances in methodology of grounded theory.* Sociological Press.

Glaser, B., & Straus, A. (1967). *The discovery of grounded theory*. Aldine.

Glober, N., Mohler, G., Huynh, P., Arkins, T., O'Donnell, D., Carter, J., & Ray, B. (2020). Impact of COVID-19 pandemic on drug overdoses in Indianapolis. *Journal of Urban Health, 97*(6), 802–807.

Gould, D. D., Watson, S. L., Price, S. R., & Valliant, P. M. (2013). The relationship between burnout and coping in adult and young offender correctional officers: An exploratory investigation. *Psychological Services, 10*(1), 37–47.

Grabosky P. (2016). *Cybercrime*. Oxford University Press.

Gramlich, J. (2019, June 11). *Only 2% of federal criminal defendants go to trial, and most who do are found guilty*. Pew Research Center. https://www.pewresearch.org/short-reads/2019/06/11/only-2-of-federal-criminal-defendants-go-to-trial-and-most-who-do-are-found-guilty/

Gramlich, J. (2022, March 3). *Two years into the pandemic, Americans inch closer to a new normal*. Pew Research Center. https://www.pewresearch.org/2022/03/03/two-years-into-the-pandemic-americans-inch-closer-to-a-new-normal

Grantham-Philips, W., Davis, T. J., & Coltrain, N. (2020, June 24). What is kettling? Here's a look into the usage and history of the controversial police tactic. *USA Today*. https://www.usatoday.com/story/news/nation/2020/06/24/kettling-controversial-police-tactic-black-lives-matter-protests/3248681001/

Graso, M. (2022). The new normal: COVID-19 risk perceptions and support for continuing restrictions past vaccinations. *PLOS One, 17*(4).

Gregorian, D. (2020). *Report: Pelosi's visit to hair salon went against coronavirus rules*. NBC News. https://www.nbcnews.com/politics/congress/report-nancy-pelosi-contravened-coronavirus-rules-getting-her-hair-blown-n1239032

Grierson, J., & Devlin, H. (2020, May 3). Hostile states trying to steal coronavirus research, says UK agency. *The Guardian*. https://www.theguardian.com/world/2020/may/03/hostile-states-trying-to-steal-coronavirus-research-says-uk-agency

Griffin, M. L., Hogan, N. L., Lambert, E. G., Tucker-Gail, K. A., & Baker, D. N. (2010). Job involvement, job stress, job satisfaction, and organizational commitment and the burnout of correctional staff. *Criminal Justice and Behavior, 37*(2), 239–255.

Grodensky, C. A., Rosen, D. L., Blue, C. M., Miller, A. R., Bradley-Bull, S., Powell, W. A., Domino, M. E., Golin, C. E., & Wohl, D. A. (2018). Medicaid enrollment among prison inmates in a non-expansion state: Exploring predisposing, enabling, and need factors related to enrollment pre-incarceration and post-release. *Journal of Urban Health, 95*(4), 454–466

Guest, G., Bunce, A., & Johnson, L. (2006). How many interviews are enough? An experiment with data saturation and variability. *Field Methods, 18*(1), 59–82.

Guyot, D. (1979). Bending granite: Attempts to change the rank structure of American police departments. *Journal of Police Science & Administration, 7*(3), 253–284.

Haffajee, R. L., & Mello, M. M. (2020). Thinking globally, acting locally—the U.S. response to Covid-19. *New England Journal of Medicine, 382*(22), e75.

Hagan, L. M. (2020). Mass testing for SARS-CoV-2 in 16 prisons and jails—six jurisdictions, United States, April–May 2020. *Morbidity and Mortality Weekly Report, 69*(33), 1139–1143.

Hale, G. (2020). *DDoS attacks on rise due to COVID-19.* Control Engineering. https://www.controleng.com/articles/ddos-attacks-on-rise-due-to-covid-19/

Halford, E. (2022). An exploration of the impact of COVID-19 on police demand, capacity and capability. *Social Sciences, 11*(7), 305.

Halford, E., Dixon, A., Farrell, G., Malleson, E., & Tilley, N. (2020). Crime and coronavirus: Social distancing, lockdown, and the mobility elasticity of crime. *Crime Science, 9*(11).

Hallas, L., Hatibie, A., Majumdar, S., Pyarali, M., & Hale, T. (2022). Variation in US states' responses to COVID-19. *Annals of Family Medicine, 20*(1).

Hammett, T. M. (2009). Sexually transmitted diseases and incarceration. *Current Opinion in Infectious Diseases, 22*(1), 77–81.

Hansen, J. A., & Lory, G. L. (2020). Rural victimization and policing during the COVID-19 pandemic. *American Journal of Criminal Justice, 45,* 731–742.

Harris, M., Allardyce, S., & Findlater, D. (2021). Child sexual abuse and COVID-19: Side effects of changed societies and positive lessons for prevention. *Criminal Behavior and Mental Health, 31*(5), 289–292.

Hawdon, J., Parti, K., & Dearden, T. E. (2020). Cybercrime in America amid COVID-19: The initial results from a natural experiment. *American Journal of Criminal Justice, 45*(4), 546–562.

Hawks, L., Woolhandler, S., & McCormick, D. (2020). COVID-19 in prisons and jails in the United States. *JAMA Internal Medicine, 180*(8), 1041.

Heil, E. C. (2012). *Sex slaves and serfs: The dynamics of human trafficking in a small Florida town.* First Forum Press.

Heil, E. C., & Nichols, A. J. (2019). *Human trafficking in the Midwest: A case study of St. Louis and the bi-state area* (2nd ed.). Carolina Academic Press.

Henry, B. F. (2020). Social distancing and incarceration: Policy and management strategies to reduce COVID-19 transmission and promote health equity through decarceration. *Health Education and Behavior, 47*(4), 536–539.

Henry, F. A., & Wachtendorf, T. (2020). Compounded social vulnerability: Parole supervision and disasters. *Corrections, 8*(4), 249–283.

Henry, N., & Powell, A. (2018). Technology-facilitated sexual violence: A literature review of empirical research. *Trauma, Violence & Abuse, 19*(2), 195–208.

Henson, B., Reyns, B. W., & Fisher, B. S. (2013). Fear of crime online? Examining the effect of risk, previous victimization, and exposure on fear of online interpersonal victimization. *Journal of Contemporary Criminal Justice, 29*(4), 475–497.

Henson, V. A., & Stone, W. E. (1999). Campus crime: A victimization study. *Journal of Criminal Justice, 27*(4), 295–307.

Herscowitz, E. (2021, September 2). *COVID mitigation efforts in state prisons called "shameful failure."* The Crime Report. https://thecrimereport.org/2021/09/02/covid-mitigation-efforts-in-state-prisons-called-shameful-failure/

Hersher, M. (2022, February 15). *States are quickly ending mask mandates. But some exceptions remain.* NBC News. https://news.yahoo.com/map-half-state-mask-mandates-132320546.html

Hess, A. J. (2020, July 2). *At least 50,904 college workers have been laid off or furloughed because of Covid-19.* CNBC. https://www.cnbc.com/2020/07/02/218-colleges-have-laid-off-or-furloughed-employees-due-to-covid-19.html

Hessick, C. B. (2021). *Punishment without trial: Why plea bargaining is a bad deal.* Abrams Press.

Hicks, M. (2020). *Fear of package theft: A survey of online retail consumers* [Unpublished master's thesis]. Middle Tennessee State University.

Hicks, M., & Stickle, B. (2021). A national perspective on retail theft prevention. In J. A. Eterno, B. Stickle, D. S. Peterson, & D. K. Das (Eds.), *Police behavior, hiring, and crime fighting: An international view* (pp. 301–310). Routledge.

Hicks, M., Stickle, B., & Harms, J. (2022). Assessing the fear of package theft. *American Journal of Criminal Justice, 47*(1), 3–22.

Hodge, T. R., Orzach, R., & Silberman, J. (2022). Higher education decision on COVID-19 vaccine mandate. *Applied Economics Letters, 30*(7), 932–936.

Hodgkinson, T., & Andresen, M.A. (2020). Show me a man or a woman alone and I'll show you a saint: Changes in the frequency of criminal incidents during the COVID-19 pandemic. *Journal of Criminal Justice, 69*, 101706.

Hoehn-Velasco, L., Silverio-Murillo, A., & Balmori de la Miyar, J. R. (2021). The great crime recovery: Crimes against women during, and after, the COVID-19 lockdown in Mexico. *Economics & Human Biology, 41*, 100991.

Holt, S., Elliffe, R., Gregory, S., & Curry, P. (2023). Social workers response to domestic violence and abuse during the COVID-19 pandemic. *British Journal of Social Work, 53*(1), 386–404.

Holt, T. J. (2007). Subcultural evolution? Examining the influence of on- and off-line experiences on deviant subcultures. *Deviant Behavior, 28*(2), 171–198.

Holt, T. J. (2013). Examining the forces shaping cybercrime markets online. *Social Science Computer Review, 31*(2), 165–177.

Holt, T. J. (2020). Computer hacking and the hacker subculture. In T. J. Holt & A. Bossler (Eds.), *The Palgrave handbook of international cybercrime and cyberdeviance* (pp. 725–742). Springer.

Holt, T., & Bossler, A. (2015). *Cybercrime in progress: Theory and prevention of technology-enabled offenses.* Routledge.

Holt, T. J., Bossler, A. M., & Seigfried-Spellar, K. C. (2022). *Cybercrime and digital forensics: An introduction.* Routledge.

Holt, T. J., Lee, J. R., Freilich, J. D., Chermak, S. M., Bauer, J. M., Shillair, R., & Ross, A. (2022). An exploratory analysis of the characteristics of ideologically motivated cyberattacks. *Terrorism and Political Violence, 34*(7), 1305–1320.

Holt, T. J., Lee, J. R., & Smirnova, O. (2023). Exploring risk avoidance practices among on-demand cybercrime-as-service operations. *Crime & Delinquency, 69*(2), 415–438.

Hong, N. (2022, February 28). Retail theft rises, and small businesses in New York pay the price. *The New York Times.* https://www.nytimes.com/2022/02/28/nyregion/new-york-stores-robberies-theft.html

Howe, M. R. (2015). *"We're more than just the guys with the keys": The professional identity of campus security at an Atlantic Canadian university.* [Unpublished bachelor's thesis]. Dalhousie University.

Hsieh, M. L., Hafoka, M., Woo, Y., van Wormer, J., Stohr, M. K., & Hemmens, C. (2015). PO roles: A statutory analysis. *Federal Probation, 79*(3), 20–37.

Hsu, L. C., & Henke, A. (2021). The effect of sheltering in place on police reports of domestic violence in the US. *Feminist Economics, 27*(1–2), 362–379.

Hu, X., Dong, B., & Lovrich, N. (2022). "We are all in this together": Police use of social media during the COVID-19 pandemic. *Policing: An International Journal, 45*(1), 106–123.

Hughes, J. E., Kaffine, D., & Kaffine, L. (2023). Decline in traffic congestion increased accident severity in the wake of COVID-19. *Transportation Research Record, 2677*(4), 892–903.

Huiskes, P., Dinis, M. A. P., & Caridade, S. (2022). Technology-facilitated sexual violence victimization during the COVID-19 pandemic: Behaviors and attitudes. *Journal of Aggression, Maltreatment & Trauma, 31*(9), 1148–1167.

Hummer, D. (2020). United States Bureau of Prisons' response to the COVID-19 pandemic. *Victims & Offenders, 15*(7–8), 1262–1276.

Humphrey, S. E., Nahrgang, J. D., & Morgeson, F. P. (2007). Integrating motivational, social, and contextual work design features: A meta-analytic summary and theoretical extension of the work design literature. *Journal of Applied Psychology, 92*(5), 1332.

Hurst, A. (2020, July 2). *Nearly 1 in 5 consumers experienced package theft since the start of the quarantine.* ValuePenguin by LendingTree. https://www.valuepenguin.com/nearly-one-in-five-consumers-experienced-package-theft-since-start-of-quarantine

Hyslip, T. S., & Holt, T. J. (2019). Assessing the capacity of DRDoS-for-hire services in cybercrime markets. *Deviant Behavior, 40*(12), 1609–1625.

Ianelli, N., & Hackworth, A. (2005). *Botnets as a vehicle for online crime.* CERT Coordination Center. https://apps.dtic.mil/sti/pdfs/AD1145899.pdf

Iliffe, G., & Steed, L. G. (2000). Exploring the counselor's experience of working with perpetrators and survivors of domestic violence. *Journal of Interpersonal Violence, 15*(4), 393–412.

Ingraham, C. (2020, September 2). COVID-19 has killed more officers this year than all other causes combined, data shows. *The Washington Post.* https://www.washingtonpost.com/business/2020/09/02/coronavirus-deaths-police-officers-2020/

Ingram, J. R. (2013). Supervisor-officer fit and role ambiguity: Re-assessing the nature of the sergeant-officer attitudinal relationship. *Policing: An International Journal of Police Strategies & Management, 36*(2), 375–398.

Ingram, J. R., & Lee, S. U. (2015). The effect of first-line supervision on patrol officer job satisfaction. *Police Quarterly, 18*(2), 193–219.

Ingram, J. R., Rockwell, A. R., Guerra, C., & Paoline, E. A., III. (2021). An examination of officer job satisfaction and workgroup cultural fit. *Policing: A Journal of Policy and Practice, 15*(3), 1713–1728.

International Association of Campus Law Enforcement Administrators. (2022). *Officer memorial.* https://www.iaclea.org/officer-memorial.

International Energy Agency (2020). *Changes in transport behaviour during the Covid-19 crisis.* https://www.iea.org/articles/changes-in-transport-behaviour-during-the-covid-19-crisis

Interpol. (2020, August 4). *Interpol report shows alarming rate of cyberattacks during COVID-19.* https://www.interpol.int/en/News-and-Events/News/2020/INTERPOL-report-shows-alarming-rate-of-cyberattacks-during-COVID-19

Jackman, T. (2020, May 19). Amid pandemic, crime dropped in many US cities, but not all. *The Washington Post.* https://www.washingtonpost.com/crime-law/2020/05/19/amid-pandemic-crime-dropped-many-us-cities-not-all/

Jackson, B. A., Vermeer, M. J. D., Woods, D., Banks, D., Goodison, S. E., Russo, J., Barnum, J. D., Gourdet, C., Langton, L., Planty, M. G., et al. (2021). *How the criminal justice system's Covid-19 response has provided valuable lessons for broader reform: Looking to the future.* RAND Corporation.

Jacobi, J. V. (2005). Prison health, public health: Obligations and opportunities. *American Journal of Law & Medicine, 31*(4), 447–478.

Jacobsen, S. K. (2015). Policing the ivory tower: Students' perceptions of the legitimacy of campus police officers. *Deviant Behavior, 36*(4), 310–329.

Jennings, W. G., & Perez, N. M. (2020). The immediate impact of COVID-19 on law enforcement in the United States. *American Journal of Criminal Justice, 45*(4), 690–701.

Jeong, A., Lai, S., & Suliman, A. (2021, November 20). Kyle Rittenhouse acquittal sparks sporadic protests and Portland clashes—but Kenosha remains peaceful. *The Washington Post.* https://www.washingtonpost.com/nation/2021/11/20/kyle-rittenhouse-verdict-protests/

Jetelina, K. K., Knell, G., & Molsberry, R. J. (2021). Changes in intimate partner violence during the early stages of the COVID-19 pandemic in the USA. *Injury Prevention, 27*(1), 93–97.

Johnson, C. (2022, August 22). *Released during COVID, some people are sent back to prison with little or no warning.* NPR. https://www.npr.org/2022/08/22/1118132380/released-during-covid-some-people-are-sent-back-to-prison-with-little-or-no-warn

Johnson, E. (2021, November 29). *Got something in self storage? What you need to know amid rising thefts.* CBC News. https://www.cbc.ca/news/canada/british-columbia/storage-locker-theft-sentinel-1.6260919

Johnson, H. (2020, March 26). *How coronavirus dramatically changed college for over 14 million students.* CNBC. https://www.cnbc.com/2020/03/26/how-coronavirus-changed-college-for-over-14-million-students.html

Johnson, L., Gutridge, K., Parkes, J., Roy, A., & Plugge, E. (2021). Scoping review of mental health in prisons through the COVID-19 pandemic. *BMJ Open, 11*, e046547.

Johnson, R. R. (2012). Police officer job satisfaction: A multidimensional analysis. *Police Quarterly, 15*(2), 157–176.

Johnson, R. R. (2015). Police organizational commitment: The influence of supervisor feedback and support. *Crime & Delinquency, 61*(9), 1155–1180.

Johnson, T. (2024). Plea bargaining in the virtual courtroom. In M. Langer, M. McConville, & L. Marsh, (Eds.), *Research handbook of plea bargaining* (pp. 379–390). Edward Elgar.

Jones, D. J. (2020). The potential impacts of pandemic policing on police legitimacy: Planning past the COVID-19 crisis. *Policing: A Journal of Policy and Practice, 14*(3), 579–586.

Jordan, M. (2020, October 19). Migrant workers restricted to farms under one grower's virus lockdown. *The New York Times.* https://www.nytimes.com/2020/10/19/us/coronavirus-tomato-migrant-farm-workers.html

Jordan, M., & Dickerson, C. (2020, April 9). Poultry worker's death highlights spread of coronavirus in meat plants. *The New York Times.* https://www.nytimes.com/2020/04/09/us/coronavirus-chicken-meat-processing-plants-immigrants.html

Jordan, T., & Taylor, P. (1998). A sociology of hackers. *The Sociological Review, 46*(4), 757–780.

Jossie, M. L., Blumstein, A., & Miller, J. M. (2022). COVID, crime & criminal justice: Affirming the call for system reform research. *American Journal of Criminal Justice, 47*(6), 1243–1259.

Junewicz, A., Sohn, I. E., & Walts, K. K. (2022). COVID-19 and youth who have experienced commercial sexual exploitation: A role for child mental health professionals during and in the aftermath of a pandemic. *Journal of the American Academy of Child & Adolescent Psychiatry, 61*(9), 1071–1073.

Kaeble, D. (2023). *Probation and parole in the United States, 2021.* Bureau of Justice Statistics.

Kang-Brown, J. (2022). *People in prison in winter 2021–2022.* Vera Institute of Justice Center on Sentencing and Corrections.

Kashif, M., Javed, M. K., & Pandey, D. (2020). A surge in cyber-crime during COVID-19. *Indonesian Journal of Social and Environmental Issues, 1*(2), 48–52.

Katrakazas, C., Michelaraki, E., Sekadakis, M., & Yannis, G. (2020). A descriptive analysis of the effect of the COVID-19 pandemic on driving behavior and road safety. *Transport Research Interdisciplinary Perspective, 7,* 100186.

Kaukinen, C. (2020). When stay-at-home orders leave victims unsafe at home: Exploring the risk and consequences of intimate partner violence during the COVID-19 pandemic. *American Journal of Criminal Justice, 45,* 668–679.

Kellough, G., & Wortley, S. (2002). Remand for plea: Bail decisions and plea bargaining as commensurate decisions. *British Journal of Criminology, 42*(1), 186–210.

Kemp, S., Buil-Gil, D., Moneva, A., Miró-Llinares, F., & Díaz-Castaño, N. (2021). Empty streets, busy internet: A time-series analysis of cybercrime and fraud trends during COVID-19. *Journal of Contemporary Criminal Justice, 37*(4), 480–501.

Kennedy, J. P., Rorie, M., & Benson, M. L. (2021). COVID-19 frauds: An exploratory study of victimization during a global crisis. *Criminology & Public Policy, 20*(3), 493–543.

Kennedy, M., & Diaz, J. (2021, November 24). *The 3 white men who killed Ahmaud Arbery are found guilty of murder.* NPR. https://www.npr.org/2021/11/24/1058240388/ahmaud-arbery-murder-trial-verdict-travis-greg-mcmichael

KhudaBukhsh, W. R., Khalsa, S. K., Kenah, E., Rempala, G. A., & Tien, J. H. (2023). COVID-19 dynamics in an Ohio prison. *Frontiers in Public Health, 11,* 1087698.

Kim, D. Y., & Phillips, S. W. (2021). When COVID-19 and guns meet: A rise in shootings. *Journal of Criminal Justice, 73,* 101783.

Kim, H., Krishnan, C., Law, J., & Rounsaville, T. (2020) *COVID-19 and US higher education enrollment: Preparing leaders for fall.* McKinsey & Company.

King, B., Patel, R., & Rishworth, A. (2021). Assessing the relationships between COVID-19 stay-at-home orders and opioid overdoses in the state of Pennsylvania. *Journal of Drug Issues, 51*(4), 648–660.

Kingson, J. A. (2020, September 16). *Exclusive: $1 billion-plus riot damage is most expensive in insurance history.* Axios. https://www.axios.com/2020/09/16/riots-cost-property-damage

Klingele, C. (2013). Rethinking the use of community supervision. *Journal of Criminal Law and Criminology, 103*(4), 1015–1070.

Koppel, S., Capellan, J. A., & Sharp, J. (2023). Disentangling the impact of COVID-19: An interrupted time series analysis of crime in New York City. *American Journal of Criminal Justice, 48*(2), 368–394.

Kornfield, M. (2021, November 24). Video of Ahmaud Arbery's killing may have led to murder conviction. *The Washington Post.* https://www .washingtonpost.com/nation/2021/11/24/arbery-video-conviction/

Koshan, J., Mosher, J., & Wiegers, W. (2020). COVID-19, the shadow pandemic, and access to justice for survivors of domestic violence. *Osgoode Hall Law Journal, 57*(3), 739–800.

Koziarski, J. (2021). The effect of the COVID-19 pandemic on mental health calls for police service. *Crime Science, 10*(1), 22.

Kristof-Brown, A. L., Zimmerman, R. D., & Johnson, E. C. (2005). Consequences of individuals' fit at work: A meta-analysis of person–job, person–organization, person–group, and person–supervisor fit. *Personnel Psychology, 58*(2), 281–342.

Kroenke, K., Spitzer, R. L., & Williams, J. B. (2001). The PHQ-9: Validity of a brief depression severity measure. *Journal of General Internal Medicine, 16*(9), 606–613.

Kronbichler, A., Kresse, D., Yoon, S., Lee, K. H., Effenberger, M., & Shin, J. I. (2020). Asymptomatic patients as a source of COVID-19 infections: A systematic review and meta-analysis. *International Journal of Infectious Diseases, 98*(1), 180–186.

Kubrin, C. E., & Bartos, B. J. (2023). The COVID-19 pandemic, prison downsizing, and crime trends. *Journal of Contemporary Criminal Justice, 40*(1), 113–137.

Kuo, S. Y. (2015). Occupational stress, job satisfaction, and affective commitment to policing among Taiwanese police officers. *Police Quarterly, 18*(1), 27–54.

Kyprianides, A., Bradford, B., Beale, M., Savigar-Shaw, L., Stott, C., & Radburn, M. (2022). Policing the COVID-19 pandemic: Police officer well-being and commitment to democratic modes of policing. *Policing and Society, 32*(4), 504–521.

Lafler v. Cooper, 566 U.S. 156 (2012).

Lallie, H. S., Shepherd, L. A., Nurse, J. R. C., Erola, A., Epiphaniou, G., Maple, C., & Bellekens, X. (2021). Cyber security in the age of COVID-19: A timeline and analysis of cyber-crime and cyber-attacks during the pandemic. *Computers & Security, 105*, 102248.

Lambert, E. G., & Hogan, N. L. (2010). Wanting change: The relationship of perceptions of organizational innovation with correctional staff job stress, job satisfaction, and organizational commitment. *Criminal Justice Policy Review, 21*(2), 160–184.

Lambert, E. G., Hogan, N. L., Griffin, M. L., & Kelley, T. (2015). The correctional staff burnout literature. *Criminal Justice Studies, 28*(4), 397–443.

Lambert, E. G., & Paoline, E. A. (2008). The influence of individual, job, and organizational characteristics on correctional staff job stress, job satisfaction, and organizational commitment. *Criminal Justice Review, 33*(4), 541–564.

Lambert, E. G., Paoline, E. A., & Hogan, N. L. (2020). The effects of inmate medical issues on correctional staff job involvement and organizational commitment. *Journal of Correctional Health Care, 26*(1), 66–82.

Lange, J., & Terry, A. T. (2020). *ACEP COVID-19 field guide.* https://www .acep.org/corona/covid-19-field-guide/special-populations/law -enforcement/

Langton, S., Dixon, A., & Farrell, G. (2021a). Small area variation in crime effects of COVID-19 policies in England and Wales. *Journal of Criminal Justice, 75*, 101830.

Langton, S., Dixon, A., & Farrell, G. (2021b). Six months in: Pandemic crime trends in England and Wales. *Crime Science, 10*(6), 1–16.

La Vigne, N. (2021, September 1). *Recidivism rates: What you need to know.* Council on Criminal Justice.

Lee, J. R. (2022). Cyberpolicing. In *Oxford research encyclopedia of criminology and criminal justice.* Oxford University Press. https://doi.org/10.1093 /acrefore/9780190264079.013.729

Lee, J. R. (2023). Understanding markers of trust within the online stolen data market: An examination of vendors' signaling behaviors relative to product price point. *Criminology & Public Policy, 22*(4), 665–693.

Lee, J. R., & Holt, T. J. (2020). Assessing the factors associated with the detection of juvenile hacking behaviors. *Frontiers in Psychology, 11*, 840.

Lee, J. R., & Holt, T. J. (2023). Assessing the correlates of cyberattacks against high-visibility institutions. *Criminal Justice Studies, 36*(3), 251–268.

Lee, J. R., Nam, Y., & Tessler, H. (2023). Understanding predictors of violent and non-violent crime victimization among Asian-American / Pacific Islanders. *Victims & Offenders, 18*(1), 194–216.

Lee, W. J., Joo, H. J., & Johnson, W. (2009). The effect of participatory management on internal stress, overall job satisfaction, and turnover intention among federal probation officers. *Federal Probation, 73*(1), 33–40.

Legal Defense Fund. (2020). *Justice denied: A call for a new grand jury investigation into the killing of Breonna Taylor.* https://www.naacpldf.org

/our-thinking/issue-report/criminal-justice/justice-denied-a-call-for
-a-new-grand-jury-investigation-into-the-killing-of-breonna-taylor/

Leka, S., Griffiths, A., Cox, T., & World Health Organization. (2003). *Work organisation and stress: Systematic problem approaches for employers, managers and trade union representatives.* WHO.

LeMasters, K., McCauley, E., Nowotny, K., & Brinkley-Rubinstein, L. (2020). COVID-19 cases and testing in 53 prison systems. *Health & Justice, 8*(1), 1–6.

LeMasters K., Ranapurwala, S., Maner, M., Nowotny, K. M., Peterson, M., & Brinkley-Rubinstein, L. (2022). COVID-19 community spread and consequences for prison case rates. *PLOS One, 17*(4), e0266772 –e0266772.

Lentz, T. S., Headley Konkel, R., Gallagher, H., & Ratkowski, D. (2022). A multilevel examination of the association between COVID-19 restrictions and residence-to-crime distance. *Crime Science, 11*(1), 1–14.

Le Page, M. (2022). Understanding omicron. *New Scientist (1971), 253*(3369), 8–9.

Lerman, A. E., Green, A. L., & Dominguez, P. (2022). Pleading for justice: Bullpen therapy, pre-trial detention, and plea bargains in American courts. *Crime and Delinquency, 68*(2), 159–182.

Leslie, E., & Wilson, R. (2020, September). Sheltering in place and domestic violence: Evidence from calls for service during COVID-19. *Journal of Public Economics, 189*, 1–38.

Levenson, M. (2021, September 5). N.F.L. will allow six social justice messages on players' helmets. *The New York Times.* https://www.nytimes.com /2021/09/05/sports/nfl-social-justice.html.

Levy, S. (1984). *Hackers: Heroes of the computer revolution.* Anchor Press / Doubleday.

Lewis J. A., & Baker S. (2013). *The economic impact of cybercrime and cyber espionage.* Center for Strategic and International Studies.

Lewis, K. R., Lewis, L. S., & Garby, T. M. (2013). Surviving the trenches: The personal impact of the job on POs. *American Journal of Criminal Justice, 38*(1), 67–84.

Lewnard, J. A., & Lo, N. C. (2020). Scientific and ethical basis for social-distancing interventions against COVID-19. *The Lancet: Infectious Diseases, 20*, 631–633.

Li, W., Lewis, N., & Vansickle, A. (2020, March 19). *This chart shows why the prison population is so vulnerable to COVID-19.* The Marshall Project. https://www.themarshallproject.org/2020/03/19/this-chart-shows-why -the-prison-population-is-so-vulnerable-to-covid-19

Lipp, N. S., & Johnson, N. L. (2023). The impact of COVID-19 on domestic violence agency functioning: A case study. *Journal of Social Issues, 79*(2), 735–746.

Liu, Y. E., LeBoa, C., Rodriguez, M., Sherif, B., Trinidad, C., del Rosario, M., Allen, S., Clifford, C., Redding, J., & Chen, W., et al. (2022). COVID-19 policies in practice and their direct and indirect impacts in Northern California jails. *Frontiers in Public Health, 13*, 854343.

Locke, E. A. (1976). The nature and causes of job satisfaction. In M. D. Dunnette (Ed.), *Handbook of industrial and organizational psychology* (pp. 1297–1343). Rand McNally.

Lockwood, A., Viglione, J., & Peck, J. H. (2023). COVID-19 and juvenile probation: A qualitative examination of emergent challenges and useful strategies. *Criminal Justice and Behavior, 50*(1), 56–75.

Loeb, S. J., & Steffensmeier, D. (2006). Older male prisoners: Health status, self-efficacy beliefs, and health-promoting behaviors. *Journal of Correctional Health Care, 12*(4), 269–278.

Lonas, L. (2022, January 12). Fauci: Omicron will "infect just about everybody." *The Hill.* https://thehill.com/policy/healthcare/589344-fauci-omicron-will-infect-just-about-everybody/

London Metal Exchange. (2022). *LEM reference prices.* https://www.lme.com/en/market-data/lme-reference-prices

Lopez, E., & Rosenfeld, R. (2021). Crime, quarantine, and the US coronavirus pandemic. *Criminology & Public Policy, 20*(3), 401–422.

Lorenzo-Redondo, E. A., & Hultquist, J. F. (2022). Covid-19: Is Omicron less lethal than Delta? *BMJ (Online), 378.*

Lovelace, H. T. (2021). Of protest and property: An essay in pursuit of justice for Breonna Taylor. *Northwestern University Law Review, 116*, 23–40.

Lucero, J. L., Lim, S., & Santiago, A. M. (2016). Changes in economic hardship and intimate partner violence: A family stress framework. *Journal of Family and Economic Issues, 37*, 395–406.

Lum, C., Koper, C. S., & Wu, X. (2021). Can we really defund the police? A nine-agency study of police response to calls for service. *Police Quarterly, 25*(3), 255–280.

Lum, C., Maupin, C., & Stoltz, M. (2020). *The impact of COVID-19 on law enforcement agencies (Wave 2).* International Association of Chiefs of Police and the Center for Evidence-Based Crime Policy, George Mason University. https://www.theiacp.org/sites/default/files/IACP_Covid_Impact_Wave2.pdf

Lum, C., Maupin, C., & Stoltz, M. (2023). The supply and demand shifts in policing at the start of the pandemic: A national multi-wave survey of the impacts of COVID-19 on American law enforcement. *Police Quarterly, 26*(4), 495–519.

Lyons, M., & Brewer, G. (2021). Experiences of intimate partner violence during lockdown and the COVID-19 pandemic. *Journal of Family Violence, 37,* 1–9.

Ma, K. F., & McKinnon, T. (2022). COVID-19 and cyber fraud: Emerging threats during the pandemic. *Journal of Financial Crime Journal, 29*(2), 433–446.

Machlin, L., Gruhn, M. A., Miller, A. B., Milojevich, H. M., Motton, S., Findley, A. M., Patel, K., Mitchell, A., Martinez, D. N., & Sheridan, M. A. (2022). Predictors of family violence in North Carolina following initial COVID-19 stay-at-home orders. *Child Abuse & Neglect, 130*(Part 1), 105376.

Malpede, M., & Shayegh, S. (2022). Staying home saves lives, really! *Letters in Spatial and Resource Sciences, 15,* 637–651.

Mandal, S., & Khan, D. A. (2020). A study of security threats in cloud: Passive impact of COVID-19 pandemic. In *Proceedings of the International Conference on Smart Electronics and Communication (ICOSEC)* (pp. 837–842). IEEE. http://doi.org/10.1109/ICOSEC49089.2020.9215374

Mandavilli, A. (2022, February 25). New C.D.C. guidelines suggest 70 percent of Americans can stop wearing masks. *The New York Times.* https://www.nytimes.com/2022/02/25/health/cdc-mask-guidance.html

Mantler, T., Veenendaal, J., & Wathen, C. N. (2021). Exploring the use of hotels as alternative housing by domestic violence shelters during COVID-19. *International Journal on Homelessness, 1*(1), 32–49.

Marcum, C. D. (2020). American corrections system response to COVID-19: An examination of the procedures and policies used in spring 2020. *American Journal of Criminal Justice, 45,* 759–768.

Marks, M. (2021, October 8). *Texas prison officials dropped mask mandates at some facilities. Worker deaths followed.* Kera News. https://www.keranews.org/news/2021-10-08/texas-prison-officials-dropped-mask-mandates-at-some-facilities-worker-deaths-followed

Marquez, N., Ward, J. A., Parish, K., Saloner, B., & Dolovich, S. (2021). COVID-19 incidence and mortality in federal and state prisons compared with the US population, April 5, 2020, to April 3, 2021. *JAMA, 326*(18), 1865–1867.

Martellozzo, E., Bleakley, P., Bradbury, P., Frost, S., & Short, E. (2022). Police responses to cyberstalking during the Covid-19 pandemic in the UK. *The Police Journal, 96*(4), 689–705.

Martin, D., Leslie, N., & Graham, W. (2023). Policing the pandemic: Front-line officers' perspectives on organisational justice. *International Journal of Police Science & Management, 25*(1), 30–41.

Martin, K. D., & Zettler, H. R. (2022). COVID-19's impact on probation professionals' views about their roles and the future of probation. *Criminal Justice Review, 47*(2), 167–184.

Martin-Howard, S. (2022). COVID-19's impact on Black, female correctional officers and justice-involved individuals at Rikers Island Jail. *Crime & Delinquency, 68*(8), 1247–1270.

Maschi, T., Kalamanofsky, A., Westcott, K., & Pappacena, L. (2015). *An analysis of United States compassionate and geriatric release laws: Towards a rights-based response for diverse elders and their families and communities.* Be the Evidence Press, Fordham University. https://tinyurl.com/mryjhftp

Maskály, J., Ivković, S. K., & Neyroud, P. (2021). Policing the COVID-19 pandemic: Exploratory study of the types of organizational changes and police activities across the globe. *International Criminal Justice Review, 31*(3), 266–285.

Maskály, J., Ivkovich, S. K., & Neyroud, P. (2022). A comparative study of the police officer views on policing during the COVID-19 pandemic in the United States. *Policing: An International Journal, 45*(1), 75–90.

Massoglia, M. (2008). Incarceration as exposure: The prison, infectious disease, and other stress-related illnesses. *Journal of Health and Social Behavior, 49*(1), 56–71.

Mathieu, J. E., & Zajac, D. M. (1990). A review and meta-analysis of the antecedents, correlates, and consequences of organizational commitment. *Psychological Bulletin, 108*(2), 171–194.

Matthay, E. C., & Schmidt, L. A. (2021). Home delivery of legal intoxicants in the age of COVID-19. *Addiction, 116*(4), 691–693.

Matz, A. K., Woo, Y., & Kim, B. (2014). A meta-analysis of the correlates of turnover intent in criminal justice organizations: Does agency type matter? *Journal of Criminal Justice, 42*(3), 233–243.

Mauer, M. (2016). A 20-year maximum for prison sentences. *Democracy: A Journal of Ideas, 39.* https://democracyjournal.org/magazine/39/a-20-year -maximum-for-prison-sentences/

Maxmen, A. (2020). The race to unravel the biggest coronavirus outbreak in the United States. *Nature, 579*(7798), 181–183.

Mayo Clinic Staff. (2022, June 11). *COVID-19: Who's at higher risk of serious symptoms?* Mayo Clinic. https://www.mayoclinic.org/diseases-conditions /coronavirus/in-depth/coronavirus-who-is-at-risk/art-20483301

McDonald, J. F., & Balkin, S. (2020). *The COVID-19 and the decline in crime.* Social Science Research Network. https://papers.ssrn.com/s013/papers .cfm?abstract_id=3567500

McKenzie, J. (1999). !nt3rh4ckt!v!ty. *Style, 33*(2), 283–298.

McNeil, A., Hicks, L., Yalcinoz-Ucan, B., & Browne, D. T. (2023). Prevalence & correlates of intimate partner violence during COVID-19: A rapid review. *Journal of Family Violence, 38*(2), 241–261.

Meikle, G. (2002). *Future active: Media activism and the internet.* Psychology Press.

Melamed, S., & Newall, M. (2020, March 17). With courts closed by pandemic, Philly police stop low-level arrests to manage jail crowding. *The Philadelphia Inquirer.* https://www.inquirer.com/health/coronavirus /philadelphia-police-coronavirus-covid-pandemic-arrests-jail -overcrowding-larry-krasner-20200317.html

Mervosh, S., Lu, D., & Swales, V. (2020, April 3). See which states and cities have told residents to stay at home. *The New York Times.* https://www .nytimes.com/interactive/2020/us/coronavirus-stay-at-home-order.html

Meyer, J. P., Stanley, D. J., Herscovitch, L., & Topolnytsky, L. (2002). Affective, continuance, and normative commitment to the organization: A meta-analysis of antecedents, correlates, and consequences. *Journal of Vocational Behavior, 61*(1), 20–52.

Meyer, M., Hassafy, A., Lewis, G., Shrestha, P., Haviland, A. M., & Nagin, D. S. (2022). Changes in crime rates during the COVID-19 pandemic. *Statistics and Public Policy, 9*(1), 97–109.

Miller, A. R., Segal, C., & Spencer, M. K. (2020). *Effects of the COVID-19 pandemic on domestic violence in Los Angeles.* Working paper 28068. National Bureau of Economic Research.

Miller, A. R., Segal, C., & Spencer, M. K. (2022). Effects of COVID-19 shutdowns on domestic violence in US cities. *Journal of Urban Economics, 131*, 103476.

Miller, E., Martin, B. D., & Topaz, C. M. (2022). New York City jails: COVID discharge policy, data transparency, and reform. *PLOS One, 17*(1), e0262255.

Miller, J. M., & Blumstein, A. (2020). Crime, justice & the COVID-19 pandemic: Toward a national research agenda. *American Journal of Criminal Justice, 45*(4), 515–524.

Miller, P. G. (2001). A critical review of the harm minimization ideology in Australia. *Critical Public Health, 11*(2), 167–178.

Minton, T. D., Zeng, Z., & Maruschak, L. M. (2021). *Impact of COVID-19 on the local jail population, January–June 2020.* U.S. Bureau of Justice Statistics.

Mitnick, K., & Simon, W. (2002). *Art of deception: Controlling the human element of security.* Wiley.

Mohler, G., Bertozzi, A. L., Carter, J., Short, M. B., Sledge, D., Tita, G. E., Uchida, C. D., & Brantingham, P. J. (2020). Impact of social distancing during COVID-19 pandemic on crime in Los Angeles and Indianapolis. *Journal of Criminal Justice, 68,* 101692.

Moise, I. K., & Piquero, A. R. (2023). Geographic disparities in violent crime during the COVID-19 lockdown in Miami-Dade County, Florida, 2018–2020. *Journal of Experimental Criminology, 19,* 97–106.

Montoya-Barthelemy, A. G., Lee, C. D., Cundiff, D. R., & Smith, E. B. (2020). COVID-19 and the correctional environment: The American prison as a focal point for public health. *American Journal of Preventative Medicine, 58*(6), 888–891.

Montross, C. (2021). *Waiting for an echo: The madness of American incarceration.* Penguin.

Moran, J. S., & Peterman, T. (1989). Sexually transmitted diseases in prisons and jails. *The Prison Journal, 69*(2), 1–6.

Morehouse, B. (2021). *The most common types of burglary in self-storage (and how to prevent it).* Janus International Group. https://www.janusintl.com /news-media/blog/preventing-self-storage-burglary

Moreira, D. N., & Da Costa, M. P. (2020). The impact of the Covid-19 pandemic in the precipitation of intimate partner violence. *International Journal of Law and Psychiatry, 71,* 101606.

Moreno, J. E. (2020, June 9). NY police union head rails against legislators, media for "vilifying" law enforcement. *The Hill.* https://thehill.com /homenews/state-watch/501899-ny-police-union-head-rails-against -legislators-media-for-vilifying-law/

Morgan, R., & Thompson, A. (2021). *Criminal victimization, 2020.* Bureau of Justice Statistics.

Mourtgos, S. M., & Adams, I. T. (2021). COVID-19 vaccine program eliminates law enforcement workforce infections: A Bayesian structural time series analysis. *Police Practice and Research, 22*(5), 1557–1565.

Mourtgos, S. M., Adams, I. T., & Nix, J. (2022). Elevated police turnover following the summer of George Floyd protests: A synthetic control study. *Criminology and Public Policy, 21*(1), 9–33.

Mrozla, T. J. (2022). Policing in the COVID-19 pandemic: Are rural police organizations immune? *Policing: An International Journal, 45*(1), 23–41.

Mueller, J. (1996). Locking up tuberculosis. *Corrections Today, 58*(6), 100.

Mugford, S. (1993) Social change and the control of psychotropic drugs: Risk management, harm reduction and "postmodernity." *Drug and Alcohol Review, 12,* 369–375.

Muhr, T. (1991). ATLAS.ti—a prototype for the support of text interpretation. *Qualitative Sociology, 14*(4), 349–371.

Murolo, A. S. (2020). Geriatric inmates: Policy and practice. *Journal of Correctional Health Care, 26*(1), 4–16.

Murolo, A. S. (2022). Does a change in statute change anything? An analysis of Virginia's geriatric parole decisions. *SN Social Sciences, 2*(4), 1–19.

Murphy, L. (2016). *Labor and sex trafficking among homeless youth.* Modern Slavery Research Project, Loyola University New Orleans.

Murray, G. R., & Davies, K. (2022). Assessing the effects of COVID-19-related stay-at-home orders on homicide rates in selected US Cities. *Homicide Studies, 26*(4), 419–444.

National Academies of Sciences, Engineering, and Medicine. (2021). *Decarcerating correctional facilities during COVID-19: Advancing health, equity, and safety.* National Academies Press.

National Conference of State Legislatures. (2020). *COVID-19: Essential workers in the states.* https://www.ncsl.org/research/labor-and-employment/covid-19-essential-workers-in-the-states.aspx

National Human Trafficking Resource Center. (2018). *2018 statistics from the national human trafficking hotline.* https://polarisproject.org/wp-content/uploads/2019/09/Polaris_National_Hotline_2018_Statistics_Fact_Sheet.pdf

National Insurance Crime Bureau. (2021a). *Catalytic converter theft skyrocketing nationwide.* https://www.nicb.org/news/news-releases/catalytic-converter-theft-skyrocketing-nationwide

National Insurance Crime Bureau. (2021b, August 31). *NICB "hot spots": Auto thefts up significantly across the country.* https://www.nicb.org/news/news-releases/nicb-hot-spots-auto-thefts-significantly-across-country

Newiss, G., Charman, S., Ilett, C., Bennett, S., Ghaemmaghami, A., Smith, P., & Inkpen, R. (2021). Taking the strain? Well-being in the COVID-19 era. *Police Journal, 95*(1), 88–108.

Newman, B. (2023). Plea bargaining with wrong reasons: Coercive plea-offers and responding to the wrong kind of reason. *Criminal Law and Philosophy, 18,* 369–393.

Newman, W. J., & Scott, C. L. (2012). *Brown v. Plata*: Prison overcrowding in California. *Journal of the American Academy of Psychiatry and the Law, 40*(4), 547–552.

Nguyen, T. T., Criss, S., Michaels, E. K., Cross, R. I., Michaels, J. S., Dwivedi, P., Huang, D., Hsu, E., Mukhija, K., Nguyen, L. H., et al. (2021). Progress and push-back: How the killings of Ahmaud Arbery, Breonna Taylor, and George Floyd impacted public discourse on race and racism on Twitter. *SSM–Population Health, 15*, 100922.

Nhan J., & Huey, L. (2013). "We don't have these laser beams and stuff like that": Police investigations as low-tech work in a high-tech world. In S. Leman-Langlois (Ed.), *Technocrime, Policing and Surveillance* (pp. 79–90). Routledge.

Nielson, K. R., Zhang, Y., & Ingram, J. R. (2022). The impact of COVID-19 on police officer activities. *Journal of Criminal Justice, 82*, 1–10.

Nir, E., & Musial, J. (2022). Zooming in: Courtrooms and defendants' rights during the COVID-19 pandemic. *Social & Legal Studies, 31*(5), 725–745.

Nivette, A. E., Zahnow, R., Aguilar, R., Ahven, A., Amram, S., Ariel, B., Burbano, M. J. A., Astolfi, R., Baier, D., Bark, H. M., et al. (2021). A global analysis of the impact of COVID-19 stay-at-home restrictions on crime. *Nature Human Behaviour, 5*(7), 868–877.

Nix, J., Adams, I., & Mourtgos, S. M. (2021, November 7). Arresting the recruitment crisis. *City-Journal*. https://www.city-journal.org/police-departments-recruitment-crisis

Nix, J., Ivanov, S., & Pickett, J. T. (2021). What does the public want police to do during pandemics? A national experiment. *Criminology & Public Policy, 20*(3), 545–571.

Nix, J., & Richards, T. N. (2021). The immediate and long-term effects of COVID-19 stay-at-home orders on domestic violence calls for service across six US jurisdictions. *Police Practice and Research, 22*(4), 1443–1451.

Nnawulezi, N., & Hacskaylo, M. (2022). Identifying and responding to the complex needs of domestic violence housing practitioners at the onset of the COVID-19 pandemic. *Journal of Family Violence, 37*(6), 915–925.

Norman, M., Ricciardelli, R., & Maier, K. (2021). In this line of work, boundaries are important. *Canadian Journal of Sociology / Cahiers canadiens de sociologie, 46*(4), 371–390.

Nouri, S., & Kochel, T. R. (2022). Residents' perceptions of policing and safety during the COVID-19 pandemic. *Policing: An International Journal, 45*(1), 139–153.

Novisky, M. A., Narvey, C. S., & Semenza, D. C. (2021). Institutional responses to the COVID-19 pandemic in American prisons. *Victims & Offenders, 15*(7–8), 1244–1261.

Nowotny, K., Bailey, Z., Omori, M., & Brinkley-Rubinstein, L. (2020). COVID-19 exposes need for progressive criminal justice reform. *American Journal of Public Health, 110*(7), 967–968.

Nowonty, K. M., & Piquero, A. R. (2020). The global impact of the pandemic on institutional and community corrections: Assessing short-term crisis management and long-term change strategies. *Victims & Offenders, 15*(7), 839–847.

Nowotny, K. M., Siede, K., & Brinkley-Rubinstein, L. (2021). Risk of COVID-19 infection among prison staff in the United States. *BMC Public Health, 21,* 1036.

Nugroho, A., & Chandrawulan, A. A. (2023). Research synthesis of cybercrime laws and COVID-19 in Indonesia: Lessons for developed and developing countries. *Security Journal, 36*(4), 651–670.

Nunphong, T., Mellow, J., Koetzle, D., & Schwalbe, C. (2023). Exploring Thailand's probationary practices since COVID-19: Changes in strategies with regards to probation supervision. *Victims & Offenders, 18*(5), 842–861.

Obidoa C., Reeves D., Warren N., Reisine S., & Cherniack M. (2011). Depression and work family conflict among corrections officers. *Journal of Occupational and Environmental Medicine, 53*(11), 1294–1301.

Officer Down Memorial Page. (2022). *ODMP's COVID-19 law enforcement memorial.* https://www.odmp.org/search/incident/covid-19

Office to Monitor and Combat Trafficking in Persons. (2020). *2020 trafficking in persons report.* U. S. Department of State.

Ollove, M. (2021, October 27). *Some states are cloaking prison COVID data.* Stateline. https://stateline.org/2021/10/27/some-states-are-cloaking-prison-covid-data/

O'Malley, R., & Holt, K. M. (2022). Cyber sextortion: An exploratory analysis of different perpetrators engaging in a similar crime. *Journal of Interpersonal Violence, 37*(1–2), 258–283.

Onyeaka, H., Anumudu, C. K., Al-Sharify, Z. T., Egele-Godswill, E., & Mbaegbu, P. (2021). COVID-19 pandemic: A review of the global lockdown and its far-reaching effects. *Science Progress, 104*(2), 1–18.

Oppel, R., Taylor, D., & Bogel-Burroughs, N. (2021, April 8). What to know about Breonna Taylor's death. *The New York Times.* https://www.nytimes.com/article/breonna-taylor-police.html

Oriola, T. B., & Knight, W. A. (2020). COVID-19, George Floyd and human security. *African Security, 13*(2), 111–115.

Osborne, S. (2020, May 3). Iran and Russia launch cyber attacks on universities desperately searching for COVID cure. *Express.* https://www.express

.co.uk/news/uk/1277156/Iran-news-coronavirus-vaccine-uk-universities
-cyber-attack-crime-russia

Ostroff, C., & Schulte, M. (2007). Multiple perspectives of fit in organizations across levels of analysis. In C. Ostroff & T. A. Judge (Eds.), *Perspectives on organizational fit* (pp. 1–65). Taylor & Francis.

Owens, C., Dank, M., Breaux, J., Banuelos, I., Farrell, A., Pfeffer, R., Bright, K., Heitsmith, R., & McDevitt, J. (2014). *Understanding the organization, operation, and victimization process of labor trafficking in the United States.* Urban Institute.

Pala, K. C., Baggio, S., Tran, N. T., Girardin, F., Wolff, H., & Gétaz, L. (2018). Blood-borne and sexually transmitted infections: A cross-sectional study in a Swiss prison. *BMC Infectious Diseases, 18,* 539.

Palmer, D. (2020). *Ransomware and DDoS attacks: Cybercrooks are stepping up their activities in the midst of coronavirus.* ZDNet. https://www.zdnet .com/article/ransomware-and-ddos-attacks-cybercrooks-are-stepping -up-their-activities-in-the-midst-of-coronavirus/

Pandolfi, S., & Chirumbolo, S. (2022). On reaching herd immunity during the COVID-19 pandemic and further issues. *Journal of Medical Virology, 94*(1), 24–25.

Paoline, E. A., III, & Gau, J. M. (2020). An empirical assessment of the sources of police job satisfaction. *Police Quarterly, 23*(1), 55–81.

Papazoglou, K., Blumberg, D. M., Schlosser, M. D., & Collins, P. I. (2020). Policing during COVID-19: Another day, another crisis. *Journal of Community Safety and Well-Being, 5*(2), 39–41.

Parsons, T. L., & Worden, L. (2021). Assessing the risk of cascading COVID-19 outbreaks from prison-to-prison transfers. *Epidemics, 37,* 100532.

Patchin, J. W., & Hinduja, S. (2023). Cyberbullying among Asian American youth before and during the COVID-19 pandemic. *Journal of School Health, 93*(1), 82–87.

Patten, R., Alward, L., & Thomas, M. (2016). The continued marginalization of campus police. *Policing: An International Journal of Police Strategy & Management, 39*(3), 566–585.

Patterson, B. L. (1992). Job experience and perceived job stress among police, correctional, and probation/parole officers. *Criminal Justice and Behavior, 19*(3), 260–285.

Payne, J., & Morgan, A. (2020). *Property crime during the COVID-19 pandemic: A comparison of recorded offence rates and dynamic forecasts (ARIMA) for March 2020 in Queensland, Australia.* SocArXiv. https://doi .org/10.31235/osf.io/de9nc

Payne, J. L., Morgan, A., & Piquero, A. R. (2020). COVID-19 and social distancing measures in Queensland, Australia, are associated with short-term decreases in recorded violent crime. *Journal of Experimental Criminology, 18*, 89–113.

Payne, J. L., Morgan, A. & Piquero, A. R. (2021). Exploring regional variability in the short-term impact of COVID-19 on property crime in Queensland, Australia. *Crime Science, 10*(7), 1–20.

Petersen, K., Redlich, A. D., & Norris, R. J. (2022). Diverging from the shadows: Explaining individual deviation from plea bargaining in the "shadow of the trial." *Journal of Experimental Criminology, 18*(2). 321–342.

Petersilia, J. (1997). Probation in the United States. *Crime and Justice, 22*, 149–200.

Petersilia, J. (2016). Realigning corrections, California style. *American Academy of Political & Social Science, 664*(1), 8–13.

Pettus-Davis, C., Kennedy, S. C., & Veeh, C. A. (2021). Incarcerated individuals' experiences of COVID-19 in the United States. *International Journal of Prisoner Health, 17*(3), 335–350.

Pfitzner N., Fitz-Gibbon K., Meyer S., & True J. (2020). *Responding to Queensland's "shadow pandemic" during the period of COVID-19 restrictions: Practitioner views on the nature of and responses to violence against women.* Monash University.

Phillips, J., Westaby, C., Ainslie, S., & Fowler, A. (2021). "I don't like this job in my front room": Practising probation in the COVID-19 pandemic. *Probation Journal, 68*(4), 426–443.

Pietrawska, B., Aurand, S. K., & Palmer, W. (2020a). COVID-19 & crime: Crime in Los Angeles & Chicago during COVID-19. *CAP Index, 3.*

Pietrawska, B., Aurand, S. K., & Palmer, W. (2020b). COVID-19 & crime: Los Angeles crime. *CAP Index, 2.*

Piquero, A. R. (2021). The policy lessons learned from the criminal justice system response to COVID-19. *Criminology & Public Policy, 20*(3), 385–399.

Piquero, A. R., Jennings, W. G., Jemison, E., Kaukinen, C., & Knaul, F. M. (2021). Domestic violence during the COVID-19 pandemic—evidence from a systematic review and meta-analysis. *Journal of Criminal Justice, 74*, 101806.

Piquero, A. R., Riddell, J. R., Bishopp, S. A., Narvey, C., Reid, J. A., & Piquero, N. L. (2020). Staying home, staying safe? A short-term analysis of COVID19 on Dallas domestic violence. *American Journal of Criminal Justice, 45*, 601–635.

Plummer, S., Ittner, T., Monreal., A. Sandelson, J., & Western, B. (2023). Life during COVID for court-involved people. *Russel Sage Foundation Journal of the Social Sciences, 9*(3), 232–251.

Polaris. (2020, April 2020). *COVID-19 exposes flaws in the H-2A visa system.* Polaris Project. https://polarisproject.org/blog/2020/04/covid-19-exposes-flaws-in-the-h2a-visa-system/

Posick, C., Rocque, M., Whiteacre, K., & Mazeika, D. (2012). Examining metal theft in context: An opportunity theory approach. *Justice Research and Policy, 14*(2), 79–101.

Powell, A., & Henry, N. (2019). Technology-facilitated sexual violence victimization: Results from an online survey of Australian adults. *Journal of Interpersonal Violence, 34*(17), 3637–3665.

Preble, K. M., Nichols, A. J., & Cox, A. (2023). Labor trafficking in Missouri: Revelations from a statewide needs assessment. *Journal of Human Trafficking, 9*(1), 15–32.

Price, M. (2018). *Everywhere and nowhere: Compassionate release in the United States.* Families Against Mandatory Minimums.

Pro, G., & Marzell, M. (2017). Medical parole and aging prisoners: A qualitative study. *Journal of Correctional Health Care, 23*(2), 162–172.

Prost, S. G., Novisky, M. A., Rorvig, L., Zaller, N., & Williams, B. (2021). Prisons and COVID-19: A desperate call for gerontological expertise in correctional health care. *The Gerontologist, 61*(1), 3–7.

Puglisi, L. B., Brinkley-Rubinstein, L., & Wang, E. A. (2023). COVID-19 in carceral systems: A review. *Annual Review of Criminology, 6*(1), 399–422.

Pyrooz, D. C., Labrecque, R. M., Tostlebe, J. J., & Useem, B. (2020). Views on COVID-19 from inside prison: Perspectives of high-security prisoners. *Justice Evaluation Journal, 3*(2), 294–306.

Quandt, K. (2020, December 8). *Incarcerated people and corrections staff should be prioritized in COVID-19 vaccination plans.* Prison Policy Initiative. https://www.prisonpolicy.org/blog/2020/12/08/covid-vaccination-plans/

Quinn, L., Clare, J., Lindley, J., & Morgan, F. (2023). The relationship between variation in price and theft rates of consumer and commodity goods over time: A systematic review. *Journal of Experimental Criminology, 19*(2), 365–395.

Rapisarda, S. S., & Byrne, J. M. (2021). The impact of COVID-19 outbreaks in the prisons, jails, and community corrections systems throughout Europe. In J. M. Byrne, D. Hummer, & S. S. Rapisarda (Eds.), *The global impact of the COVID-19 pandemic on institutional and community corrections* (pp. 283–290). Routledge.

Ravi, K. E., Rai, A., & Schrag, R. V. (2022). Survivors' experiences of intimate partner violence and shelter utilization during COVID-19. *Journal of Family Violence, 37*(6), 979–990.

Reaves, B. A. (2015). *Campus law enforcement, 2011–2012.* Bureau of Justice Statistics.

Reuters, T. (2022, February 25). *Sweden's no-lockdown COVID strategy was broadly correct, commission suggests.* CBC. https://www.cbc.ca/news/world/sweden-report-coronavirus-1.6364154

Rhineberger-Dunn, G., & Mack, K. Y. (2020). Predicting burnout among juvenile detention and juvenile probation officers. *Criminal Justice Policy Review, 31*(3), 335–355.

Ricciardelli, R., Czarnuch, S., Carleton, R. N., Gacek, J., & Shewmake, J. (2020). Canadian public safety personnel and occupational stressors: How PSP interpret stressors on duty. *International Journal of Environmental Research and Public Health, 17*(13), 4736.

Richards, T. N., Nix, J., Mourtgos, S. M., & Adams, I. T. (2021). Comparing 911 and emergency hotline calls for domestic violence in seven cities: What happened when people started staying home due to COVID-19? *Criminology & Public Policy, 20*(3), 573–591.

Rief, R. M., & Clinkinbeard, S. S. (2020). Exploring gendered environments in policing: Workplace incivilities and fit perceptions in men and women officers. *Police Quarterly, 23*(4), 427–450.

Riggle, R. J., Edmondson, D. R., & Hansen, J. D. (2009). A meta-analysis of the relationship between perceived organizational support and job outcomes: 20 years of research. *Journal of Business Research, 62*(10), 1027–1030.

Riley, E. (2021, July 12). *Compassionate release and the pandemic: A policy failure?* The Crime Report. https://thecrimereport.org/2021/07/12/compassionate-release-and-the-pandemic-a-policy-failure/

Ritchey, F. J. (2000). *The statistical imagination: Elementary statistics for the social sciences.* McGraw-Hill.

Rizzo, J. R., House, R. J., & Lirtzman, S. I. (1970). Role conflict and ambiguity in complex organizations. *Administrative Science Quarterly, 15*(2), 150–163.

Robalo, T. L. A. S., & Abdul Rahim, R. B. B. (2023). Cyber victimization, restorative justice, and victim-offender panels. *Asian Journal of Criminology, 18*(1), 61–74.

Roe, G. (2005). Harm reduction as paradigm: Is better than bad good enough? The origins of harm reduction. *Critical Public Health, 15*(3), 243–250.

Rogers, K. (2021, December 24). *Why you should upgrade your mask as the Omicron variant spreads.* CNN. https://www.cnn.com/2021/12/24/health /cloth-mask-omicron-variant-wellness/index.html

Rosenfeld, R., & Lopez, E., Jr. (2020). Pandemic, social unrest, and crime in U.S. cities. *Federal Sentencing Reporter, 33*(1–2), 72–82.

Rossner, M. (2021). Remote rituals in virtual courts. *Journal of Law and Society, 48*(3), 334–361.

Sacks, M., & Ackerman, A. R. (2012). Pretrial detention and guilty pleas: If they cannot afford bail they must be guilty. *Criminal Justice Studies, 25*(3), 265–278.

Saks, A. M., & Ashforth, B. E. (1997). A longitudinal investigation of the relationships between job information sources, applicant perceptions of fit, and work outcomes. *Personnel Psychology, 50*(2), 395–426.

Saladié, Ò., Bustamante, E., & Gutiérrez, A. (2020). COVID-19 lockdown and reduction of traffic accidents in Tarragona province, Spain. *Transportation Research Interdisciplinary Perspectives, 8*, 100218.

Saloner, B., Parish, K., Ward, J. A., DiLaura, G., & Dolovich, S. (2020). COVID-19 cases and deaths in federal and state prisons. *JAMA, 324*(6), 602–603.

Salyers, M. P., Fukui, S., Rollins, A. L., Firmin, R., Gearhart, T., Noll, J. P., Williams, S., & Davis, C. J. (2015). Burnout and self-reported quality of care in community mental health. *Administration and Policy in Mental Health and Mental Health Services Research, 42*, 61–69.

Sanga, S., & McCrary, J. (2021). The impact of the coronavirus lockdown on domestic violence. *American Law & Economics Review, 23*(1), 137–163.

Santaularia, N. J., Osypuk, T. L., Ramirez, M. R., & Mason, S. M. (2022). Violence in the Great Recession. *American Journal of Epidemiology, 191*(11), 1847–1855.

Saunders, M. J., & Evans, C. A. (2020). COVID-19, tuberculosis, and poverty: Preventing a perfect storm. *European Respiratory Journal, 56*(1).

Sawyer, W. (2022, January 11). *New data: The changes in prisons, jails, probation, and parole in the first year of the pandemic.* Prison Policy Initiative . https://www.prisonpolicy.org/blog/2022/01/11/bjs_update/

Schilling, R., & Wang, W. (2023). Cyberbullying victimization and the COVID-19 pandemic: A routine activity perspective. *Journal of School Violence, 22*(4), 517–528.

Schleimer, J. P., McCort, C. D., Tomsich, E. A., Pear, V. A., De Biasi, A., Buggs, S., Laqueur, H. S., Shev, A. B., & Wintemute, G. J. (2021). Physical distancing, violence, and crime in US cities during the coronavirus pandemic. *Journal of Urban Health, 98*(6), 772–776.

Schneider, D., Harknett, K., & McLanahan, S. (2016). Intimate partner violence in the great recession. *Demography, 53*(2), 471–505.

Schneider, R. A., & Zottoli, T. M. (2019). Disentangling the effects of plea discount and potential trial sentence on decisions to plead guilty. *Legal and Criminological Psychology, 24*(2), 288–304.

Schuler, R. S., Aldag, R. J., & Brief, A. P. (1977). Role conflict and ambiguity: A scale analysis. *Organizational Behavior and Human Performance, 20*(1), 111–128.

Schulhofer, S. J. (1992). Plea bargaining as disaster symposium: Punishment. *Yale Law Journal, 101*(8), 1979–2010.

Schwalbe, C. S., & Koetzle, D. (2021). What the COVID-19 pandemic teaches about the essential practices of community corrections and supervision. *Criminal Justice and Behavior, 48*(9), 1300–1316.

Schwartzapfel, B., & Blankinger, K. (2021, December 22). *Omicron has arrived. Many prisons and jails are not ready.* The Marshall Project. https://www.themarshallproject.org/2021/12/22/omicron-has-arrived-many-prisons-and-jails-are-not-ready

Schwarz, C. (2017). *Human trafficking in the Midwest: Service providers' perspectives on sex and labor trafficking.* Anti-Slavery and Human Trafficking Initiative. https://kuscholarworks.ku.edu/handle/1808/23853

Scott, R. E., & Stuntz, W. J. (1992). Plea bargaining as contract symposium: Punishment. *Yale Law Journal, 101*(8), 1909–1968.

Searcy, C., Michelson, G., & Castka, P. (2022, March 15). Modern slavery in global supply chains: The impact of Covid-19. *California Review of Management.* https://cmr.berkeley.edu/2022/03/modern-slavery-in-global-supply-chains-the-impact-of-covid-19/

Segura, A., Henkhaus, M., Banyard, V., Obara, L. M., & Jefferson, G. C. (2023). Rethinking dating and sexual violence prevention for youth during the pandemic: Examining program feasibility and acceptability. *Journal of Interpersonal Violence, 38*(3–4), 4114–4137.

Seiter, R. P. (2008). *Corrections: An introduction.* Pearson Prentice Hall.

Shammas, B., Cheng, A., Hassan, J., & Beachum, L. (2022, February 15). Average of new U.S. coronavirus cases falls below Delta peak. *The Washington Post.* https://www.washingtonpost.com/nation/2022/02/15/covid-omicron-variant-live-updates/

Sharma, D., Li, W., Lavoie, D., & Lauer, C. (2020). *Prison populations drop by 100,000 during pandemic.* The Marshall Project. https://www.themarshallproject.org/2020/07/16/prison-populations-drop-by-100-000-during-pandemic

Shilling, F., & Waetjen, D. (2020). *Special report (update): Impact of COVID19 mitigation on numbers and costs of California traffic crashes.* Road Ecology Center, UC Davis.

Shjarback, J., & Magny, O. (2022). Cops and COVID: An examination of California officers' perceptions and experiences while policing during a pandemic. *Policing: An International Journal, 45*(1), 59–74.

Short, E., Bradbury, P., Martellozzo, E., Frost, S., & Bleakley, P. (2022). Front-line response: Exploring the impact of COVID-19 on stalking behaviours. *Journal of Police and Criminal Psychology, 37*(3), 540–548.

Sidebottom, A., Ashby, M., & Johnson, S. D. (2014). Copper cable theft: Revisiting the price-theft hypothesis. *Journal of Research in Crime and Delinquency, 51*(5), 684–700.

Sidebottom, A., Belur, J., Bowers, K., Tompson, L., & Johnson, S. D. (2011). Theft in price-volatile markets: On the relationship between price and copper theft. *Journal of Research in Crime and Delinquency, 48*(3), 396–418.

Simmons, C., Cochran, J. K., & Blount, W. R. (1997). The effects of job-related stress and job satisfaction on probation officers' inclinations to quit. *American Journal of Criminal Justice, 21*(2), 213–229.

Simpson, P. L., & Butler, T. G. (2020). Covid-19, prison crowding, and release policies. *British Medical Journal, 369*, m1551.

Simpson, P. L., Levy, M., & Butler, T. (2021). Incarcerated people should be prioritised for Covid-19 vaccination. *British Medical Journal, 373*, n859.

Simpson, P. L., Simpson, M., Adily, A., Grant, L., & Butler, T. (2019). Prison cell spatial density and infectious and communicable diseases: A systematic review. *British Medical Journal Open, 9*(7), e026806.

Sims, K. M., Foltz, J., & Skidmore, M. E. (2021). Prisons and COVID-19 spread in the United States. *American Journal of Public Health, 111*(8), 1534–1541.

Sivashanker, K., Rossman, J., Resnick, A., & Berwick, D. M. (2020). Covid-19 and decarceration. *British Medical Journal, 369*, m1865.

Skeem, J. L., & Manchak, S. (2008). Back to the future: From Klockars' model of effective supervision to evidence-based practice in probation. *Journal of Offender Rehabilitation, 47*(3), 220–247.

Slate, R. N., & Johnson, W. W. (2013). Stressors experienced by state and federal probation officers. In M. K. Miller & B. H. Bornstein (Eds.), *Stress, trauma, and wellbeing in the legal system* (pp. 197–215). Oxford University Press.

Sloan, J. J. (1992). The modern campus police: An analysis of their evolution, structure, and function. *American Journal of Police, 11*(2), 85–104.

Sloan, J. J., Lanier, M. M., & Beer, D. L. (2000). Policing the contemporary university campus: Challenging traditional organizational models. *Journal of Security Administration, 23*(1), 1–20.

Smith, L. (2020, August 7). Lewis Hamilton is demanding change. *The New York Times.* https://www.nytimes.com/2020/08/07/sports/autoracing/lewis-hamilton-formula-1-diversity.html

Smyth, C., Cullen, P., Breckenridge, J., Cortis, N., & Valentine, K. (2021). COVID-19 lockdowns, intimate partner violence and coercive control. *Australian Journal of Social Issues, 56*(3), 359–373.

Snider, D. E., & Hutton, M. D. (1989). Tuberculosis in correctional institutions. *JAMA, 261*(3), 436–437.

Snowdon, Q. (2021, February 2). Storage soars: Local storage units see spike in burglaries in 2020. *Sentinel.* https://sentinelcolorado.com/orecent-headlines/storage-soars-local-storage-units-see-spike-in-burglaries-in-2020/

Sorenson, S. B., Sinko, L., & Berk, R. A. (2021). The endemic amid the pandemic: Seeking help for violence against women in the initial phases of COVID-19. *Journal of Interpersonal Violence, 36*(9–10), 4899–4915.

Spitzer, R. L., Kroenke, K., Williams, J. B., & Löwe, B. (2006). A brief measure for assessing generalized anxiety disorder: The GAD-7. *Archives of Internal Medicine, 166*(10), 1092–1097.

Spradley J. P. (1979). *The ethnographic interview.* Holt, Rinehart & Winston.

Stanistreet, P., Elfert, M., & Atchoarena, D. (2021). Education in the age of COVID-19: Understanding the consequences. *International Review of Education, 66*(5), 627–633.

Statista. (2023, September 21). *Number of internet users worldwide from 2005 to 2024.* https://www.statista.com/statistics/273018/number-of-internet-users-worldwide/

Stein, S., & Jacobs, J. (2020, March 16). *Cyber-attack hits U.S. health agency amid COVID-19 outbreak.* Bloomberg. https://www.bloomberg.com/news/articles/2020-03-16/u-s-health-agency-suffers-cyber-attack-during-covid-19-response

Steinmetz, K. F. (2015). Craft(y)ness: An ethnographic study of hacking. *British Journal of Criminology, 55*(1), 125–145.

Steinmetz, K. F. (2017). Ruminations on warning banners, deterrence, and system intrusion research. *Criminology & Public Policy, 16*(3), 725–735.

Steinmetz, K. F., Schaefer, B. P., & Green, E. L. (2017). Anything but boring: A cultural criminological exploration of boredom. *Theoretical Criminology, 21*(3), 342–360.

Stickle, B. (2015). Examining public willingness-to-pay for burglary prevention. *Crime Prevention and Community Safety, 17*(2), 120–138.

Stickle, B. (2017). *Metal scrappers and thieves: Scavenging for survival and profit*. Palgrave Macmillan.

Stickle, B. (2020a). *Package theft in a pandemic*. Jill Dando Institute of Security and Crime Science, University College London.

Stickle, B. (2020b). Street scavengers and street culture. In J. I. Ross (Ed.), *Handbook on street culture* (pp. 170–185). Routledge.

Stickle, B., & Felson, M. (2020). Crime rates in a pandemic: The largest criminological experiment in history. *American Journal of Criminal Justice, 45*(4), 525–536.

Stickle, B., Hicks, M., Stickle, A., & Hutchinson, Z. (2020). Porch pirates: Examining unattended package theft through crime script analysis. *Criminal Justice Studies: A Critical Journal of Crime, Law, and Society, 33*(2), 79–95.

Stickle, B., Pietrawska, B., & Aurand, S. K. (2023). Crime during COVID-19: The impact on retail. In M. Deflem (Ed.), *Crime and social control in pandemic times* (pp. 87–104). Emerald Publishing.

Stogner, J., Miller, B. L., & McLean, K. (2020). Police stress, mental health, and resiliency during the COVID-19 pandemic. *American Journal of Criminal Justice, 45*, 718–730.

StorageCafe. (2022). *Self-storage industry trends*. https://www.storagecafe.com/self-storage-industry-statistics/

Strodel, R., Dayton, L., Garrison-Desany, H. M., Eber, G., Beyrer, C., Arscott, J., Rubenstein, L., & Sufrin, C. (2021). COVID-19 vaccine prioritization of incarcerated people relative to other vulnerable groups: An analysis of state plans. *PLOS One, 16*(6), e0253208.

Studt, E. (1972). *Surveillance and service in parole: A report of the parole action study*. Institute of Government and Public Affairs, University of California, Los Angeles.

Sudre, C. H., Murray, B., Varsavsky, T., Graham, M. S., Penfold, R. S., Bowyer, R. C., Pujol, J. C., Klaser, K., Antonelli, M., Canas, L. S., et al. (2021). Attributes and predictors of long COVID. *Nature Medicine, 27*(4), 626–631.

Summers, D. (2020). *Denver's theft up in 2020, outpaces last five years*. Fox 31 Denver. https://kdvr.com/news/denvers-theft-up-in-2020-outpaces-last-five-years/

Sun, L. (2020, April 21). CDC director warns second wave of coronavirus is likely to be even more devastating. *The Washington Post*. https://www.washingtonpost.com/health/2020/04/21/coronavirus-secondwave-cdcdirector/

Surprenant, C. W. (2020). *COVID-19 and pretrial detention*. Mercatus Center, George Mason University.

Syamsuddin, R., Fuady, M. I. N., Prasetya, M., & Umar, K. (2021). The effect of the COVID-19 pandemic on the crime of theft. *International Journal of Criminology and Sociology, 10*, 305–312.

Tankebe, J. (2014). *Rightful authority: Exploring the structure of police self-legitimacy.* Social Science Research Network. https://ssrn.com/abstract=2499717

Tankebe, J. (2019). In their own eyes: An empirical examination of police self-legitimacy. *International Journal of Comparative and Applied Criminal Justice, 43*(2), 99–116.

Tankebe, J., & Meško, G. (2015). Police self-legitimacy, use of force, and pro-organizational behavior in Slovenia. In G. Meško & J. Tankebe (Eds.), *Trust and legitimacy in criminal justice* (pp. 261–277). Springer.

Tartaglia, M. (2014). Private prisons, private records. *Boston University Law Review, 94*(5), 1689–1744.

Taxman, F. S. (2010). Probation and diversion: Is there a place at the table and what should we serve? *Victims and Offenders, 5*(3), 233–239.

Taylor, D. (2021, May). A timeline of what has happened in the year since George Floyd's death. *The New York Times.* https://www.nytimes.com/2021/05/25/us/george-floyd-protests-unrest-events-timeline.html

Taylor, P. A. (1999). *Hackers: Crime in the digital sublime.* Psychology Press.

Taylor, P. A. (2005). From hackers to hacktivists: Speed bumps on the global superhighway? *New Media & Society, 7*(5), 625–646.

Testa, A., & Fahmy, C. (2021). Family member incarceration and coping strategies during the COVID-19 pandemic. *Health & Justice, 9*, 1–10.

Thomas, J. C., Levandowski, B. A., Isler, M. R., Torrone, E., & Wilson, G. (2008). Incarceration and sexually transmitted infections: A neighborhood perspective. *Journal of Urban Health, 85*(1), 90–99.

Thomas, J. C., & Sampson, L. Y. (2005). High rates of incarceration as a social force associated with community rates of sexually transmitted infection. *Journal of Infectious Diseases, 191*(Suppl. 1), S55–S60.

Thompson, A., & Tapp, S. (2022). *Criminal victimization, 2021.* Bureau of Justice Statistics.

Thornburg, E. G. (2020). Observing online courts: Lessons from the pandemic. *Family Law Quarterly, 54*(3), 181–244.

Tinto, E. K., & Roberts, J. (2020). Expanding compassion beyond the COVID-19 pandemic. *Ohio State Journal of Criminal Law, 18*(2), 575–604.

Todres, J., & Diaz, A. (2020). COVID-19 and human trafficking—the amplified impact on vulnerable populations. *JAMA Pediatrics, 175*(2), 123–124.

Tolan, C. (2021, September 30). *Compassionate release became a life-or-death lottery for thousands of federal inmates during the pandemic.* CNN. https://cnn.it/3VWNClH

Toman, E. L., Cochran, J. C., & Cochran, J. K. (2018). Jailhouse blues? The adverse effects of pretrial detention for prison social order. *Criminal Justice and Behavior, 45*(3), 316–339.

Torkington, S. (2021, July 7). *The pandemic has changed consumer behavior forever—and online shopping looks set to stay.* World Economic Forum. https://www.weforum.org/agenda/2021/07/global-consumer-behaviour-trends-online-shopping/

Trinkner, R., Tyler, T. R., & Goff, P. A. (2016). Justice from within: The relations between a procedurally just organizational climate and police organizational efficiency, endorsement of democratic policing, and officer well-being. *Psychology, Public Policy, and Law, 22*(2), 158–172.

Turgeman-Goldschmidt, O. (2008). Meanings that hackers assign to their being a hacker. *International Journal of Cyber Criminology, 2*(2), 382–396.

Tyagi, E., & Manson, J. (2021, August 12). *Prison staff are refusing vaccines. Incarcerated people are paying the price.* UCLA COVID Behind Bars Project. https://uclacovidbehindbars.org/prison-staff-vaccine-refusals

Udwadia, Z. F., Vora, A., Tripathi, A. R., Malu, K. N., Lange, C., & Raju, R. S. (2020). COVID-19–tuberculosis interactions: When dark forces collide. *Indian Journal of Tuberculosis, 67*(4), 155–162.

Ulmer, J., & Bradley, M. (2006). Variation in trial penalties among serious violent offenses. *Criminology, 44*(3), 631–670.

U.S. Department of Justice. (2022, October 15). *Current and former Louisville, Kentucky police officers charged with federal crimes related to death of Breonna Taylor.* https://www.justice.gov/opa/pr/current-and-former-louisville-kentucky-police-officers-charged-federal-crimes-related-death

U.S. Department of State. (2020). *Trafficking in persons report* (20th ed.).

Vadala, D. (2021). *Prosecuting the police: How America's criminal justice system has failed.* Trinity College.

Van Gelder, N., Peterman, A., Potts, A., O'Donnell, M., Thompson, K., Shah, N., & Oertelt-Prigione, S. (2020). COVID-19: Reducing the risk of infection might increase the risk of intimate partner violence. *EClinicalMedicine, 21*, 100348.

Vanlaar, W. G. M., Woods-Fry, H., Barrett, H., Lyon, C., Brown, S., Wicklund, C., & Robertson, R. D. (2021). The impact of COVID-19 on road safety in Canada and the United States. *Accident Analysis & Prevention, 160*, 106324.

Van't Hoff, G., Fedosejeva, R., & Mihailescu, L. (2009). Prison's preparedness for pandemic flu and the ethical issues. *Public Health, 123*(6), 422–425.

Vella, R., Giuga, G., Piizzi, G., Alunni Fegatelli, D., Petroni, G., Tavone, A. M., Potenza, S., Cammarano, A., Mandarelli, G., & Marella, G. L. (2022). Health management in Italian prisons during COVID-19 outbreak: A focus on the second and third wave. *Healthcare, 10*(2), 282.

Vermeer, M. J. D., Woods, D., & Jackson, B. A. (2020). *Would law enforcement leaders support defunding the police? Probably if communities ask police to solve fewer problems.* Rand Corporation.

Vest, N., Johnson, O., Nowotny, K., & Brinkley-Rubinstein, L. (2021). Prison population reductions and COVID-19: A latent profile analysis synthesizing recent evidence from the Texas state prison system. *Journal of Urban Health, 98*(1), 53–58.

Vigderman, A. (2020, September 24). *Package theft remained near "peak levels" throughout the summer: One-in-five households victimized in the last 90 days.* Security.org. http://www.cheapwhitecabinets.com/index-650.html

Viglione, J., Alward, L. M., & Lockwood, A. (2021). Impact of COVID-19 on community corrections in the United States. *Perspectives, 4*(4), 44–52.

Viglione, J., Alward, L. M., Lockwood, A., & Bryson, S. (2020). Adaptations to COVID-19 in community corrections agencies across the United States. *Victims & Offenders, 15*(7–8), 1277–1297.

Viglione, J., & Nguyen, T. (2022). Changes in the use of telehealth services and use of technology for communication in US community supervision agencies since COVID-19. *Criminal Justice and Behavior, 49*(12), 1727–1745.

Viglione, J., Peck, J. H., & Frazier, J. D. (2023). COVID-19 and courts: An exploration of the impacts of the pandemic on case processing and operations. *Victims & Offenders, 18*(5), 818–841.

Virginia Department of Corrections. (2011). *Geriatric conditional release requirements.* https://vadoc.virginia.gov/

Virginia Department of Corrections. (2017, September). *State responsible offender population trend reports, 2011–2015.* https://vadoc.virginia.gov/media/1343/vadoc-offender-population-trend-report-2011-2015.pdf

Virginia Department of Corrections. (2020a). *Monthly population summary, June 2020.* https://vadoc.virginia.gov/media/1574/vadoc-monthly-offender-population-report-2020-06.pdf

Virginia Department of Corrections. (2020b, January). *State responsible offender population trend reports, 2015–2019.* https://vadoc.virginia.gov/media/1473/vadoc-offender-population-trend-report-2015-2019.pdf

Virginia Department of Corrections. (2021). *Monthly population summary, June 2021.* https://vadoc.virginia.gov/media/1702/popsummaryjune2021 .pdf

Virginia Parole Board. (2013). *Releasing geriatric offenders: Presentation to the Senate Finance Committee Public Safety.* http://sfc.virginia.gov/pdf /Public%20Safety/2013/091713%20N02%20Parole%20Boa rd%20to% 20PS%20Sub.pdf

Virginia Parole Board. (2014). *Report on the response of the Virginia Parole Board to the impact of the aging of Virginia's population.* https://www .vda.virginia.gov/2015email_pdfdocs/Virginia%20Parole%20Board% 20Aging%20Report%202-12-15.pdf

Visca, D., Ong, C. W. M., Tiberi, S., Centis, R., D'Ambrosio, L., Chen, B., Mueller, J., Mueller, P., Duarte, R., Dalcolmo, M., Sotgiu, G., Migliori, G. B., & Goletti, D. (2021). Tuberculosis and COVID-19 interaction: A review of biological, clinical, and public health effects. *Pulmonology, 27*(2), 151–165.

Vogels, E. A. (2021). *The state of online harassment.* Pew Research Center. https://www.pewresearch.org/internet/2021/01/13/the-state-of-online -harassment/

Vose, B., Cullen, F. T., & Lee, H. (2020). Targeted release in the COVID-19 correctional crisis: Using the RNR model to save lives. *American Journal of Criminal Justice, 45,* 769–779.

Wada, J. C., Patten, R., & Candela, K. (2010). Betwixt and between: The perceived legitimacy of campus police. *Policing: An International Journal of Police Strategies & Management, 33*(1), 114–131.

Walke, H. T., Honein, M. A., & Redfield, R. R. (2020). Preventing and responding to COVID-19 on college campuses. *JAMA, 324*(17), 1727–1728.

Wall, D. S. (2001). *Cybercrimes and the internet.* Routledge.

Wall, D. S. (2007). *Cybercrime: The transformation of crime in the information age.* Polity Press.

Wallace, D., Eason, J. M., Walker, J., Towers, S., Grubesic, T. H., & Nelson, J. R. (2021). Is there a temporal relationship between COVID-19 infections among prison staff, incarcerated persons and the larger community in the United States? *International Journal of Environmental Research and Public Health, 18*(13), 6873.

Wallace, D., White, M. D., Gaub, J. E., & Todak, N. (2018). Body-worn cameras as a potential source of de-policing: Testing for camera-induced passivity. *Criminology, 56*(3), 481–509.

Wang, J., Fung, T., & Weatherburn, D. (2021). The impact of the COVID-19, social distancing, and movement restrictions on crime in NSW, Australia. *Crime Science, 10,* 24.

Watson, C., Warmbrod, K. L., Vahey, R. A., & Beyrer, C. (2020). *COVID-19 and the US criminal justice system: Evidence for public health measures to reduce risk*. Johns Hopkins Center for Health Security.

Weber, R. P. (1990). *Basic content analysis* (2nd ed.). Sage.

Weil, J. Z. (2021, October 28). D.C.'s Black Lives Matter Plaza, created overnight, is now a permanent multimillion-dollar concrete installation. *The Washington Post*. https://www.washingtonpost.com/dc-md-va/2021/10/28/black-lives-matter-plaza-dc/

Weine, S., Kohrt, B. A., Collins, P. Y., Cooper, J., Lewis-Fernandez, R., Okpaku, S., & Wainberg, M. L. (2020). Justice for George Floyd and a reckoning for global mental health. *Global Mental Health, 7*, e22.

Weinstein, J. (2020, October 7). COVID-19's impact on campus law enforcement operations. *Campus Safety*. https://www.campussafetymagazine.com/news/covid-19s-impacts-on-campus-law-enforcement-operations/

Wesley, R. W., & Beyer, B. B. (2021). *COVID-19 review series, part three*. Office of the Inspector General, State of California.

West, H. C., Sabol, W. J., & Greenman, S. J. (2010). *Prisoners in 2009*. Bureau of Justice Statistics.

Western, B., Braga, A. A., Davis, J., & Sirois, C. (2015). Stress and hardship after prison. *American Journal of Sociology, 120*(5), 1512–1547.

Wetzel, J. E., & Davis, J. M. (2020). The response to the COVID19 crisis by the Pennsylvania Department of Corrections. *Victims & Offenders, 15*(7–8), 1298–1304.

White, D. R. (2019). *Police officer self-legitimacy: The role of value congruence* [Unpublished doctoral dissertation]. Southern Illinois University at Carbondale.

White, D. R., Kyle, M. J., & Schafer, J. (2020). Police officer self-legitimacy: The role of organizational fit. *Policing: An International Journal, 43*(6), 993–1006.

White, D. R., Kyle, M. J., & Schafer, J. A. (2021). Police self-legitimacy and democratic orientations: Assessing shared values. *International Journal of Police Science & Management, 23*(4), 431–444.

White, D. R., Kyle, M. J., & Schafer, J. A. (2022). Police officers' job satisfaction: Combining public service motivation and person-environment fit. *Journal of Crime and Justice, 45*(1), 21–38.

White, D. R., Schafer, J., & Kyle, M. (2022). The impact of COVID-19 on police training academies. *Policing: An International Journal, 45*(1), 9–22.

White, L. M., Aalsma, M. C., Holloway, E. D., Adams, E. L., & Salyers, M. P. (2015). Job-related burnout among juvenile probation officers:

Implications for mental health stigma and competency. *Psychological Services, 12*(3), 291–302.

White, M. D., & Fradella, H. F. (2020). Policing a pandemic: Stay-at-home orders and what they mean for the police. *American Journal of Criminal Justice, 45,* 702–717.

Whiteacre, K., Medler, L., Rhoton, D., & Howes, R. (2008). *Indianapolis metals theft project: Metals theft database pilot study.* Community Research Center, University of Indianapolis.

Whitehead, J., & Lindquist, C. (1985). Job stress and burnout among probation/parole officers: Perceptions and causal factors. *International Journal of Offender Therapy and Comparative Criminology, 29*(2), 109–119.

Widra, E. (2020, December 21). *Since you asked: Just how overcrowded were prisons before the pandemic, and at this time of social distancing, how overcrowded are they now?* Prison Policy Initiative. https://www.prison-policy.org/blog/2020/12/21/overcrowding/

Widra, E. (2021, December 16). *Since you asked: What information is available about COVID-19 and vaccinations in prison now?* Prison Policy Initiative. https://www.prisonpolicy.org/blog/2021/12/16/covid_data/

Widra, E. (2022, February 10). *State prisons and local jails appear indifferent to COVID outbreaks, refuse to depopulate dangerous facilities.* Prison Policy Initiative. https://www.prisonpolicy.org/blog/2022/02/10/february2022_population/

Widra, E., & Hayre, D. (2020, June 25). *Failing grades: State responses to COVID-19 in jails and prisons.* Prison Policy Initiative. https://www.prisonpolicy.org/reports/failing_grades.html

Widra, E., & Herring, T. (2020, August 14). *Half of states fail to require mask use by correctional staff.* Prison Policy Initiative. https://www.prisonpolicy.org/blog/2020/08/14/masks-in-prisons/

Wilford, M. M., & Khairalla, A. (2019). Innocence and plea bargaining. In V. A. Edkins & A. D. Redlich (Eds.), *A system of pleas: Social science's contribution to the real justice system* (pp. 132–152). Oxford University Press.

Wilford, M. M., & Redlich, A. D. (2018). Deciphering the guilty plea: Where research can inform policy. *Psychology, Public Policy, and Law, 24*(2), 145–146.

Wilford, M. M., Sutherland, K. T., Gonzales, J. E., & Rabinovich, M. (2021). Guilt status influences plea outcomes beyond the shadow-of-the-trial in an interactive simulation of legal procedures. *Law and Human Behavior, 45*(4), 271–286.

Wilford, M. M., Zimmerman, D. M., Yan, S., & Sutherland, K. T. (2021). Innocence in the shadow of COVID-19: Plea decision making during a pandemic. *Journal of Experimental Psychology: Applied, 27*(4), 739–750.

Williams, B., & Abraldes, R. (2007). Growing older: Challenges of prison and reentry for the aging population. In R. Greifinger (Ed.), *Public health behind bars: From prisons to community* (pp. 56–72). Springer.

Williams, B. A., Stern, M. F., Mellow, J., Safer, M., & Greifinger, R. B. (2012). Aging in correctional custody: Setting a policy agenda for older prisoner health care. *American Journal of Public Health, 102*(8), 1475–1481.

Williamson, K. D. (2021). The ORC invasion. *National Review, 73*(21), 29–32.

Willis, J. G. (2015) *Exploring the dispositions of effective university police officers* [Unpublished doctoral dissertation]. Northern Kentucky University.

Wilson, C. P., & Wilson, S. A. (2011). Perceived roles of campus law enforcement: A cognitive review of attitudes and beliefs of campus constituents. *Professional Issues in Criminal Justice, 6*(1–2), 1–12.

Wolak, J., & Finkelhor, D. (2016). *Sextortion: Findings from a survey of 1,631 victims.* Crimes Against Children Research Center, University of New Hampshire.

Wolak, J., Finkelhor, D., Walsh, W., & Treitman, L. (2018). Sextortion of minors: Characteristics and dynamics. *Journal of Adolescent Health, 62*(1), 72–79.

Wolfe, D., & Dale, D. (2020). *All of the times President Trump said Covid-19 will disappear.* CNN. https://edition.cnn.com/interactive/2020/10/politics/covid-disappearing-trump-comment-tracker/

Wolfe, M. I., Xu, F., Patel, P., O'Cain, M., Schillinger, J. A., St. Louis, M. E., & Finelli, L. (2001). An outbreak of syphilis in Alabama prisons: Correctional health policy and communicable disease control. *American Journal of Public Health, 91*(8), 1220–1225.

Wolfe, S. E., & Nix, J. (2016). The alleged "Ferguson Effect" and police willingness to engage in community partnership. *Law and Human Behavior, 40*(1), 1–10.

Wolfe, S. E., & Nix, J. (2017). Police officers' trust in their agency: Does self-legitimacy protect against supervisor procedural injustice? *Criminal Justice and Behavior, 44*(5), 717–732.

Wong, A. K., & Balzer, L. B. (2022). State-level masking mandates and COVID-19 outcomes in the United States: A demonstration of the causal roadmap. *Epidemiology, 33*(2), 228–236.

World Health Organization. (2020, December 11). *Call for action: Managing the infodemic.* https://www.who.int/news/item/11-12-2020-call-for-action-managing-the-infodemic

Wylie, L. E., Knutson, A. K., & Greene, E. (2018). Extraordinary and compelling: The use of compassionate release laws in the United States. *Psychology, Public Policy, and Law, 24*(2).

Xiong, C., Walsh, P., & Olson, R. (2021, April 21). Derek Chauvin cuffed after murder, manslaughter convictions in death of George Floyd. *Minneapolis Star Tribune*. https://www.startribune.com/derek-chauvin-cuffed-after -murder-manslaughter-convictions-in-death-of-george-floyd/600047825/

Yan, S., & Bushway, S. D. (2018). Plea discounts or trial penalties? Making sense of the trial-plea sentence disparities. *Justice Quarterly, 35*(7), 1226–1249.

Yar, M. (2013). *Cybercrime and society*. Sage.

Yu, A., Sappor, J., Nickels, L., & Cecil, R. (2021, June 24). *Impact of COVID-19 pandemic on industrial metal markets: One year on*. S&P Global Market Intelligence. https://www.spglobal.com/marketintelligence/en/news -insights/research/impact-of-covid-19-pandemic-on-industrial-metals -markets-one-year-on

Zahran, S., Shelley, T. O., Peek, L., & Brody, A. N. D. (2009). Natural disasters and social order: Modeling crime outcomes in Florida. *International Journal of Mass Emergency and Disasters, 27*(1), 26–52.

Zhang, H. (2022). The influence of the ongoing COVID-19 pandemic on family violence in China. *Journal of Family Violence, 37*, 733–743.

Zhang, S. X. (2012). *Looking for hidden population: Trafficking of migrant laborers in San Diego County*. National Institute of Justice.

Zhao, J., Thurman, Q., & He, N. (1999). Sources of job satisfaction among police officers: A test of demographic and work environment models. *Justice Quarterly, 16*(1), 153–173.

Index

167; policy implications, 185–86; violation of during emergencies, 185, 186. *See also* carceral facilities; decarceration; Virginia

Paul, Rand, 106

peer-group-based crimes, 4, 25

Pelosi, Nancy, 106

person-environment interactions, 92

phone and app-related reporting systems, 58

plea bargaining, 13, 126–46; as backbone of the criminal justice system, 126, 144; coercive nature of, 126; false guilty pleas, 127, 128, 132; guilty pleas, 127–30; and innocence, 127–28, 130; main effect diagnostics, *139*; perceptions of COVID-19 risk, 130, 138, 140–43; pretrial detention, 127–30, 144–45; release status of defendant, 126–27, 128; sentencing range, 128; shadow-of-the-trial theory, 127–28; simulation, 132–33; study on influence of COVID-19, 132–44, *136, 137, 139, 140*; theoretical basis of, 127–31; and time period, 137–41, *139, 140*; willingness to accept a plea (WTAP) scores, 133–42, *137, 138, 139, 140*. *See also* carceral facilities; criminal justice system

police-recorded crime data, 16, 23

police violence, 104, 109–12; at left-wing protests, 114

pre-pandemic crime patterns, 18–19, 29, 36

pretrial detention, 127–30, 144–45, 202

price-theft hypothesis, 39

Prison Policy Initiative, 169, 171

prison staff: strain and stressors on, 157–58; as vectors for COVID-19, 152–53, 171

probation and parole officers (PPOs), 13, 192–210; caseloads, 196, *197*, 200; coworker support, 204–5, 207–8; face-to-face/personal connections with clients, 11, 193–94, 201–2, 208; family concerns about COVID-19, 202–3; increased stress during COVID-19, 200–204; individual-level coping mechanisms, 204–8; lack of drug testing during COVID-19, 11, 194, 201; measures of mental health, 197–99; revised roles of, 192–94, 203–4, 208; traditional work expectations of unchanged, 195; work-from-home policies, impact on, 194, 200–201, 207, 209. *See also* community supervision

property crimes, 3, 30–45; commercial burglary, 30, 43–44, 45; crime opportunity structure and routine activity theory, 33; employees not available for protection, 36–37, 40, 43; metal theft, 39–40; overall crime drop, 4, 32–33; package theft, 30, 40–42, 44; patterns of change, 20; residential burglary, 30, 42–45; retail theft, 30, 33–37; storage locker theft, 38–39; theft and burglary during COVID-19, 30, 33–44; vandalism, 44; vehicle theft and theft from vehicles, 37–38. *See also* theft

prosecutors, 127–28

prosocial theories, 26–27

protests of the summer of 2020, 2, 12–13, 20, 104–5

racism, systemic, 110–13, 123

recidivism, 176, 185–86

remote work, 36, 46, 88, 214; and cybercrime, 220–21; and labor trafficking, 75; and PPOs, 208–9

PERSPECTIVES
ON CRIME AND JUSTICE

Open, inclusive, and broad in focus, the series covers scholarship on a wide range of crime and justice issues, including the exploration of understudied subjects relating to crime, its causes, and attendant social responses. Of particular interest are works that examine emerging topics or shed new light on more richly studied subjects. Volumes in the series explore emerging forms of deviance and crime, critical perspectives on crime and justice, international and transnational considerations of and responses to crime, innovative crime reduction strategies, and alternate forms of response by the community and justice system to disorder, delinquency, and criminality. Both single-authored studies and collections of original edited content are welcome.

Series Editor
Joseph A. Schafer is a professor of criminology and criminal justice at Arizona State University. His research considers issues of police behavior, police organizations, and citizen perceptions of crime. He is the author, coauthor, or coeditor of several books, including *Effective Leadership in Policing: Successful Traits and Habits* and *Contemporary Research on Police Organizations*, and he has written more than fifty scholarly journal articles and more than two dozen book chapters and essays.